GAMMA GLOBULINS

STRUCTURE AND BIOSYNTHESIS

Fifth FEBS Meeting

Volume 15

GAMMA GLOBULINS Structure and Biosynthesis

Volume 16

BIOCHEMICAL ASPECTS OF ANTIMETABOLITES AND OF DRUG HYDROXYLATION

Volume 17

MITOCHONDRIA Structure and Function

Volume 18

ENZYMES AND ISOENZYMES Structure, Properties and Function

FEDERATION OF EUROPEAN BIOCHEMICAL SOCIETIES
FIFTH MEETING, PRAGUE, JULY 1968

GAMMA GLOBULINS

STRUCTURE AND BIOSYNTHESIS

Volume 15

Edited by

F. FRANĚK

Czechoslovak Academy of Science
Prague, Czechoslovakia

D. SHUGAR

Polish Academy of Sciences
Warsaw, Poland

 1969

ACADEMIC PRESS · London and New York

ACADEMIC PRESS INC. (LONDON) LTD.
Berkeley Square House
Berkeley Square
London, W1X 6BA

U.S. Edition published by
ACADEMIC PRESS INC.
111 Fifth Avenue
New York, New York 10003

SBN: 12-640850-5
Library of Congress Catalog Card Number: 79-98909

Printed in Great Britain by
Spottiswoode, Ballantyne and Co. Ltd
London and Colchester

Foreword

It is for me a particular honour and pleasure to introduce the Symposium "Gamma globulins, structure and biosynthesis", because it was here in Prague, almost 40 years ago, where I became interested in the chemical aspects of immunology. At that time next to nothing was known about the chemical nature of antibodies. Although they were found in the globulin fraction of the immune sera, it was not yet clear whether they were indeed proteins of the globulin type, or whether they were substances of unknown nature contaminated by globulins. In 1930, together with my colleague F. Breinl, we analysed the precipitate formed by horse hemoglobin and its rabbit antibody, and found that the bulk of the precipitate consisted of a protein similar to normal serum globulin, and that the amount of this globulin corresponded to two or more globulin molecules per hemoglobin molecule. Repetition of this experiment with an arsanil-azoprotein antigen showed that the ratio of serum globulin molecules per phenylarsonate residues in the precipitate increased with an increase in the number of hapten residues per antigen molecule. This finding, and the analysis of the non-antigen portion of the precipitate, led us to the conclusion that the antibodies are indeed serum globulins. In 1937 Tiselius found that antibodies migrated electrophoretically as gamma globulins. We are not yet quite sure whether all proteins found in the gamma globulin fraction are antibodies. However, most of them have the chemical and serological properties of typical antibodies and are at present designated as immunoglobulins.

One of the most remarkable properties of the immunoglobulins is their great stability. We all know that they differ from the labile complement complex, and also from many of the enzymes, by their resistance to a temperature of 55 °C. I will never forget an experiment in which we exposed azoprotein-antibody precipitates to pH values from 1 to 12, hoping that dissociation of the antigen-antibody complex at some pH value might result in the separation and isolation of antibodies. It seemed to me quite improbable that the antibodies should maintain their biological activity outside the physiological pH range close to pH 7. To my great surprise, we found that the precipitate at pH 1-2 released soluble, biologically active antibodies free of azoprotein antigen. I mention this experiment because it demonstrates impressively the great stability of the specific combining sites of antibodies.

In spite of numerous physical and chemical analyses during the years from 1930 to 1959, very little insight was gained into the structure of antibodies. The tremendous development of immunochemistry during the last decade was started in 1959 by the work of R. R. Porter in London, who succeeded in cleaving the antibody molecule by means of papain into fragments which we designate at present as Fab and Fc. Shortly thereafter, it became clear from the work of Edelman and collaborators in 1961, and Porter in 1962, that the typical gamma G antibody molecule consists of two heavy and two light chains. This discovery led to an enormous increase in experimental work on the nature of immunoglobulins. Immunoglobulins are at present in the centre of chemical, immunological and genetic research.

We are very fortunate that one of the contributors to this Symposium is Prof. Porter who, in his fundamental experiments, has initiated a stupendous advance in our knowledge on the structure of immunoglobulins. Finally, I would like to assure the Prague organizers, Prof. Hořejší and Dr. Franĕk, that participants who came from other countries appreciated very much their efforts in making this Symposium successful.

Department of Chemistry,   F. HAUROWITZ
Indiana University,
Bloomington, Indiana, U.S.A.

Contents

FEBS Symposium, Volume 15, 1969, pp. 1-12

Heterogeneity and Biosynthesis of Antibodies*

F. HAUROWITZ

Department of Chemistry, Indiana University, Bloomington, Indiana, 47401, U.S.A

My work on antibodies began here in Prague. In cooperation with my colleague F. Breinl [1] we found that antibodies have the physical and chemical properties of serum globulins, and that they are, essentially, globulins. The lack of any prosthetic group in the antibody globulins led us to the conclusion that the combination of antigen with antibody must be attributed to a complementary shape of the peptide chains in the antibody molecule. We could at that time not believe that the organism should contain pre-existent antibody molecules for the many hundreds of synthetic chemical determinants used by Landsteiner. For this reason we postulated that the antigen acts as a matrix or a template and interferes in the process of globulin formation in such a way that complementarily-shaped globulins (antibodies) are formed [1, 2]. While our postulates concerning globulin nature and complementarity of the antibodies are still valid, the template nature of the antigen was difficult to reconcile with modern views on protein biosynthesis, particularly with the role of DNA in determining amino acid sequences and with the postulate that the primary sequence of the amino acids determines the folding, i.e. the shape or conformation of the protein molecule.

As I mentioned above, our assumption of a template role of the antigen was based on the belief that the organism could not contain preformed antibodies for hundreds or thousands of synthetic antigenic determinants. Investigations of the last few years have revealed that the organism indeed does contain many different types of γ globulins, and that the γ globulins isolated from an individual blood serum are always a heterogeneous mixture of many different globulins. The differences affect particularly the N-terminal half of the light chains and the Fd portion of the heavy chains. The immunoglobulins of a normal human or animal serum are apparently a mixture of many globulins which differ from each other in the amino acid sequence of the variable portions of their heavy and light chains.

* The experimental work of our laboratory was generously supported by grants GMO 1852 of the National Institutes of Health and GB 7850 of the National Science Foundation, and by contracts of Indiana University with the Office of Naval Research (Nonr CO178-AO1) and the Atomic Energy Commission (AT 11-1)-209.

It may be useful to estimate the extent of heterogeneity. We know at present that at least 30 amino acid residues of the light (L) chains can be replaced by one or two, in rare cases also by three or more, different amino acids. Theoretically, this would give 2^{30} ($\approx 10^9$) variations for single-step mutations resulting in replacement by only one amino acid. Two-step mutations would yield 3^{30} ($\approx 10^{14}$) variants. Although many of these changes may take place outside the specific combining sites of the antibody molecules, they would still affect the conformation of the combining sites by causing alterations in the conformation of adjacent parts of the peptide chain. If only 0·1% of all possible single-step variants were stable, we would still have 10^6 variants of the L chain and, probably, a similar number of variants of the H chain, yielding 10^{12} different combinations of L and H chains. Even if only one millionth of these LH combinations were stable, there would be still 10^6 different types of immunoglobulins. One can reasonably expect that in this enormous number of immunoglobulin molecules there would always be at least a few molecules with combining sites complementary to a given antigenic determinant.

As for the morphological aspects of antibody formation, we know that immunoglobulins are formed predominantly in lymphocytes and plasma cells. Neither of these two cell types contains significant amounts of antigen. Most of the injected antigen is found in macrophages which are large phagocytic cells, quite different from lymphocytes and plasma cells [3, 4]. Fischman and Adler [5] have found that an extract of normal macrophages which had been incubated *in vitro* with antigen induces antibody formation in normal lymphoid cells. Since the extract loses its activity when it is exposed to ribonuclease, its immunogenic activity depends on the presence of intact RNA. It is not yet clear whether the immunogenically-active compound is RNA or a complex formed by RNA and the antigen. We know from experiments with azoprotein antigens, which contain isotopically-labelled determinant groups, that the radioactive determinant is concentrated in the cytoplasmic granules and in other insoluble material, even if the injected azoprotein was completely soluble in the body fluids. Most probably the radioactive determinant groups, such as azophenyl-sulfonate or azophenylarsonate residues are transferred from their soluble protein carriers to RNA or to nucleoproteins. This "processed" antigen seems to be responsible for the immunogenic action of macrophages after their incubation with the antigen. According to this view, antibody formation would be a cooperative process depending on the activity of two cell types, and consisting of (a) the processing of the antigen in phagocytic cells (macrophages) and (b) the immunogenic action of the antigen-containing macrophages in lymphoid cells, and formation of antibody in the latter cells.

Only few lymphoid cells are involved in antibody formation after a single administration of the antigen; the number of antibody-forming cells is much larger in the secondary reaction. This has frequently been attributed to a mysterious "memory" of the cells which were primed in the first administration of antigen. In investigations with Richter and Zimmerman [6] we have found that a single injection of bovine serum albumin or ovalbumin into a rabbit, causes continuous production of antibody over periods of many months even though the amount of antibody is too small to be detected by the precipitin test. The "memory" cells are, evidently, cells which continue to produce antibodies over long periods of time and, therefore, secrete antibody from their surface. The rapid and intense antibody formation in the secondary response is apparently caused by the rapid binding of the injected antigen to the primed cells, i.e. to the formation of antigen-antibody complexes on the surface of these cells. The formation of these complexes acts, evidently, as a stimulus for division and multiplication of these cells which is paralleled by an increase in antibody formation. I do not see any necessity to invoke a mysterious "memory" of the cells as explanation for their ability to form antibody against a previously injected antigen. As we have shown, the cells have never lost this ability. It has been merely increased by the re-injection of the antigen.

Since the generation time of the lymphoid cells is approximately 8 hours, continuous mitotic divisions should result in rapid dilution of the antigen, and in its loss within a few weeks. It appeared difficult to reconcile this conclusion with the production of antibody over many months after a single injection of antigen [6]. However, investigations in which lymphocytes with chromosome markers were transferred to individuals of the same species revealed that many of the small lymphocytes have life-times of several months and, in some instances, persist in the circulation for years [7, 8]. It is not yet known whether these long-living cells are involved in antibody formation. However, experiments with isotopically-labelled antigens have shown that the decrease in the isotope content in the spleen proteins of the injected rabbits parallels approximately the decrease in the antibody content of the sera of the same animals [6].

For many years it has been assumed that the inter-relation between antigen and antibody would be similar to that between substrate and enzyme. In both instances mutual close fit is a pre-requisite for interaction. Since enzymes are usually homogeneous and have a definite, invariable structure, it was our hope that this would also be the case in antibodies. For this reason, we have attempted to isolate antibodies, to purify them and to determine their chemical structure by analytical methods. The results of the analytical work reveal that even the purest antibody preparations are mixtures of a large number of similar but not identical antibody molecules. Their heterogeneity is demonstrated by the presence of numerous bands when the heavy and light chains of the antibody preparations are exposed to gel electrophoresis in starch or in acrylamide [9]. We used in these investigations two antibodies, one of them (anti-As) directed against the azophenylarsonate anion, the other (anti-R_4N) directed against the azophenyl-N-trimethylammonium cation [9]. Since Koshland and Englberger

[10] found that the amino acid composition of the hapten-specific antibodies shows small but significant differences, we expected to find differences in the peptide maps of the two antibodies. However, no differences were detectable [9].

We have repeated our experiments with chicken anti-As and anti-R_4N antibodies. Although the chicken antibodies combined with As-BSA or R_4N-BSA in the same way as the analogous rabbit antibodies, the peptide maps of chicken anti-R_4N and rabbit anti-R_4N were quite different [11]. No difference was found between the peptide maps of chicken anti-As and anti-R_4N. Evidently, their specific combining sites are just as heterogeneous as those of the analogous rabbit antibodies. Although the amino acid composition of chicken anti-As or anti-R_4N was quite different from the amino acid composition of the analogous rabbit antibodies, only small differences were found between the amino acid compositions of the two chicken antibodies [12].

The heterogeneity revealed by gel electrophoresis, by the identity of peptide maps of antibodies of different specificity, and by the occurrence of some of the amino acids in fractions rather than in integers of residues per molecule of antibody, demonstrate clearly that each of the analyzed antibody preparations, in spite of its serological purity, is highly heterogeneous. The failure to find differences with the highly sensitive method of "fingerprinting" leads to the further conclusion that the heterogeneity involves also the specific combining sites of the antibody molecules [9, 11]. This conclusion, at first sight, seems to contradict the postulate that the conformation of a molecule is dictated by its amino acid sequence. However, this postulate does not exclude the possibility that conformations approximately complementary to a given antigenic determinant can be accomplished by different amino acid sequences. We know from the cross-reactivity of antibodies directed against certain antigenic determinants, that these antibodies combine also with determinants of similar but not identical structure. Evidently, only approximate complementarity is necessary for the combination of antigen with antibody.

Although the anti-As and anti-R_4N antibodies were serologically highly specific, they are still heterogeneous. Gel electrophoresis reveals the presence of at least two different heavy (H) and eight different light (L) chains, i.e. the possibility of 16 different combinations of the symmetrical structure LHHL of the typical 7S antibodies of molecular weight 160,000. Some of the rabbit sera were found to be heterozygous and to contain the allotypes b4 and b5, others the allotypes a1 and a2, a1 and a3, or a2 and a3. This would increase the number of different H chains from 2 to 6, and the number of L chains from 8 to 16, resulting in a maximum of $6 \times 16 = 96$ different H_2L_2 molecules. In evaluations of this type it must be borne in mind that the number of allotypes is certainly much higher than the numbers given above since the latter are based on the present limits of serological detectability. There is hardly any doubt that new allotypes will be detected during the next few years.

How can we reconcile this heterogeneity with our present view on protein biosynthesis in general, and particularly with theories on antibody formation? Let us start with the assumption that antibody biosynthesis does not differ from the synthesis of other proteins and that the amino acid sequence of each antibody molecule is determined by the trinucleotide sequence of the mRNA molecule, and this again by the complementary sequence in the analogous DNA. We would then need more than 100 genes directing the synthesis of the heterogeneous population of more than 100 different antibodies directed against the azophenylarsonate residue, and a similar number for the anti-ammonium antibodies. Oudin [13a] has designated antibodies produced in a single individual against a definite antigenic determinant as idiotypes. We do not yet know whether these hundreds of anti-As idiotypes are formed in each single antibody-forming cell, or whether each of the different anti-As antibodies is formed in another cell. Although the latter explanation seems to be more attractive, formation of a hundred or more anti-As antibodies in a single cell is also reconcilable with the enormous number of genes in the DNA of a mammalian cell. The amount of DNA in a mammalian lymphoid cell is so large [13b] that 1% of the DNA could still contain 30,000 different genes for the same number of heavy chain, and also the same number of genes for the light chain; thus it could determine the amino acid sequences of approximately $30,000 \times 30,000$ or approximately 10^9 antibody molecules. Even if each antigenic determinant would give rise to the formation of approximately a hundred antibodies of the same idiotype, the cell would still be able to produce antibodies directed against 10^7 different antigenic determinants.

The maximum number of antibody-forming sites in a cell can be estimated by measuring the amount of immunoglobulin formed in a culture of a definite number of lymphoid cells, and estimating the time required for the assembly of amino acids in the peptide chains which combine to form the 7S immuno-globulin molecule. Experiments of this type have revealed that the number of immunoglobulin molecules produced in a lymphoid cell is approximately 120 per minute corresponding to 240 H chains [14]. The time required for the formation of the heavy chains is approximately one minute, that required for the light chains only one half minute [15]. The combination of heavy and light chains takes place spontaneously within a few seconds. Since the cell produces approximately 240 molecules of H chains per minute and since the time required for the formation of the complete 7S globulin molecule is approximately one minute, it is clear that the cell must contain approximately 240 H chain forming sites (mRNA molecules) whose nucleotide sequences are determined by the transcription of the same number of cistrons (genes). Evidently, only a very small portion of the total DNA is translated into mRNA and involved in antibody formation in a cell which is producing antibody. If it is remembered that 1% of the total DNA contains 30,000 cistrons for the formation of heavy and light chains, the 240 cistrons involved in antibody formation in a single cell would form only 0.8% of the DNA involved in immunoglobulin formation, or 0.008% of the total DNA of the cell. The number of cistrons involved may be much smaller because one cistron may produce more than one molecule of mRNA per minute.

We do not yet know whether the antibody-forming cell can produce only one type of antibody, or several types, or even all types of antibodies. Since the potentiality of the cell may be different before and after contact with the antigen, it is necessary to consider each of these two types of lymphoid cells separately. It is usually assumed that the immunocyte (immunocompetent cell) which has not yet had any contact with the antigen, and which we may call the virgin immunocyte, reacts with the antigen only slowly whereas the primed immunocyte produces antibody much faster. This criterion is of doubtful value since Litt [16] has recently demonstrated that antibody formation can be detected 7.5 minutes after the first administration of the antigen when the highly sensitive method of hemolytic plaque formation is applied. In view of these results it is questionable whether a lag period exists, and whether the early or late appearance of antibody can be used as a criterion to differentiate virgin immunocompetent cells from primed cells.

Numerous attempts have been made to determine whether an antibody-forming cell, in an organism injected with two different antigens or with an antigen containing two different determinants, produces antibody directed against only one type of antigenic determinant or antibodies against two or more different determinants. The results of these experiments are contradictory. However, most experimenters agree that the majority of cells produce antibodies against only one type of antigenic determinant, and that cells producing antibodies directed against two or more different determinants are rare.

Unfortunately, the results obtained do not allow us to decide whether the antibody-forming cells, even if they produce only one type of antigen, were unipotent or multipotent *before* contact with the antigen. We cannot exclude the possibility that multipotent virgin cells, after contact with one antigen, become inaccessible to other antigens, thus lose their multipotentiality, and become unipotent. Szilard [17] has translated this idea into the language of genetics by postulating that the immunocompetent cells originally are multipotent, that their potentiality to produce specific antibodies is usually repressed, but is *derepressed* by the action of an antigen. They would thus acquire unipotentiality after contact with the antigen.

If the antigen acts as a derepressor, what then is the nature of the repressor? As I mentioned earlier, we have shown that the primed cells continue to form antibody for periods of many months. It is imaginable that each of the cistrons of the nuclear DNA in the virgin immunocyte is transcribed *once* into mRNA, that each of the single mRNA molecules formed is then translated into an immunoglobulin (antibody) molecule, but that in the virgin cell most of the immunoglobulin molecules remain bound to mRNA and thus block further transcription and translation. These cistrons (genes) would thus remain "silent". Injection of the antigen would result in combination with the cell-bound antibody, would thus activate the blocked mRNA and trigger the formation of more antibody.

Recently, Jerne [18] has revived Ehrlich's old theory [19] of preformed receptors. According to this view, the organism produces receptors complementarily adjusted to a large number of antigens which it has never encountered before. After administration of the antigen, the closely fitting receptors are detached from the cell, regenerated at an increased rate, and secreted into the serum as antibodies. The antigen would merely select the cell which forms the closely fitting receptor and would stimulate its regeneration. Although it appeared for a long time difficult to believe that the cell should indeed produce preformed "receptors" for the numerous synthetic haptens described by Landsteiner, Ehrlich's view of preformed receptors and Jerne's similar view are rendered much more attractive by the enormous heterogeneity of the normal immunoglobulin population. Each of these immunoglobulins would act as an antibody if its combining site happened to fit closely to an antigenic determinant. While these views are shared by many if not most immunologists, there is no agreement about the reasons for the heterogeneity of the immunoglobulin population.

It has been mentioned earlier that the Bence-Jones proteins, which form the light chains of immunoglobulins produced in myeloma cells, differ from each other in some of the amino acid positions, and that the replacements can frequently be explained by single-step mutations, i.e. by the change of a single nucleotide in the trinucleotide which acted as a codon for the variable amino acid. It was the purpose of the computations which I presented earlier to demonstrate that the redundance of DNA in the mammalian cell is so large that tens of thousands of different heavy and light chains could be produced in a single cell. Since we know that the much less extensive variability of hemoglobin and other proteins is produced by mutations in the germ-line during long periods of evolution, it was obvious to consider germ-line mutations over periods of millions of years as the cause of the heterogeneity of the immunoglobulins. Burnet in 1959 made the additional assumption that each cell is unipotent and can produce only one type of antibody; the daughter cells of such a cell would then form a clone of unipotent cells; this is the basis of Burnet's clonal selection theory [20]. In its original form it would require an enormous number, not only of different immunoglobulin molecules, but also of different lymphoid cells. The assumption of unipotentiality is difficult to reconcile with the observation that in some mice injected with sheep red blood cells *all* lymphoid cells of the spleen produce antibody directed against sheep red blood cells [26]. This result supports the view that the cells originally were multipotent and that they acquired the ability to produce antibodies of identical specificity after exposure of the organism to the administered antigen. Various hypotheses have been advanced to avoid the assumption of multipotentiality of the immunocytes.

Most of these hypotheses are based on Lederberg's assumption that the cells which produce antibodies undergo frequent *somatic mutations* [21]. The idea of hypermutability appeared to Burnet so attractive that he abandoned his original clonal selection theory and postulated positive and negative selective action of the antigen in a population of cells which continually undergo rapid, random mutations [22]. Very little is known on the occurrence and the mechanism of somatic mutations. Various investigators have proposed various mechanisms of somatic mutation, for instance crossing over between a master gene and a scrambler gene, or crossing over between parts of a single gene [23-25]. Since somatic cells cannot be mated, the classical experiment of genetics cannot be applied to decide whether somatic mutations do indeed take place.

One of the most serious objections raised against the assumption of somatic mutation in immunoglobulins is the great stability of the allotypes during the life of an organism and their transmittance from mother cell to daughter cells according to Mendelian laws of inheritance. Each of the allotypes is determined by a particular amino acid sequence in either the light or the heavy chain, different from analogous amino acid sequences in other allotypes. If the immunoglobulin-producing cells would undergo rapid, random mutations, one would expect changes in the allotypes. Such changes have never been observed, nor have changes in the allotypes been observed in myeloma proteins, although the myeloma cells undergo repeated division and rapid multiplication. Since the allotypes A1, A2, and A3 of the heavy chains of rabbit immunoglobulins occur in H chains of the γ, the μ and the α type, it has been concluded that formation of these allotypes must precede duplication of those genes which mutate and thus give rise to variety [27a], and that a special mechanism would then be necessary to prevent crossing over and genetic drift. It must be admitted that the stability of the allotypes in highly variable peptide chains is difficult to reconcile with classical genetics. However, it must not be forgotten that the allotypes are determined by those amino acid sequences which happen to be detectable by serological methods, and that we do not yet know whether they differ essentially from other amino acid sequences controlled by apparently non-allelic genes.

There is no doubt that the mutations which produce differences in allotypes or differences between individual myeloma proteins are germ-line mutations, i.e. rare mutations of the germ cells which occur during evolution over millions of years [27b, 27c]. Germ-line mutations may also be responsible for all the other differences in the amino acid sequences of the heavy and light chains of the immunoglobulins. The differences between immunoglobulin molecules, their heterogeneity in a single individual, might be attributed to repeated duplication of an ancestral gene over periods of millions of years, and errors or mutational changes during duplication [27b, 28]. A process of this type would explain the redundance in the DNA of a single cell of genes for the production of 10^4–10^5 different heavy chains and a similar number of light chains.

Objections raised against the multiple-gene hypothesis are based particularly on the presence of a variable N-terminal half and an invariant or common C-terminal half in the Bence-Jones proteins. The different variability of the two halves of the light chains appeared to be irreconcilable with the dogma "one gene—one peptide chain". Some investigators postulated the existence of a common gene for the invariant C-terminal amino acid sequences. The assumption of two genes for the two halves of the light chain complicates matters; additional assumptions are necessary to explain the combination of the two halves of the light chains. It is also possible that the amino acid sequence of the entire light chain, like that of other peptide chains, is determined by a single cistron (gene) and a single mRNA template, and that the portion of the gene which determines the amino acid sequence of the N-terminal half of the light chains, undergoes mutations much more frequently than that portion of the DNA which determines the C-terminal amino acid sequence. We do not know at present why one half of the gene should have a higher mutations rate. One might speculate that the numerous cistrons which supply the code for the amino acid sequence of the light chains are arranged in spirals and that one side of this spiral might be stabilized by combination with histone, whereas the other side, consisting of the variable part, would be free and more susceptible to changes by radiation or by mutagens. Other geometrical models can easily be constructed. All of these are speculative as long as we do not know the conformation of the genes involved in immunoglobulin formation.

Although we may not need to invoke random somatic mutations as the reason for the heterogeneity of the immunoglobulin population, it is necessary to emphasize that the immunoglobulin-forming cells undergo important changes during their maturation. Their precursor in the bone marrow has been designated as stem cell. It is an immature cell which is either converted into a large blast cell or may be identical with the blast cells. The blast cells undergo further changes on maturation and may finally become either red blood cells, lymphoid cells, or other types of white blood cells. The lymphoid cells, after contact with the antigen, are converted into plasma cells which by some authors are considered as terminal cells, which cannot multiply. I mention here these phenomena because they demonstrate clearly important changes in the structure of the cells involved in immunoglobulin formation. The morphological changes are accompanied by important changes in function. The lymphoid cells of the newborn animal produce only traces of immunoglobulin; the ability to form immunoglobulins is acquired only a few weeks after birth. Changes of this type are designated as *differentiation*. Unfortunately, very little is known about the mechanism of differentiation.

The question may be asked whether differentiation does not involve changes similar to those produced by mutations. The changes observed in differentiation are frequently much more drastic than those caused by mutagens or by radiation. They may involve the formation of highly specialized muscle or nerve cells from quite different precursor cells. However, differentiation, in contrast to mutation, involves maturation, i.e. predictable orderly changes towards a state of higher specialization of the cell. Differentiation is a continuous process whereas mutations are rare events which take place randomly.

The stem cell, the precursor of the antibody-forming cells, cannot yet produce antibodies; but it contains probably all the structural genes for the numerous immunoglobulins which are later formed in the mature lymphoid cells. Differentiation of the stem cells and their daughter cells, the lymphoblasts, results in the production of lymphoid cells which may still possess the genes for all immunoglobulins although most of these genes are probably repressed. As mentioned earlier, we do not yet know whether the next product of differentiation, the virgin immunocytes, are multipotent, or whether they differentiate further and then have the ability to produce only one type of antibody, or a few types of similar antibodies.

We may finally ask, what is the role of the antigen in antibody formation? If we agree that antibody formation proceeds in the same way as the formation of other proteins, we may narrow down the question by asking whether the antigen interferes in DNA replication, in the transcription of DNA into mRNA, or in the translation of the latter into the amino acid sequence of the nascent peptide chain. As pointed out elsewhere [29], action of the antigen in the first two phases of protein biosynthesis is extremely improbable because we do not know of any particular affinity of the antigen to the coding DNA cistron or to the homologous mRNA molecule. It is much more probable that the antigen interferes in the translation phase, either directly [29, 30] or, more probably, by combination with traces of cell-bound immunoglobulins which have combining sites complementary to the antigen, and therefore act as repressors for further formation of the same antibody. Administration of the antigen would result in combination with these repressors, release them from the cell, and stimulate further translation of the derepressed mRNA template and secretion of antibody from the cell. The essential role of the antigen would be that of a derepressor as first postulated by Szilard [17] and later, in modified form, by Nezlin [31], Finch [32], and others.

In summary, the great variability of the immunoglobulins, the occurrence of various classes, subclasses and allotypes of immunoglobulins can be explained by repeated duplications of an ancestral gene [28] and numerous mutations in the germ-line during a period of several hundred millions of years [27a, b, c]. The ability of the immunocytes to produce many different antibodies, and the great heterogeneity of these antibodies can be attributed either to somatic mutations, or to the presence in the genome of the immunocompetent cells of numerous genes required for the production of the heavy and light chains of all types of antibodies. It has not yet been possible to decide whether the genome of the antibody-forming cells contains genes for thousands of heavy and thousands of light chains, or whether it is necessary to invoke the occurrence of somatic mutations. My own preference for the multiple genes hypothesis is based on (a) *the difficulty of reconciling somatic mutations with the great stability of the allotypes* of heavy and light chains; (b) *the formation of antibody a few minutes after the administration of antigen* [16]; and (c) the orderliness and *predictability of antibody formation* which is compatible with the orderliness and predictability of differentiation, but not with the randomness of mutations. The antigen, according to this view, derepresses the repressed production of the homologous antibody, and thus initiates the differentiation of the immunocompetent cells, possibly by converting multipotent precursor cells into more highly differentiated cells which are either unipotent or able to produce only a few types of antibodies.

REFERENCES

1. Breinl, F. and Haurowitz, F., *Hoppe-Seyler's Z. physiol. Chem.* **192** (1930) 45.
2. Haurowitz, F., *Hoppe-Seyler's Z. physiol. Chem.* **245** (1936) 23.
3. Cheng, H. F., Dicks, M., Shellhamer, R. H., Brown, E. S., Roberts, A. N. and Haurowitz, F., *Proc. Soc. exp. Biol. Med.* **106** (1961) 93.
4. Haurowitz, F., *Ergeb. Mikrobiol. Immunitaetsforsch. exp. Therap.* **34** (1961) 1.
5. Fischman, M. and Adler, F. L., *J. exp. Med.* **117** (1963) 595.
6. Richter, M., Zimmerman, S. and Haurowitz, F., *J. Immun.* **94** (1965) 938.
7. Gowans, J. L. and McGregor, D. D., *Prog. Allergy* **9** (1965) 1.
8. Norman, A., Sasaki, M. S., Ottoman, R. E. and Fingerhut, A. G., *Science, N.Y.* **147** (1965) 745.
9. Knight, K. L., Lopez, M. A. and Haurowitz, F., *J. biol. Chem.* **241** (1966) 2286.
10. Koshland, M. E. and Englberger, F. M., *Proc. natn. Acad. Sci. U.S.A.* **50** (1963) 61.
11. Gold, E. F., Cordes, Sh., Lopez, M. A., Knight, K. L. and Haurowitz, F., *Immunochemistry* **3** (1966) 433.
12. Kamat, G., Lopez, M. A., Vötsch, W., Tharp, E. and Haurowitz, F., unpublished experiments.
13a. Oudin, J., *Proc. R. Soc. Ser. B,* **166** (1966) 207.
13b. Gurvich, A. E. and Nezlin, R. S., *Usp biol. Khim.* **7** (1966) 150.

14. Van Furth, R., Schuit, H. R. E. and Hijmans, W., *Immunology* **11** (1968) 1.
15. Shapiro, A. L., Scharff, M. D., Maizel, J. V. and Uhr, J. W., *Proc. natn. Acad. Sci. U.S.A.* **56** (1966) 216.
16. Litt, M., *Cold Spring Harb. Symp. quant. Biol.* **32** (1967) 477.
17. Szilard, L., *Proc. natn. Acad. Sci. U.S.A.* **46** (1960) 293.
18. Jerne, N. K., *Cold Spring Harb. Symp. quant. Biol.* **32** (1967) 591.
19. Ehrlich, P., *Proc. R. Soc.* Ser. B, **66** (1900) 424.
20. Burnet, F. M., "The Clonal Selection Theory of Acquired Immunity", Vanderbilt University Press, 1959.
21. Lederberg, J., *Science, N.Y.* **129** (1959) 1649.
22. Burnet, F. M., *Nature, Lond.* **203** (1964) 451.
23. Smithies, O., *Science, N.Y.* **157** (1967) 267.
24. Edelman, G. M. and Gally, J. A., *Proc. natn. Acad. Sci. U.S.A.* **57** (1967) 353.
25. Whitehouse, H. L. K., *Nature, Lond.* **215** (1967) 371.
26. Moller, G., *J. exp. Med.* **127** (1968) 291.
27a. Lennox, E. S. and Cohn, M., *A. Rev. Biochem.* **36** (1967) 365.
27b. Ceppellini, R., Genetica delle Immunoglobuline, Assoc. Genetica Italiana, 1966.
27c. Dreyer, W. J., Gray, W. R. and Hood, L., *Cold Spring Harb. Symp. quant. Biol.* **32** (1967) 353.
28. Hill, R. L., Delaney, R., Lebovitz, H. E. and Fellows, R. E., *Proc. R. Soc.* Ser. B, **166** (1966) 159.
29. Haurowitz, F., "Immunochemistry and the Biosynthesis of Antibodies", J. Wiley and Sons, New York, 1968.
30. Haurowitz, F., *Cold Spring Harb. Symp. quant. Biol.* **32** (1967) 559.
31. Nezlin, R. S., "Biokhimya Antit'el", Nauka, Moscow, 1966.
32. Finch, I. R., *Nature, Lond.* **201** (1964) 1288.

FEBS Symposium, Volume 15, 1969, pp. 13-19

Recent Studies on the Structure of the Heavy Chain of Immunoglobulins

R. R. PORTER

Department of Biochemistry, University of Oxford, Oxford, England

There is general agreement that all the immunoglobulins have a basic structure of 2 heavy chains and 2 light chains held together by disulphide bonds. In IgG the molecule is a monomer in solution, in IgM a pentomer held together by disulphide bonds, and in IgA a dimer or larger aggregates, probably held only by non-covalent bonds.

Extensive sequence studies have been carried out, particularly on the Bence-Jones proteins. These are proteins excreted in the urine of some patients with myelomatosis, a cancer of lymphoid tissue, and have been shown to be free light chains from the myeloma protein present in the patients' serum [1]. From preliminary studies, Hilschmann and Craig [2] drew the conclusion that the C-terminal half of the chain was of identical sequence in a given light chain type but that the N-terminal half differed from one protein to the next. This conclusion has been fully supported by the much more extensive information now available. Though the evidence is much less complete, the same phenomenon appears to occur also in the heavy chain. Thus in one species there are two types of light chain characterized by the sequence of the C-terminal half of the chain, but each with a variable N-terminal half. There are also some 10 or 20 kinds of heavy chain in which the sequence of the C-terminal part is characteristic of the class and subclass to which they belong, but each seems to vary in N-terminal section.

This is a most remarkable phenomenon, unique to the immunoglobulins, and the very reasonable conclusion has been drawn that it is the origin of the many different forms of the steric structure of the antibody-combining site, and hence of the wide range of antibody specificity. It would appear to follow that each given antibody specificity and combining affinity would be characterized by a unique sequence in the variable parts of both the heavy and light chains. Direct proof of this is hard to obtain, however, because of the extreme subtlety of antibody specificity. To persuade an animal to make an antibody of one precise specific affinity for a well-characterized antigen seems to be impossible and the fractionation of a mixture of very similar antibodies is equally difficult. The

13

most hopeful approach seems to be work with myeloma proteins, now being found to show antibody-like activity [3]. These proteins appear to have a unique structure, and correlation with specificity may be possible, unless more than one myeloma protein is found to have a given specificity, as seems possible. This will again make it difficult to distinguish the sequences essential for activity from those varying for other reasons. Needless to say, there is very great interest in finding out not only the correlation between sequences and specificity but also in determining the biological origin of this apparently infinite variety of similar, but not identical, proteins. Many of the papers this morning will be concerned with this aspect of the problem. As most of the emphasis of these papers will be on the work with the light chains, I wish to summarize briefly the work so far available on the heavy chain.

The work on the structure of the heavy chain was slower in starting, partly because of the greater difficulty of getting sufficient myeloma protein compared to the easily available Bence-Jones protein, and partly due to its greater size. The heavy chain contains some 450 residues and can be obtained in two halves following papain hydrolysis of the whole molecule, or alternatively broken down, as most now prefer, by the splitting of the isolated heavy chain into several fragments by cyanogen bromide at the methionine residue. There seem to be 4 to 6 methionine residues in the heavy chain of the several classes and subclasses of immunoglobulin which have been examined and hence a relatively small number of fragments can be obtained. These are aligned by comparing the products obtained from the whole chain and from the Fc and Fd position of the chain and by isolation of methionine-containing peptides to give the overlapping sequences. The solution of the sequences has then been obtained by isolation of peptides from digestion with trypsin, chymotrypsin and other enzymes, using the well-established methods.

These methods have been applied to both the Fd and the Fc fractions of the γ chain from rabbit sera, and to the heavy chain of several human myeloma proteins. The major objective has been to establish the nature and extent of the variable section of the heavy chain relative to the light chain in the myeloma protein and to see how far this was applicable to the γ chain of normal rabbits.

In the work with the myeloma proteins, the positions of the methionine appear as shown in Fig. 1. These are three γ chains of the same subclass but Daw and Cor are Gma^+f^- while Eu is Gma^-f^+. Thorpe and Deutsch [6] have shown that Gma^+ and Gma^- myelomas differ in a methionine peptide present in a^- but absent in a^+. It therefore seems highly likely that the additional methionine in the Fc section of Eu relative to Daw and Cor is the position of an allotype-related peptide, and evidence to this effect has been obtained. There is, however, some difference between the sequences of these peptides reported from the two laboratories [7]. The two other methionine residues in the Fc are the same and there is evidence that they are also found in the γ chain of IgG from several subclasses in different species and hence are likely to be characteristic of all γ chains. The methionines in the Fd section are clearly in different positions and show that this is a variable region. It can also be seen that a half cystine in position 22 in both Daw and Cor is joined to another at positions 96 and 79 respectively, another indication of variability up to at least position 96. Similarity, though not identity, of sequence nearer the carboxyl end suggested that there is in fact a deletion of 17 residues in Cor relative to Daw between positions 30 to 70. The position of the enzymic splitting in these three

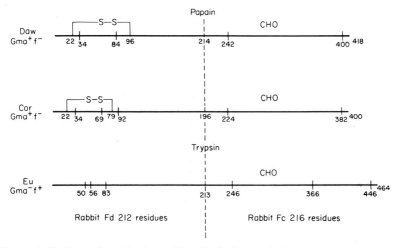

Figure 1. Position of methionine residues in the heavy chain of three human myeloma proteins IgG 1. Daw and Cor taken from Press and Piggot [4]. Eu calculated from molecular weights of CNBr fragments [5]. A mean amino acid residue weight of 110 has been assumed.

myelomas and in rabbit IgG occurs always in the middle of the heavy chain, presumably because only a short section here is approachable by the enzymes. The exact sequences of this section are now known, as are the main positions of splitting by papain trypsin and pepsin [8-12]. The most extensive sequence available is that of Daw, and is shown in Fig. 2.

Press (unpublished) has isolated identical peptides from the Cor γ chain and the same sequences have been reported for Eu [12] and for another γG1 myeloma [10]. Clearly this region has a constant sequence in IgG of this subclass. There is also general agreement on the position of the four interchain disulphide bonds. The sequence of the N-terminal section is available from the work of Press and her colleagues, who have published the results for the residues 1–84 in Daw γ chain [13]. This has been extended to give a partial sequence for most of the Fd section for both Cor and Daw and, though still incomplete, it is clear that there are obvious differences beyond residue 110, showing that the

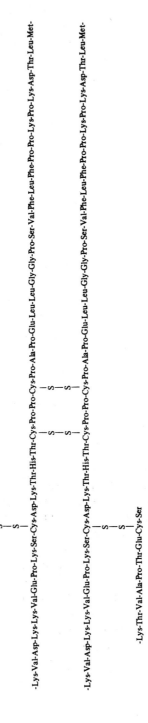

Figure 2. Sequence containing the inter-heavy chain disulphide bonds of a pathological human IgG 1. From [9].

variable section is rather greater than the 107 residue section found in Bence-Jones proteins. Complete sequences of the Fd section of many myeloma γ chains will be needed to define precisely the length and degree of variability of the heavy chains. It is, however, already apparent that the length of the variable section is similar to that now well established for Bence-Jones proteins. Extension of these studies will bring out the correlation of sequence with subclass and allotype, sufficient data being already available to show that this exists—for example, the varying sequences of the C-terminal 18 amino acids in human subclasses [14] and the variation of sequence around the interchain disulphide bonds of different subclasses [10, 15].

Similarly, it might be expected that sequence studies of myeloma proteins of a given specific affinity, as are now being found, would reveal a correlation between sequence and specificity. This may well prove possible, and I understand that work with several mouse myeloma proteins with a specific affinity for the dinitrophenyl group has been started at St. Louis and elsewhere. Some uncertainty has arisen, however, from the relative ease with which these specific myeloma proteins have been found. On a random basis it would not be expected that anti-DNP activity would occur frequently; neither would any selection in favour of that specificity be expected as no naturally occurring cross-reacting antigen is known. More information may clarify this point and it will be of great interest to know if sequences characteristic of DNP specificity can be detected. The recent papers of Eisen and his colleagues [16, 17] have shown that a given specificity (anti-DNP) can be associated with varying chemical composition and therefore sequence. It is apparent that information from a number of myeloma proteins with a given specificity may be necessary before the characteristic features will become apparent.

An alternative approach is to work with antibody produced by immunization of normal animals and to compare this sequence with that of IgG from the pooled serum of immunized animals. With this approach, averages from two complex populations are being compared and only the salient features might be apparent. The difficulty lies, of course, in the complexity of the material handled. The IgG of normal animals is likely to be a mixture of many thousand antibodies mostly present in trace amounts, and if they do vary substantially in sequence in the variable section then it might be impossible to find any coherent sequence in this key section. In fact, this does not appear to be so. It has been found [18, 19] that if the lysine residues in the Fd section of heavy chain from IgG of pooled rabbit sera are reacted with trifluoracetic acid, subsequent digestion with trypsin at the six arginine residues leads to the formation of six peptides which can be isolated. They are sufficiently distinctive in composition to be aligned by comparison with the known sequences of human myeloma heavy chain. They are clearly not derived from overlapping sections of the chain and together appear to account for at least 90% of the sequence of the Fd section. A seventh peptide with arginine C-terminal was expected but was found only recently and appears to be quite small (S. A. Jackson, unpublished). The sequence of the N-terminal 34 residues [20] and of the C-terminal 150 residues (R. F. Fruchter and S. A. Jackson, unpublished) is nearly completed, leaving about 50 positions unknown. They are accounted for by a well-defined peptide of 31 residues, of which part of the sequence is known, and another poorly characterized peptide of 39 residues which is believed to include a substantial part of the N-terminal 34 section. Though incomplete, there seems to be a reasonable prospect of obtaining a majority sequence along the whole Fd section. Many replacement positions have been identified, some of which, near the N-terminus, appear to correlate with allotype [20]. Another, near the C-terminal, also appears to be allotype related [21] but in the heavy chain from the IgG of an allotypically homozygous rabbit a variety of other replacement positions have been found and it is certain that many more remain to be identified which are not related to allotype. It should also be emphasized that a replacement present in less than 20% of the molecules could be missed. With these reservations, however, the progress in establishing a sequence across this variable area was surprising. Most surprising was the consistent isolation of a pure peptide of 26 residues length in 50–80% yield, though the results with the myeloma proteins suggest that it includes the C-terminal end of the variable section.

These results raise several questions, the most obvious perhaps being to ask again whether myeloma proteins are really representative of the different forms of immunoglobulin present in the normal animal. The incomplete data on Daw and Cor suggest variation in sequence in not less than 30 positions, some of it being accounted for by an insertion in Daw relative to Cor. If the assumption is made that the variable sections of the light and heavy chains are comparable, then 60–70 variable positions would be expected to be found as the data accumulate, with perhaps up to five alternative residues in some positions. A complexity of this order in a mixture of many thousand myeloma proteins, such as normal IgG is thought to be, seems incompatible with the comprehensible sequence which appears to be emerging in the rabbit Fd section. However, there have been several suggestions that the Bence-Jones protein may be divided into groups which differ obviously from each other but are rather similar within one group [22-24]. If this is correct, and one group is dominant in normal IgG, as occurs for the subclasses, a reconciliation of the data from the rabbit IgG and myeloma proteins may be possible.

A comparison of the structure of the Fd section of the anti-DNP antibody with that of normal IgG has been carried only as far as analysis of the major tryptic peptides (after reaction of the lysine with trifluoracetic acid). No differences sufficiently large to be considered significant in these mixed sequences were found, though in a related study, using antibodies of different specificity, Koshland [25] reported that significant differences were detectable. There are a number of major discrepancies between the results of Koshland and those of Cebra *et al.* [18, 19]. However, if the basic sequence can be completed and peptides arising from variants positioned against this, it should be possible to repeat the work with a purified antibody and identify any characteristic sequences which exist. This should give some guide as to the structural basis of antibody specificity, should help to decide how far myeloma proteins are characteristic of normal immunoglobulins, and perhaps give a hint as to the mechanism of synthesis of specific antibodies.

REFERENCES

1. Edelman, G. M. and Gally, J. A., *J. exp. Med.* **116** (1962) 207.
2. Hilschmann, N. and Craig, L. C., *Proc. natn. Acad. Sci. U.S.A.* **56** (1965) 602.
3. Eisen, H. N., Little, J. R., Osterland, C. K. and Simms, E. S., *Cold Spring Harb. Symp. quant. Biol.* **32** (1967) 75.
4. Press, E. M. and Piggot, P. J., *Cold Spring Harb. Symp. quant. Biol.* **32** (1967) 45.
5. Edelman, G. M., *in* "Gamma Globulins," Nobel Symposium 3 (edited by J. Killander), Almqvist and Wiksell, Stockholm, 1967, p. 89.
6. Thorpe, N. O. and Deutsch, H. F., *Immunochemistry* **3** (1966) 329.
7. Waxdal, M. J., Konigsberg, W. H. and Edelman, G. M., *Biochemistry, N.Y.* **7** (1968) 1967.
8. Smyth, D. S. and Utsumi, S., *Nature, Lond.* **216** (1967) 332.
9. Steiner, L. A. and Porter, R. R., *Biochemistry, N.Y.* **6** (1967) 3957.
10. Frangione, B. and Milstein, C., *Nature, Lond.* **216** (1967) 939.
11. Givol, D. and de Lorenzo, F., *J. biol. Chem.* **243** (1968) 1886.
12. Gall, W. E., Cunningham, B. A., Waxdal, M. J., Konigsberg, W. H. and Edelman, G. M., *Biochemistry, N.Y.* **7** (1968) 1973.
13. Press, E. M., *Biochem. J.* **104** (1967) 30C.
14. Prahl, J. W., *Biochem. J.* **105** (1967) 1019.
15. Pink, J. R. L. and Milstein, C., *Nature, Lond.* **216** (1967) 941.
16. McGuigan, J. and Eisen, H. N., *Biochemistry, N.Y.* **7** (1968) 1919.
17. McGuigan, J., Simms, E. S. and Eisen, H. N., *Biochemistry, N.Y.* **7** (1968) 1929.
18. Cebra, J. J., Givol, D. and Porter, R. R., *Biochem. J.* **107** (1968) 69.
19. Cebra, J. J., Steiner, L. A. and Porter, R. R., *Biochem. J.* **107** (1968) 79.
20. Wilkinson, J. M., this volume, p. 183.
21. Prahl, J. W. and Porter, R. R., *Biochem. J.* **107** (1968) 753.
22. Smithies, O., *Science, N.Y.* **157** (1967) 267.
23. Niall, H. D. and Edman, P., *Nature, Lond.* **216** (1967) 262.
24. Milstein, C., *Nature, Lond.* **216** (1967) 330.
25. Koshland, M. E., *Cold Spring Harb. Symp. quant. Biol.* **32** (1967) 119.

FEBS Symposium, Volume 15, 1969, pp. 21-41

Structure and Variability of Immunoglobulin Light Chains

F. W. PUTNAM

Division of Biological Sciences,
Indiana University, Bloomington,
Indiana, 47401, U.S.A.

Immunoglobulins are members of the large family of γ globulins and are either endowed with known antibody activity or are related to antibodies in chemical structure and hence in antigenic specificity [1]. Their usual heterogeneity obstructs determination of their structure by present methods of protein chemistry. In multiple myeloma, a tumor of the plasma cells which are normally a site of antibody biosynthesis, and in macroglobulinemia, large amounts of homogeneous immunoglobulins are secreted into the serum and incomplete immunoglobulins (Bence-Jones proteins) may be excreted in the urine. These abnormal proteins lack demonstrated antibody activity but are classified as immunoglobulins because of their similarity in site of synthesis, polypeptide chain structure, and antigenic specificity [2]. The homogeneity of these abnormal proteins permits their amino acid sequence analysis, unlike normal γ globulins and the natural mixture of antibodies. However, the abnormal proteins, though serving as a model for structural study of antibody γ globulins, appear to differ in amino acid sequence for each patient.

Because such almost infinite variability in primary structure is unique to the immunoglobulins it is thought to be related to antibody specificity. Though indirect, this is still the best evidence for the hypothesis that specific antibodies differ from each other in amino acid sequence. This is the crux of the antibody problem and leads to the paradox; either protein structure is not invariant and is not uniquely determined by pre-existing genes, or there must be already present in the genetic make-up of vertebrate animals sufficient immunoglobulin genes to provide for an almost unlimited number of antibodies. To solve this problem, knowledge is needed of the exact structure of immunoglobulins; at present this is best obtainable by study of the abnormal globulins.

CLASSIFICATION OF IMMUNOGLOBULINS

The structural relationships of abnormal globulins, normal γ globulin, and antibodies, are manifested as common antigenic determinants. Hence, by use of antisera specific for abnormal globulins, normal human γ globulins were classified into six major subgroups [3-5]. These later were related to the polypeptide chain structures (Fig. 1) and were shown to occur generally in vertebrate species. All six subgroups and many subtypes thereof are produced by healthy individuals, but patients with plasma cell disorders usually make only a single kind, often in large amounts and invariably characteristic for the individual.

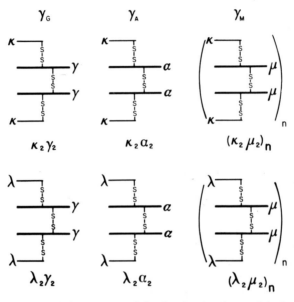

Figure 1. Polypeptide chain structure of the three major classes of the immunoglobulins (γG, γA, and γM). Alternatively, the three immunoglobulin classes may be designated by the abbreviation Ig, i.e. IgG, IgA, and IgM [1]. The light chains are denoted κ and λ and the heavy chains γ, α, or μ. The chain formula is given under each subgroup. (From Fig. 1, Putnam [6]).

A major breakthrough in the structural study of immunoglobulins came from recognition of their multichain structure and from dissociation of the molecules into the two kinds of polypeptide chains, light and heavy [7-9]. The chains are so designated because of their molecular weight, about 23,000 and 50,000 respectively. In vertebrates, all three major classes of immunoglobulins (γG, γA, and γM or alternatively, IgG, IgA, and IgM) appear to consist of a pair of identical heavy chains and a pair of identical light chains linked together through interchain disulfide bonds (Fig. 1). The heavy chains carry the antigenic determinants characteristic of the class; they differ in structure and are designated the γ, α, or μ chains [1]. The light chains determine the antigenic type, K or L and are called κ or λ respectively [1]. Significant homologous

relationships in structure exist between κ and λ chains and probably also among the three kinds of heavy chains. Although the latter differ distinctly from light chains, certain general principles may govern the biosynthesis and structure of both kinds of chains and they seem to have had a common evolutionary origin.

The subclassification of human γ globulins initially depended on two facts about the immunochemistry of Bence-Jones proteins; first, that these proteins are antigenically related to normal human γ globulin, second, that there are two antigenically distinct types, κ and λ. By use of antisera to Bence-Jones proteins it was shown that all human γ globulins are either of κ or λ type and that healthy individuals produce both types in a ratio of about two to one [3-5]. The Bence-Jones protein, which differs in structure for each patient, is either of the κ or λ type; it is equivalent to the light polypeptide chain of the serum myeloma globulin of the patient and is related structurally to all normal light chains of the corresponding type. Whereas the Bence-Jones protein is usually homogeneous and has a unique amino acid sequence [10], normal light chains are heterogeneous and possibly represent as many as a thousand kinds of κ and λ chains, each differing in amino acid sequence. Thus, amino acid sequence may be determined readily on Bence-Jones proteins, but only with difficulty and much uncertainty for normal γ globulins.

Only part of the heterogeneity of γ globulins is explained by the classification into six subgroups shown in Fig. 1. In man there are minor classes such as γD and γE and also four subclasses of γ heavy chains, γG1, γG2, γG3, and γG4, which differ in structure at restricted points. There are also allelic variants for both the light and heavy chains. For example, in man more than 20 known Gm-genetic antigens are associated with the subclasses of the γ heavy chain [11], and several Inv hereditary types of κ light chains occur. Analogous allotypes are found in other species.

Light chain preparations from normal γ globulin of all species are resolved electrophoretically into about ten distinct and regularly spaced components, each differing from the next by a unit electrical charge. Purified preparations of normal κ or λ chains and allotypic forms of the normal chain are just as heterogeneous; thus, there appear to be at least 40 distinct forms of light chains in man, and probably many more. Light chain preparations from specific antibodies are also heterogeneous except for those from antibodies associated with chronic cold agglutinin disease. However, the Bence-Jones proteins from man or the mouse usually migrate as a single band that may correspond in mobility to any of the normal bands.

The principal structural features of γG globulin are shown in more detail in the schematic drawing of Fig. 2. This summarizes information on the sequence of κ and λ light chains obtained in our laboratory [13-16], the enzymatic cleavage of γG globulins studied by Porter and others [17], and the structural studies of γ heavy chains by Hill *et al.* [18], Edelman *et al.* [19] and Porter's group [8]. As Fig. 2 indicates, it has been established that the Bence-Jones protein of a given myeloma patient is identical to the light chain of his serum myeloma globulin and is structurally related to one of the two types of light chains (kappa or lambda) [7, 9]. The same is true for the Bence-Jones protein and the light chain of the macroglobulin from patients with macroglobulinemia [20]. Hence, hereafter the terms Bence-Jones protein and light chain will be

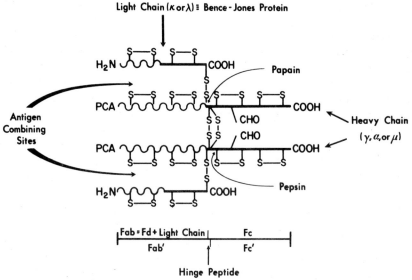

Figure 2. Schematic diagram drawn to scale of the linear polypeptide chain structure of γG globulin. γA and γM globulins probably have an analogous structure. Two identical half-molecules are symmetrically arranged; each contains a light chain and a heavy chain. The position and number of the intrachain disulfide bonds are correctly shown in the light chains but are hypothetical in the heavy chains. Human γG has two, but rabbit γG has only one heavy-heavy interchain bond at the location shown. Papain cleaves the heavy chain on the NH_2-terminal side and pepsin on the COOH-terminal side of this bond yielding fragments Fab, and Fc or (Fab')$_2$ described in the text. CHO denotes a carbohydrate prosthetic group attached at the location shown. The variable portion of the sequence is symbolized by wavy lines and the constant portion by straight lines. The location and relative length of these regions are correctly shown in light chains but are hypothetical in heavy chains. (From Fig. 2, Putnam [12]).

used synonymously. However, although the myeloma patient makes a single kind of light chain differing in amino acid sequence from one patient to another, a healthy individual may make a thousand kinds of light chains of both the κ and λ types, all of which likewise presumably differ in amino acid sequence.

As indicated in Fig. 2, antibodies are divalent and have two combining sites, one located in each Fab piece. Each site apparently involves combination of the antigen with a portion of both the light and heavy chains. We believe that the variation in amino acid sequence that occurs in the NH_2-terminal half of both light and heavy chains is involved in antibody specificity. Here, the variable portion of the sequence is represented by the wavy lines, and the constant portion by the straight lines. The univalent Fab piece of antibody contains a single intact light chain and about one half of the heavy chain. Except for changes in amino acid sequence associated with genetic factors, all the variability in the primary structure of γ globulins appear to be located in this piece. Hence, we assume the variability in sequence is related to antibody specificity.

The linear diagrams of the polypeptide chain structure of γ globulins, of course, do not represent the full structure of the molecule, which can only be obtained by a combination of X-ray crystallography and complete amino acid sequence analysis.

PRIMARY STRUCTURE OF LIGHT CHAINS

The remaining discussion will largely be concerned with studies of the amino acid sequence of human κ and λ Bence-Jones proteins and their relationship to the normal light and heavy chains of man and other species. The purpose is not to present the procedures for determining the sequence or the proof of structure, but rather to summarize present knowledge of the primary structure of κ and λ light chains and to interpret this in terms of the structural evolution of these chains and their present-day function. The questions to be raised are what is the structural relationship between κ and λ chains in the same species and among different species, and likewise among light and heavy chains, and what can be deduced from this with regard to the genetic origin and evolutionary development of light and heavy chains, for the preceding figures suggest that such structural relationships do exist. It is first necessary to consider the remarkable variation in primary structure that is found on comparison of the amino acid sequences of the Bence-Jones proteins excreted by different individuals with multiple myeloma. These proteins are equivalent to the light chains of the abnormal globulin in the serum of the patients, and they share many structural features with normal human light chains including identity in sequence in the carboxyl-terminal half of all light chains of the same antigenic type.

Human light chains have structural features that are probably shared by the light chains of most other vertebrate species. The unique structural characteristic of light chains—also the one most difficult to explain by current genetic theory—is that both kappa and lambda chains are almost exactly divisible into an NH_2-terminal half, which is variable in amino acid sequence, and a COOH-terminal half that is almost invariant in sequence. These are designated the variable and constant regions in Fig. 3, which gives the complete amino acid sequence for one human lambda light chain (Bence-Jones protein Sh) and also indicates positions of identity or of variance for two other human lambda light chains (Ha and Bo). In the constant region the last 105 residues of the three

2

proteins are identical in sequence, whereas in the variable region 53 positions are different in any two or in all three of the proteins [13, 14].

Whereas proteins of the same kind within a species are believed to have a common amino acid sequence except for polymorphic variants under genetic

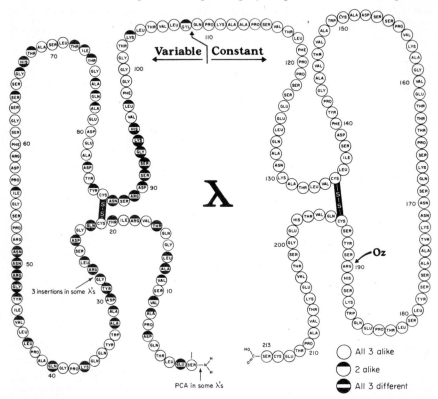

Figure 3. Amino acid sequence of the human λ-type Bence-Jones protein Sh. Positions given in white circles are identical in the human λ-type Bence-Jones proteins Ha and Bo. Where the circle is black at the top, two of the three λ chains have the same amino acid but differ from the third. All three proteins differ in positions where the circles are black at the top and bottom. (From Fig. 4, Putnam [6]).

control, the Bence-Jones protein from each patient has a unique sequence. Thus far, no two Bence-Jones proteins of the same antigenic type from the same species have been found to be identical. In the three human λ proteins illustrated in Fig. 3 the differences in sequence range from 40 to 53 (Table 1). In human κ-type Bence-Jones proteins 73 loci of variation in the NH_2-terminal region have been discovered, and the sequence differences observed between any two proteins have ranged from 16 to 60 (Table 1). This contrasts with the single amino acid replacements found in the abnormal human hemoglobins and resembles the structural differences observed between proteins of similar kind from divergent species. Furthermore, the amino acid substitutions observed in more than 50 abnormal human hemoglobins are consistent with a one-base mutation in the corresponding codon, whereas in the above λ proteins the ratio of minimum one-base changes to two-base changes is about two to one and there are many transversions as well as transitions.

Human λ light chains (and likewise human and mouse κ chains) may differ not only in sequence in the variable region, but also in length. Unlike the specimen illustrated, most λ chains in man and other species begin with a blocked amino group (probably pyrrolidone-carboxylic acid, a cyclized form of

Table 1. Number of amino acid differences between human kappa, mouse kappa and human lambda Bence-Jones proteins.

	λ_{Sh}	λ_{Ha}	λ_{Bo}	κ_{M41}	κ_{M70}	κ_{Ag}	κ_{Roy}	κ_{Cum}
λ_{Sh}	0	53	49	128	130	135	136	139
λ_{Ha}	53	0	40	132	126	134	134	134
λ_{Bo}	49	40	0	130	129	134	136	137
κ_{M41}	128	132	130	0	47	82	84	101
κ_{M70}	130	126	129	47	0	91	91	94
κ_{Ag}	135	134	134	82	91	0	16	55
κ_{Roy}	136	134	136	84	91	16	0	60
κ_{Cum}	139	134	137	101	94	55	60	0

*Modified from Putnam et al. [10] and Dayhoff and Eck [21].

glutamine, denoted PCA), whereas κ chains generally have an unblocked NH_2-terminal group, usually aspartic acid. Insertions of three amino acid residues after position 27 occur in the sequence of the human λ-type proteins Ha and Bo. At about the same place four residues are inserted in the mouse κ-type Bence-Jones protein M70 [22, 23] and six in the human κ chain Cum [24]. Thus, the length of light chains may vary from 213 to 221 residues. This leads to a difficulty in systematic numbering which has been resolved by using as a reference the numbering for λ chains given for protein Sh in Fig. 3 and for κ chains that are given later for protein Ag in Fig. 4, for these were the first proteins of each antigenic type for which the sequence was reported [13-16].

A third feature shared by all light chains so far studied is the presence of two intrachain disulfide bonds, each forming a loop of about 60 amino acids (see Figs. 3 and 4). These are symmetrically distributed; one is within the variable half and the other in the constant half of the chain. Thus, the two halves of the molecule exhibit bilateral symmetry suggestive of two similar subunits despite the great difference in amino acid sequence of the two regions. This apparent symmetry should result in a gross similarity in conformation of the two halves of the chain and has led to the idea that light chains originated by duplication of an ancestral gene coding for about 110 amino acid residues [10, 18].

Another general feature of light chains is the presence of a cysteine residue at the COOH-terminus which, through formation of an interchain disulfide bond, provides a link to the heavy chain. In most species this cysteine is the last residue in κ chains and is penultimate in λ chains. Through disulfide bonding it may

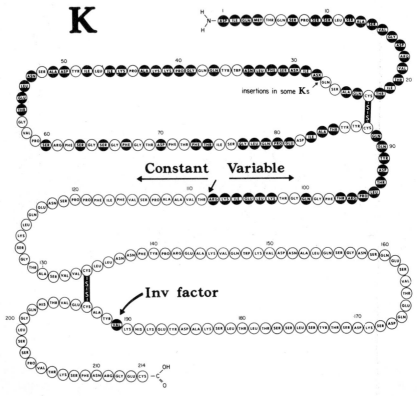

Figure 4. Amino acid sequence of the human kappa Bence-Jones protein Ag. The black circles mark the 73 variable loci where different amino acids have been found in other human kappa Bence-Jones proteins. The sequence at positions 28 to 32 is provisional. Data obtained from Titani *et al.* [15, 16], Hilschmann [24], Whitley and Putnam [28], Cunningham *et al.* [29], Niall and Edman [30], Milstein [31], and Hood *et al.* [32]. It is uncertain whether position 108 is part of the variable region or the site of a genetic variation like that observed at the Inv locus. Modified from Putnam [6].

cause dimerization of free light chains excreted in the urine as Bence-Jones proteins.

Although the three human λ-type Bence-Jones proteins illustrated in Fig. 3 have an identical sequence for the last 105 residues, as does a fourth [25], four possible loci of variation have been reported in the carboxyl half of other human λ chains. In λ chains of the Oz(+) serological system lysine replaces the arginine at position 190 in Oz(−) λ chains [26]. Ser-153 is replaced by glycine in some λ chains [27], and preliminary results suggest that Ala-144 may be replaced by valine and Lys-172 by asparagine [25]. It is not known whether these interchanges are controlled by allelic genes or whether they represent a limited variability in sequence in the carboxyl half of λ chains. This may provide a critical test for several hypotheses of the genetic origin of the structural variability of light chains.

STRUCTURAL VARIATION IN KAPPA CHAINS

Like λ chains, κ chains differ in many positions in the NH_2-terminal portion but are essentially invariant in sequence in the COOH-terminal half. Nearly complete amino acid sequences have been reported for four human κ-type Bence-Jones proteins designated Ag [15, 16], Roy [24], Cum [24], and Mil [22]. A fifth (Tew) has almost been completed [28], and the sequence of the variable region of one κ light chain from a human γG globulin is known [29]. Two mouse κ-type Bence-Jones proteins have been almost completely sequenced [22, 23]. All these proteins exhibit the characteristics described above for human λ chains, namely, an almost equal division into variable and constant regions, variation in chain length owing to insertions at about residue 27, the presence of two intrachain disulfide loops each of about 60 residues, and a COOH-terminal cysteine which provides a link to the heavy chain. These features are illustrated in a different alignment of the disulfide loops in Fig. 4 which depicts the amino acid sequence of the human κ-type Bence-Jones protein Ag in comparison with a mouse κ chain and a human λ chain. In human κ chains, 73 variable loci have been identified in the NH_2-terminal portion, which ends at residue 108, but only one in the COOH-terminal half. The latter, associated with the Inv genetic factor, is located at position 191 and thus is analogous to the Oz factor located at position 190 in human λ chains. Residue 191 is valine if the human κ chain is Inv(b+) but is leucine if the κ protein is Inv(a+).

From the number of sequence differences in the three human κ Bence-Jones proteins listed in Table 1, it is evident that some κ chains are more similar in structure than others, and thus that subtypes may exist.

The extent of the variation in the primary structure of κ chains is illustrated in Table 2 by comparison of the amino acid sequence of the first 18 to 22 residues of 25 individual human Bence-Jones proteins or separated light chains, all of the κ type, for which data have been reported [15, 16, 24, 28-32]. Several of the proteins are identical in this initial sequence though differing further along the chain. Altogether for the 25 specimens, 17 different sequences have been recorded for the first 18 residues. These 17 sequences differ from each other by as many as nine residues and as few as one.

Three subtypes of NH_2-terminal sequence are evident. Type I, representing 13 specimens, ıs like protein Ag. Type II (three examples) differs from Ag in up to

13 positions in the first 22. Type III, comprising nine specimens, differs from both of the kappa subtypes I and II in almost half the positions in the sequence illustrated. These subtypes are sometimes designated κ_I, κ_{II}, and κ_{III}. There is no parallel for such remarkable differences in amino acid sequence of proteins having a similar function and cellular site of synthesis, except for polymorphic proteins controlled by separate genes.

Table 2. Amino-terminal sequence of human kappa chains.

Sub-type		1	5	10	15	20
I	Ag	Asp-Ile-Gln-Met-Thr-Gln-Ser-Pro-Ser-Ser-Leu-Ser-Ala-Ser-Val-Gly-Asp-Arg-Val-Thr-Ile-Thr				
	Others	Val		Thr Thr	Val Leu Arg	Ile Ala
		Leu		Phe		
II	Tew	Val		Leu	Pro Val Thr Pro	Glu Pro Ala Ser Ser
	Others		Leu Thr			
III	Fr4	Glu Val Leu		Gly Thr	Leu Pro Glu	Ala Leu Ser
	Others	Lys Met		Asx	Met	
				Ala		
Number of Different Residues		3 2 3 2	1 1 2 1 6	3 1 2 4 2	3 2 2 2 3	2 2 3

The sequence is given on the top line for protein Ag[15]. Below each position are summarized all of the different residues reported in 24 other human κ chains, including work of Hilschmann [24], Whitley and Putnam [28], Cunningham et al. [29], Niall and Edman [30], Milstein [31], and Hood et al. [32].

At the bottom of Table 2 is listed the number of different residues thus far observed at each position. There are only four remaining invariant positions in the first 22 of human κ chains, and the number of different residues at one position may be as high as four or six. This seems to rule out any simple mechanism of somatic hypermutation such as multiple recombination between just two genes. About one quarter of the interchanges listed in the table would require a double mutation in the corresponding codons. The presence of many two-step changes indicates a high frequency of mutation but does not provide a decisive test whether the variability in sequence arose entirely by an evolutionary process resulting in many separate light chain genes carried in the germ line, or whether somatic hypermutation arising from gene recombination [33] or some other mechanism is the origin.

The three specimens of subtype II κ chains, for which almost complete sequences have been determined, are very similar in primary structure. For example, they differ at only two positions in the first 24 residues illustrated in Table 2, and, excluding possible amide differences, these three light chains are identical for at least 35 consecutive residues. This long stretch of identity is illustrated in Fig. 5 giving the sequence for subtype II κ proteins Tew, Mil, and Cum from residues 54 through 88 in comparison to the sequences of three subtype I κ chains. Each of the latter differs from subtype II in 14 of the 35 positions illustrated and they differ from each other in from 3 to 8 positions. This obvious subdivision into several kinds of κ chains dispels the idea that all the sequence variation in light chains results either from random

κ_II (positions 54–70)

	54						60								70	
TEW	ARG	ALA	SER	GLY	VAL	PRO	ASP	ARG	PHE	SER	GLY	SER	GLY	THR	ASP	PHE
MIL	ARG	ALA	SER	GLY	VAL	PRO	ASN	ARG	PHE	SER	GLY	SER	GLY	THR	ASX	PHE
CUM	ARG	ALA	SER	GLY	VAL	PRO	ASP	ARG	PHE	SER	GLY	SER	GLY	THR	ASP	PHE

κ_I (positions 54–70)

	54						60								70	
ROY	LEU	GLU	ALA	GLY	VAL	PRO	SER	ARG	PHE	SER	GLY	SER	GLY	THR	ASP	PHE
AG	LEU	GLU	THR	GLY	VAL	PRO	SER	ARG	PHE	SER	GLY	PHE	GLY	THR	ASP	PHE
EU	LEU	GLX	SER	GLY	VAL	PRO	SER	ARG	ILE	GLY	SER	GLY	THR	GLX	PHE	

κ_II (positions 72–88)

	72								80							
TEW	THR	LEU	LYS	ILE	SER	ARG	VAL	GLU	ALA	VAL	GLY	VAL	TYR	TYR	CYS
MIL	THR	LEU	LYS	ILE	SER	ARG	VAL	GLX	ALA	VAL	GLY	VAL	TYR	TYR	CYS
CUM	THR	LEU	LYS	ILE	SER	ARG	VAL	GLU	ALA	ASX	GLY	VAL	TYR	TYR	CYS

κ_I (positions 72–88)

	72								80							
ROY	THR	PHE	THR	ILE	SER	SER	LEU	GLN	PRO	GLU	ASP	ILE	ALA	THR	TYR	TYR	CYS
AG	THR	PHE	THR	ILE	SER	GLY	LEU	GLN	PRO	GLU	ASP	ILE	ALA	THR	TYR	TYR	CYS
EU	THR	LEU	THR	ILE	SER	SER	LEU	GLX	PRO	GLX	ASX	PHE	ALA	THR	TYR	TYR	CYS

Figure 5. Amino acid sequence of three subtype II (K_II) and three subtype I (K_I) human kappa chains from position 54 through 88. The subtype II proteins are identical throughout the 35 residues shown. Many differences from them and from each other occur in this region for subtype I kappa chains. Data from Whitley and Putnam [28]. Dreyer et al. [22], Hilschmann [24], Titani et al. [15], and Cunningham et al. [29].

mutation or from somatic recombination between just one pair of master and scrambler genes.

The first observations from limited sequence data on κ chains suggested that the great majority of interchanges at any position were compatible with single base mutations in the codons corresponding to the exchanged residues. As more complete sequence data became available, it appeared that about one quarter of the interchanges in κ chains [12] and about one third of those in λ chains [14] would require a double mutation in the corresponding codons. However, if the

Lack of Linkage in Sequence of Kappa Chains.

Subtype		89	90	91	92	93	94	95	96	97	98	99	100	101	102	103	104	105	106	107	108	191
κI	Ag	Gln	Gln	Tyr	Asp	Thr	Leu	Pro	Arg	Thr	Phe	Gly	Gln	Gly	Thr	Lys	Leu	Glu	Ile	Lys	Arg	- - - Val
	Roy			Phe		Asn			Leu				Gly			Val	Asp	Phe				Leu
	Eu					Ser	Asx	Ser	Lys	Met						Val			Val		Gly	- - - Val
κII	Mil	Met		Ala		Leu	Gln		Thr	Leu			Gly			Asn			Val			- - - Val
	Cum	Met	Arg	Leu	Glu	Ile				Tyr												- - - Val
	Tew	Met		Ala		Leu	Gln		Ala	Ile									Arg			- - - Val
Number of Different Residues		2	2	4	2	5	5	2	5	2	1	1	2	1	1	3	2	2	3	1	2	2

Figure 6. Amino acid sequence of three subtype II (κ_{II}) and three subtype I (κ_I) human kappa chains from position 89 through 108 and also showing the Inv locus, position 191. Data from the same sources as in Fig. 5.

comparison is restricted to proteins within a given kappa subtype, many fewer of the interchanges are incompatible with single base mutations. Thus, all the interchanges shown for subtype II κ chains in Fig. 5 accord with single base changes, as do all but two of those within the subtypes for the sequences given in Table 2 for the NH_2-terminal region of κ chains. This fits with the idea of multiple genes with early branching into three subtypes that continued to undergo point mutations.

The preceding observations that the great majority of interchanges within kappa subtypes are explicable by single point mutations is less true, however, in the region between the first disulfide bridge and the beginning of the constant portion of κ chains. This is a highly variable portion of the molecule, and there is no linkage between the sequence here and that in the beginning of the κ chains, nor with the valine-leucine substitution associated with the Inv factor. In Fig. 6 the sequence is given from position 89 through 108 for three κ chains of subtype I and three of subtype II. Here there are about as many differences within subtypes as between subtypes (an average of 8 in 20 residues). The region from 91 through 96 is highly variable; at half of the positions in this hexapeptide, there are five possible amino acids and four at another. Thereafter, two of the subtype II κ proteins are more like Ag, a subtype I protein, than are the other members of the latter subtype. Of these six proteins only Roy differs in being Inv(a+) and having leucine at position 191. Only Eu, the light chain of a γGl myeloma globulin, has glycine in place of arginine at position 108 which, rather than 107, is now regarded as the termination of the variable region of κ chains.

STRUCTURAL RELATIONSHIPS OF KAPPA
AND LAMBDA CHAINS

The evolutionary relationships of human κ and λ chains is manifested by their striking similarity in primary structure [6, 10]. For comparison of two proteins of different length the amino acid sequences are aligned with the introduction of gaps in one or the other so as to achieve maximum identity. Each gap implies an earlier event of codon deletion in the evolutionary differentiation of the genes for the respective proteins. Maximum structural homology of the κ and λ light chains of man is obtained by the introduction of five gaps in the λ chain and of four insertions in the κ chain at the positions identified in Fig. 7. Some κ and λ chains also have insertions of three to six residues in the region of positions 27 to 32. The homology in sequence illustrated in Fig. 7 for the κ-type protein Ag and the λ-type protein Sh applies in the variable region only to the two proteins being compared, whereas in the constant region it holds for all human κ and λ chains except for substitutions owing to the Inv and Oz determinants and other similar factors.

In the alignment shown, 209 positions in the two proteins are compared directly; of these 84 or almost 40% are identical. Thus, the degree of sequence homology of this pair of human κ and λ chains is similar to that exhibited by the α and β chains of human hemoglobin (45%). In addition to positions of identity there are many positions where the pairs of amino acids are chemically homologous, such as leucine and isoleucine. Conservation of the main polypeptide chain structure of human κ and λ chains is shown by the retention of the two intrachain disulfide bridges that determine their two-fold internal symmetry. The distribution of positions of identity is seemingly random throughout the human κ and λ chains and, in this pairing, it is almost equally divided between the constant and variable portions. However, the number of positions of identity common to all human κ and λ chains in the constant region (about 40) is nearly twice the number of positions common to the variable region in the eight Bence-Jones proteins (five κ and three λ) for which nearly complete sequence data are available. The number of differences in amino acid sequence between three human kappa and three human lambda Bence-Jones proteins in pairwise combinations of κ and λ types is given in matrix form in Table 1. The number is remarkably constant, ranging only from 134 to 139 despite the great variation in sequence within the group of κ chains and within the group of λ chains. As might be expected if the primitive genes for kappa and lambda light chains diverged owing to independent mutation, there is a strong tendency for mutable (i.e. variable) positions in λ chains to coincide with those in κ

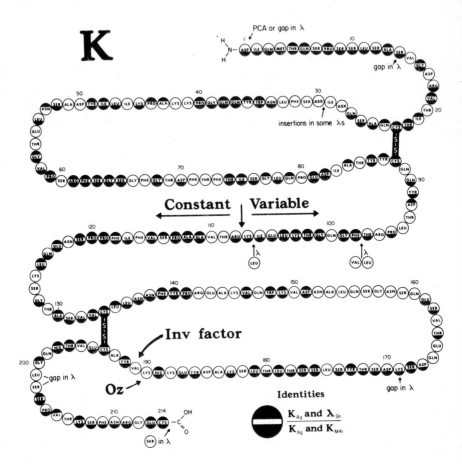

Figure 7. Homology in amino acid sequence of human κ and λ light chains and mouse κ chains. The identities in sequence of the human kappa Bence-Jones protein Ag and the human lambda Bence-Jones protein Sh are indicated by black in the upper half of the circle for each residue. The identities in sequence of the human κ Bence-Jones protein Ag and the mouse κ Bence-Jones protein M41 are indicated by black in the lower half of the circle. No adjustments in alignment have been made for the κ chains of the two species except that some mouse κ chains (e.g. M70) and some human κ chains (e.g. Cum) have four and six residues, respectively, inserted at about the same position as the insertions in human λ chains. Data for the human κ chain Ag from Titani *et al.* [15, 16], for mouse κ from Gray *et al.* [23], and for human λ from Wikler *et al.* [13]. Modified from Putnam *et al.* [10].

chains. This is illustrated by the proximity of the interchanges associated with the Inv and Oz factors.

SPECIES DIFFERENCES IN KAPPA LIGHT CHAINS

Because of the infrequency of multiple myeloma, sequence data are available only for the κ- and λ-type Bence-Jones proteins of man and the κ-type Bence-Jones proteins of two tumor lines (M41 and M70) in the BALB/c strain of mouse. Many resemblances are found in the light chains of the two species, as

108

SH	LYS	LEU	THR	VAL	LEU	GLY	GLN	PRO	LYS	ALA	ALA
BO	LYS	LEU	THR	VAL	LEU	ARG	GLN	PRO	LYS	ALA	ALA
HA	GLN	LEU	THR	VAL	LEU	ARG	GLN	PRO	LYS	ALA	ALA
X	ARG	LEU	THR	VAL	LEU	SER	GLN	PRO	LYS	ALA	ALA

HUMAN λ (label for first table)

EU	LYS	VAL	GLX	VAL	LYS	GLY		THR	VAL	ALA	ALA
ROY	LYS	VAL	ASP	PHE	LYS	ARG		THR	VAL	ALA	ALA
CUM	LYS	LEU	GLU	ILE	ARG	ARG		THR	VAL	ALA	ALA
AG	LYS	LEU	GLU	ILE	LYS	ARG		THR	VAL	ALA	ALA

HUMAN κ (label for second table)

M41	LYS	LEU	GLU	ILE	LYS	ARG		ALA	ASP	ALA	ALA
M70	LYS	LEU	GLU	ILE	LYS	ARG		ALA	ASX	ALA	ALA

MOUSE κ (label for third table)

Figure 8. Amino acid sequence of four human λ, four human κ, and two mouse κ light chains at the juncture of the variable and constant regions. A gap is inserted in the kappa chains to attain maximum homology with the lambda chains. Data from Wikler *et al.* [13], Putnam *et al.* [14], Milstein *et al.* [25], Cunningham *et al.* [29], Hilschmann [24], Titani *et al.* [15], and Gray *et al.* [23].

well as differences characteristic of the species, the antigenic type, and the individual. All these points are illustrated in Fig. 8 which shows a short stretch of sequence at the switch point in four human λ, four human κ, and two mouse κ light chains. Each of these three kinds of proteins has a region of constant sequence beginning with Gln-109 in human λ, Thr-109 in human κ, and Ala-109 in mouse κ chains. The Ala-Ala sequence is identical in all ten proteins. Other residues such as the lysine at position 103 or the leucine at position 104 are present in most of the proteins but are replaced in several that show individual variation at these loci.

Like the human kappa protein Ag, M41 has 214 residues so these two light chains of man and the mouse can be compared directly without any insertions or deletions in the sequence. When this is done (Fig. 7), 132 positions or 62% of the total are identical, including superimposition of all five half-cystine residues in each chain. *These two κ-type light chains of different species have an identical sequence in their first 14 residues, whereas three-quarters of the 24 other human κ-type light chains studied differ from them by one or more residues in the same length of sequence.* In order to obtain the most homologous alignment with

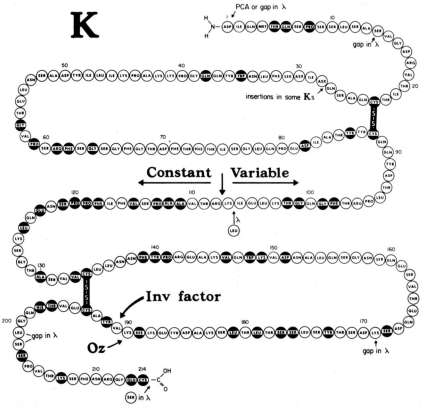

Figure 9. Conservation of light chain structure. The amino acid sequence of the human κ Bence-Jones protein Ag is given. Residues coded black are identical in the κ chains of man and mouse and the λ chains of man when all the available data are compared with the same alignment as in Fig. 7. Data obtained from the same sources as Figs. 7 and 8.

human λ chains, deletions and insertions must be placed at the same locations in mouse κ chains as in human κ chains. Furthermore, the κ chains of the two species are more closely related in amino acid sequence than are the κ and λ chains of man (Fig. 7, and Table 1). Thus, the interspecies homology of κ chains is greater than the intraspecies homology of κ and λ chains. From Fig. 7 it is evident that all three types of light chains must be very much alike in their general conformation and three-dimensional structure. It may be concluded that these light chains, and probably all immunoglobulin light chains, originated from a common ancestral gene that duplicated and gave rise to independently-mutating primordial genes of the κ and λ type prior to the species differentiation of higher vertebrates.

Besides the elements of size and the location of disulfide bridges, other aspects of the structure of light chains have been retained from species to species and in κ and λ types within man. Approximately one quarter of the residues (i.e. 53) are identical in the κ chains of man and mouse and in κ and λ chains of man when all the available data are compared in Fig. 9 using the same alignment as in Fig. 7. These residues occur twice as frequently in the COOH-half of the chain as in the NH_2-terminal half. They are widely distributed throughout the chain and, except for the half-cystines involved in disulfide bonds, they appear to exhibit no particular structural function. Next to half-cystine the most frequently conserved residues are proline, tryptophan, histidine, phenylalanine, and tyrosine, all of which contain ring structures. The conservation of proline is undoubtedly related to its strong influence on the polypeptide chain conformation such as the interruption of helical segments of a chain.

SPECIES DIFFERENCES IN LIGHT CHAIN CLASSES

Proof for the existence of two classes of light chains in normal humans is based on sequence analysis of the κ- or λ-type Bence-Jones proteins excreted by myeloma patients and the finding of the corresponding NH_2- and COOH-terminal sequences in pooled normal light chains. These sequences are so characteristic that they can be used to identify the classes of light chains in other species. Kappa chains generally have a free α-amino group and end with cysteine, whereas λ chains are usually blocked at the amino end and have cysteine in the penultimate position.

Limited sequence data on the NH_2- and COOH-termini of the pooled light chains of various species suggest that most higher vertebrates and probably also sharks have two light chain classes corresponding to human kappa and lambda [32]. The ratio of κ to λ chains varies with the species; some species such as the horse apparently have only a single class of light chain. The variability in sequence makes species comparison difficult at the NH_2-terminus. However, as judged from the COOH-terminus, the species differences are restricted and result from the permutation of only a small number of alternative residues (Table 3). The pig has two additional residues at the COOH-terminus of a kind of light chain that Hood et al. [32] designate as kappa; however, Franěk designates this as the π chain because its dominant amino-terminal group is alanine and thus both its NH_2- and COOH-terminal characteristics differ from human kappa. The pig λ chain, however, has a blocked NH_2-terminus like human λ, and thus has also a high degree of similarity in the sequence around the disulfide bridges of human and pig λ chains [35]. Although 15-20% of rabbit light chains begin with PCA and presumably are of the λ type [37], most begin with alanine and have three disulfide bridges, two of which seem to be in the NH_2-terminal half [36]. Like the π chains of the pig, this may constitute a third class of light chains. Mice make κ chains predominantly so that a λ-type Bence-Jones protein is rarely excreted. Hood *et al.* [32] have speculated on the selective forces involved in the production of different light chain ratios by different species.

Table 3. Alternative residues in the COOH-terminus of the light chains of different species. Amino acid residues are listed for other species only where they differ from human light chains. Pig kappa (or pi) chains have the COOH-terminal sequence Asx·Glx·Cys·Glx·Ala. From data of Hood *et al.* [32] and Doolittle [36].

Kappa			*Lambda*			
Human	Gly-Glu-Cys	Human	Val-Ala-Pro-Thr-Glu-Cys-Ser			
Other	Asn Asp	Other	Leu Thr	Ser		Ala
species	Ser Gly	species		Ser	Ala	Pro

From comparison of the sequence of the 216 amino acid residues of the rabbit Fc fragment and the 214 residues of the human κ Bence-Jones protein Ag (with insertion of gaps to give an alignment with the maximum number of identical and similar residues) Hill *et al.* [18] found 42 identical residues at the same position; this is equivalent to 25% of the positions compared. An equal number of residues in the two apparently diverse chains were chemically homologous. This striking homology in sequence suggested an evolutionary relationship between the light and heavy chains of immunoglobulins. An example is given in Fig. 10, which shows the consecutive sequences of 18 residues beginning with half-cystine in each of the four chains. Seven of the columns contain identical residues; in others there are identities for two or three of the chains for a total identity of 62%. Although the similarity in sequence is not as strong throughout the four chains, other segments do have a high degree of homology [10, 18]. There is also a weak homology within the rabbit Fc fragment and within the mouse and human light chains that suggests all of these chains arose by duplication of a primitive gene coding for about 110 amino acids. Tentative phylogenetic trees for the immunoglobulins have been drawn on the basis of this structural homology [18, 21].

Although Fig. 10 depicts the homology of human κ and λ light chains to the COOH-terminal half or Fc fragment of the rabbit γ chains, there is also a similarity in the sequence of human light chains and the Fd piece of the human γG1 chain [38] and with the Fd portion of the rabbit γ chain [39, 40]. Corresponding similarities of these heavy chains to the kappa light chains of the mouse must exist and likewise to the κ and λ light chains of other species. Indeed, one of the most important approaches to the structural study of immunoglobulins lies in the elucidation of the sequences of separated components of normal light chains, as is being undertaken by Franěk *et al.* [34, 35]. This will enable the comparison of the variation *within* species to the structural differences *among* species and thus afford a better assessment of the evolutionary development of light chains.

	135	140	150
Human λ	*Cys-Leu-Ile*-Ser-Asp-*Phe-Tyr-Pro*-Gly-Ala-Val-Thr-*Val*-Ala-*Trp-Lys*-Ala-*Asp*		
Human κ	*Cys-Leu-Leu-Asn-Asn-Phe-Tyr-Pro*-Arg-Glu-Ala-Lys-*Val*-Gln-*Trp-Lys*-Val-*Asp*		
Mouse κ	*Cys*-Phe-*Leu-Asn-Asn-Phe-Tyr-Pro*-Lys-*Asp Ile*-Asn-*Val*-Lys-*Trp-Lys*-Ile-*Asp*		
Rabbit F$_c$	*Cys*-Met-*Ile*-Asp-Gly-*Phe-Tyr-Pro*-Ser-*Asp-Ile*-Ser-*Val*-Gly-*Trp*-Glu-Lys-*Asp*		

Figure 10. Comparison of homologous segments of the amino acid sequences of human and mouse light chains and rabbit Fc heavy chain fragment. The numbering system refers to the human λ chain. Data obtained from [13, 15, 18].

The theme I have attempted to emphasize throughout is that the evolutionary relationships among light and heavy chains of the same and different species are manifested by the homology in primary structure that persists despite the variability in amino acid sequence even within the same type of chain from one species. As a consequence, large disulfide loops containing about 60 amino acids are characteristic features of both light and heavy chains. These loops dominate the conformation of the chains, as is depicted elsewhere in molecular models [6, 10]; the loops also impart internal symmetry and seem to have important roles in antibody function. This type of comparative structural study suggests that the genes for both light and heavy chains evolved from a common ancestral gene coding for about 110 amino acids.

ACKNOWLEDGEMENT

Sequence data on human kappa and lambda light chains from the author's laboratory have previously been published in collaboration with K. Titani, M. Wikler, T. Shinoda, H. Köhler, and E. J. Whitley, Jr., to whom I am also indebted for discussion of the ideas presented in this article. This work was supported by research grant CA-08497 from the National Cancer Institute, National Institutes of Health, USPHS.

REFERENCES

1. Nomenclature for Human Immunoglobulins, *Bull. Wld. Hlth Org.* **30** (1964) 447.
2. Putnam, F. W., *in* "The Proteins", Vol. III (edited by H. Neurath), Academic Press, New York, 1965, p. 153.
3. Mannik, M. and Kunkel, H. G., *J. exp. Med.* **116** (1962) 859.
4. Migita, S. and Putnam, F. W., *J. exp. Med.* **117** (1963) 81.
5. Fahey, J. L., *J. Immun.* **91** (1963) 483.
6. Putnam, F. W., *in* "Gamma Globulins", Nobel Symposium 3 (edited by J. Killander), Almqvist and Wiksell, Stockholm, 1967, p. 45.
7. Edelman, G. M. and Gally, J. A., *J. exp. Med.* **116** (1962) 207.
8. Porter, R. R., *Biochem. J.* **105** (1967) 417.
9. Bernier, G. M., Tominaga, K., Easley, C. W. and Putnam, F. W., *Biochemistry, N.Y.* **4** (1965) 2072.
10. Putnam, F. W., Titani, K., Wikler, M. and Shinoda, T., *Cold Spring Harb. Symp. quant. Biol.* **32** (1967) 9.
11. Natvig, J. B., Kunkel, H. G. and Gedde-Dahl, Jr., T., *in* "Gamma Globulins", Nobel Symposium 3 (edited by J. Killander), Almqvist and Wiksell, Stockholm, 1967, p. 313.
12. Putnam, F. W., *Science, N.Y.* **163** (1969) 633.
13. Wikler, M., Titani, K., Shinoda, T. and Putnam, F. W., *J. biol. Chem.* **242** (1967) 1668.
14. Putnam, F. W., Shinoda, T., Titani, K. and Wikler, M., *Science, N.Y.* **157** (1967) 1050.
15. Titani, K., Whitley, Jr., E. J. and Putnam, F. W., *Science, N.Y.* **152** (1966) 1513.
16. Putnam, F. W., Titani, K. and Whitley, Jr., E. J., *Proc. R. Soc. Ser. B,* **166** (1966) 124.
17. Porter, R. R., *Biochem. J.* **73** (1959) 119.
18. Hill, R. L., Delaney, R., Fellows, R. E. and Lebovitz, H. E., *Proc. natn. Acad. Sci. U.S.A.* **56** (1966) 1762.
19. Edelman, G. M., Gall, W. E., Waxdal, M. J. and Konigsberg, W. H., *Biochemistry, N.Y.* **7** (1968) 1950.
20. Putnam, F. W., Kozuru, M. and Easley, C. W., *J. biol. Chem.* **242** (1967) 2435.
21. Dayhoff, M. O. and Eck, R. V., "Atlas of Protein Sequence and Structure, 1967-68", National Biomedical Research Foundation, Silver Spring, 1968.
22. Dreyer, W. J., Gray, W. R. and Hood, L., *Cold Spring Harb. Symp. quant. Biol.* **32** (1967) 353.
23. Gray, W. R., Dreyer, W. J. and Hood, L., *Science, N.Y.* **155** (1967) 828.
24. Hilschmann, N., *Hoppe-Seyler's Z. physiol. Chem.* **348** (1967) 1077.
25. Milstein, C., Frangione, B. and Pink, J. R. L., *Cold Spring Harb. Symp. quant. Biol.* **32** (1967) 31.
26. Appella, E. and Ein, D., *Proc. natn. Acad. Sci. U.S.A.* **57** (1967) 1449.
27. Ponstingl, H., Hess, M., Langer, B., Steinmetz-Kayne, M. and Hilschmann, N., *Hoppe-Seyler's Z. physiol. Chem.* **348** (1967) 1213.
28. Whitley, Jr., E. J. and Putnam, F. W., unpublished results.
29. Cunningham, B. A., Gottlieb, P. D., Konigsberg, W. H. and Edelman, G. M., *Biochemistry, N.Y.* **7** (1968) 1973.

30. Niall, H. D. and Edman, P., *Nature, Lond.* **216** (1967) 262.
31. Milstein, C., *Proc. R. Soc.* Ser. B, **166** (1966) 138.
32. Hood, L., Gray, W. R., Sanders, B. G. and Dreyer, W. J., *Cold Spring Harb. Symp. quant. Biol.* **32** (1967) 133.
33. Smithies, O., *Science, N.Y.* **157** (1967) 267.
34. Franěk, F., *in* "Gamma Globulins", Nobel Symposium 3 (edited by J. Killander), Almqvist and Wiksell, Stockholm, 1967, p. 221.
35. Franěk, F., Keil, B., Novotný, J. and Šorm, F., *Eur. J. Biochem.* **3** (1968) 422.
36. Doolittle, R. F., *Proc. natn. Acad. Sci. U.S.A.* **55** (1966) 1195.
37. Rüde, E. and Givol, D., *Biochemistry, N.Y.* **107** (1968) 449.
38. Press, E. M. and Piggot, P. J., *Cold Spring Harb. Symp. quant. Biol.* **32** (1967) 45.
39. Cebra, J. J., Givol, D. and Porter, R. R., *Biochem. J.* **107** (1967) 69.
40. Cebra, J. J., Steiner, L. A. and Porter, R. R., *Biochem. J.* **107** (1967) 79.

FEBS Symposium, Volume 15, 1969, pp. 43-56

The Variability of Human Immunoglobulin G

C. MILSTEIN

M.R.C. Laboratory of Molecular Biology, Cambridge, England

One of the key problems in investigations of the molecular basis of the immune response is the mechanism by which the immunological system can synthesize an indefinite number of different antibody molecules and yet retain the basic structure characteristic of all antibodies. The structural complexity of normal immunoglobulins and specific antibodies has stimulated renewed interest in those homogeneous proteins that are found in mice and in men in association with myelomatosis and certain related lympho-proliferative disorders. Sequence studies on these proteins have provided much detailed information about immunoglobulin structure and in particular have shown that large stretches of immunoglobulin molecules have a relatively conservative structure. Such an arrangement fulfils ideally the biological functions of antibodies, which must be unique in their specific recognition of an indefinite number of antigens and yet conserve those general properties (such as the capacity to fix, complement and to attach to or traverse, specific biological membranes) which are characteristic of the class of antibodies to which they belong.

The heterogeneity of immunoglobulins is the result of three types of amino acid sequence variability: (1) the isotypic variants, which are common to all individuals of the same species and differentiate classes and types of immuno-globulins; (2) the allotypic variants, which distinguish polymorphic forms of immunoglobulins not present in all members of a given species; and (3) the idiotypic variants, which characterize individual antibodies and myeloma proteins (reviewed in [1]).

The arrangement of the disulphide bridges of the immunoglobulin chains provides a startling picture of these variations. The earlier observation that κ light chains contain two disulphide bridges [2], one type specific and the other variable, each including about 60 residues [3, 4], encouraged the study of the intrachain bridges in other chains. A similar arrangement of bridges was detected in λ chains [5] also involving 60-residue loops [6, 7]. Recent studies on heavy chains support the idea that the 60-residue loop is the basic building block of all immunoglobulin chains.

The similar distribution of two loops of about 60 residues in light chains and in Fc fragments of the four types of human [34] and of rabbit [8] IgG is further emphasized by the observation that the loops in rabbit are separated by about 45 residues. This has now been shown to be true also in human $\gamma 4$ chain [9].

The similarity between Fd fragments and light chains is even more marked. To find out how much of the Fd portion was invariant we applied the method originally used in light chains—that is to search for the common S-S bridges. The first sequence we found to be common to IgGl Fd fragments was the peptide including the Cys involved in heavy-light chains binding [10]. A larger invariant portion of Fd was indicated by the isolation of the intrachain bridge peptide present in human Fd fragments of several myeloma proteins [11, 12]. It was very similar to the cystine peptide involved in the folding of the invariant C-terminal loop of light chains and for this reason we like to think that it involves a loop of about 60 residues. The bridged peptide seems to be identical in different myelomas of the same type and adds support to the suggestion [10] that Fd shares the overall general structure of light chains, containing a C-terminal half common to all fragments of the same type, and an N-terminal half peculiar to each myeloma. In addition, similarities between some sequences of pooled Fd rabbit and human light chains have also been observed [13].

Thus, a common structure of the four IgG heavy chains seems to consist essentially of a type-specific section made up of three loops of about 60 residues each (as shown in Fig. 1). A fourth disulphide-bridged loop, similar to the light chain variable loop found in a few proteins [11, 12], is likely to be part of the variable portion of the heavy chains, in an analogous fashion to that found in light chains. However, the variable loop of Fd is still speculative. Furthermore, the occurrence of additional bridges in Fd is not excluded. The work of Press and Piggot [14] on protein Daw indeed suggests that this is a distinct possibility.

In contrast with the close similarity of the intrachain bridges of heavy chains, the interchain bridges are different in the four subtypes (Fig. 1). Although we do not yet have a definite picture of the $\gamma 2$ interchain bridges, we can say that it is different from the other three. Only two bridges bind the $\gamma 1$ [11, 15] and $\gamma 4$ [12] heavy chains, while $\gamma 3$ [16] and $\gamma 2$ (Frangione and Milstein, unpublished) have additional bridges. Differences in the sequence around the two homologous interchain cystine residues in the different chain types are also apparent (Fig. 2). These differences in the interchain bridges provide a clear-cut structural difference between the types of heavy chains. This has in fact been used by Frangione to develop a method for the chemical typing of heavy chains which is now in use in our laboratory.

Since disulphide bridges define the proximity of points along the peptide chains, it is pertinent to ask if the variation of disulphide bridges is correlated with major variations in the three-dimensional structure of the different IgGs.

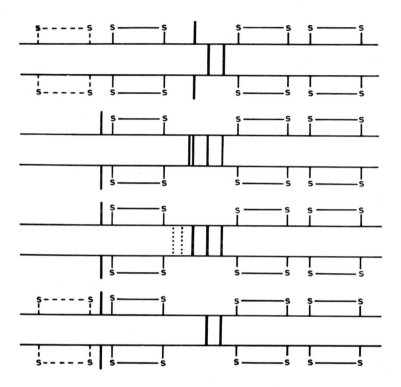

Figure 1. A schematic representation of the homologous interchain disulphide bridges and the variations in the interchain links in heavy chains of the four types of human IgG-myeloma proteins. This scheme is partly based on the results of work on the disulphide bridges of heavy chains made in collaboration with Frangione and Pink published in references 7, 9, 10, 11, 12 and 16. The disulphide bridges of other γ1-myeloma proteins are discussed in references 14, 15 and 26. The scheme includes unpublished results of γ3 and γ4 proteins, performed in collaboration with B. Frangione.

The interchain bridges are indicated by thick vertical lines. The dotted vertical lines of γ3 indicate that the location of those two bridges is not precisely known [16]. The open vertical lines show the point of attachment of the light chains. The evidence that the interheavy chain bridges occur in a parallel fashion is only inferred from the results on γ3 proteins [16].

The distribution of the intrachain loops (each involving a 60 residues loop) is mainly derived by comparison with light chains [2-6] and rabbit Fc fragment [8]. The dotted intrachain disulphide bridge isolated only in γ1 and γ4 proteins is considered to be variable within a single heavy chain type.

This is difficult to say at the moment. For example, the difference in the location of the point of attachment of the light chains on the heavy chains, dramatic as it appears (perhaps 100 residues along the chain), may in the three-dimensional structure be a minor re-adjustment of a few key bond angles. In fact, the "γ4-like" point of attachment, as placed in Fig. 1, is brought nearer in space from the γ1 point of attachment by the common Fd intrachain disulphide bridge. On the other hand, the presence of multiple cross links between the heavy chains of IgG3 might conceivably have a dramatic effect on the flexibility of the two arms of the Y-shaped IgG [17, 18] and thus influence the potential antibody activity of the molecule.

Homologous sequences around the interchain bridges in γGl-, γG2-, γG3- and γG4-myeloma proteins

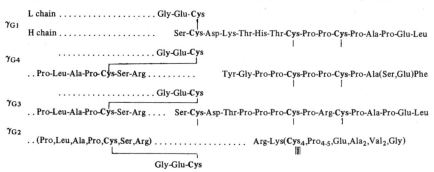

Figure 2. Homologous sequences around the interchain bridges of γG1-, γG2-, γG3- and γG4-myeloma proteins. For references see Fig. 1.

The structural nature of the isotypic variants of heavy and light chains is thus at least partly defined, although the biological implication of the differences is not well understood. The structural nature of the idiotypic variants, on the other hand, is much more of a question and in order to discuss this point further I would like to present some recent results which I have obtained with pathological κ chains and with normal human light chains.

THE NATURE OF THE VARIABILITY OF THE
N-TERMINAL HALF OF κ CHAINS

The observations leading to the proposal of two types of human N-terminal halves of κ chains [19] was the basis for the revival [20] of a previously abandoned idea [21] that the variability of κ chains was originated by somatic recombination of two basic sequences. However, I was able to show that the number of basic sequences in human κ chains was not less than three [22]. I have now collected more data which further supports the existence of the three basic sequences. Furthermore, sequence studies on other Bence-Jones proteins, published recently or unpublished and shown in Tables 1 and 2, are in agreement

Table 1. Partial sequence of the N-terminal half of Bence-Jones protein Bel (type KI).

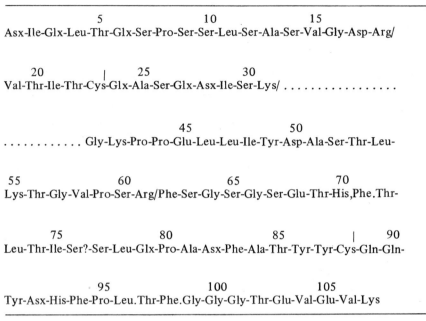

```
                    5                    10                    15
Asx-Ile-Glx-Leu-Thr-Glx-Ser-Pro-Ser-Ser-Leu-Ser-Ala-Ser-Val-Gly-Asp-Arg/

     20         |      25                   30
Val-Thr-Ile-Thr-Cys-Glx-Ala-Ser-Glx-Asx-Ile-Ser-Lys/ . . . . . . . . . . . . . . . .

                                     45                   50
. . . . . . . . . . . Gly-Lys-Pro-Pro-Glu-Leu-Leu-Ile-Tyr-Asp-Ala-Ser-Thr-Leu-

     55              60              65                   70
Lys-Thr-Gly-Val-Pro-Ser-Arg/Phe-Ser-Gly-Ser-Gly-Ser-Glu-Thr-His,Phe.Thr-

          75              80              85        |         90
Leu-Thr-Ile-Ser?-Ser-Leu-Glx-Pro-Ala-Asx-Phe-Ala-Thr-Tyr-Tyr-Cys-Gln-Gln-

             95              100             105
Tyr-Asx-His-Phe-Pro-Leu.Thr-Phe.Gly-Gly-Gly-Thr-Glu-Val-Glu-Val-Lys
```

The overlaps of the tryptic peptides marked with a line (/) are based on homology. Dots (.) indicate that the overlap within the tryptic peptide is based on homology. The question mark (?) indicates that the identification of the residue was uncertain.

Table 2. Partial sequence of Bence-Jones proteins Fr 4, Rad and B6 used to establish the basic sequence III in κ light chains. Part of these sequences have been published previously [21]. The numbering of residues is based on homology with other proteins.

```
            5                10                15               20
Fr 4  Glu(Ile,Val,Leu)Thr-Gln-Ser-Pro-Gly-Thr-Leu-Ser-Leu-Ser-Pro-Gly-Glu-Arg/Ala-Thr-Leu-
Rad   Glu-Ile-Val-Leu-Thr-Gln-Ser-Pro-Gly-Thr-Leu-Ser-Leu-Ser-Pro-Gly-Asp-Arg/Ala-Thr-Leu-
B6    (Glx,Ile,Val,Leu,Thr,Glx,Ser,Pro,Gly,Thr,Leu,Ser,Leu,Ser,Pro,Gly,Glu,Arg)

                                            65                70             75
Ser-Cys-Arg/ - - - - - - - - / - -Phe-Ser-Gly-Ser-Gly-Ser-Gly(Thr,Asp,Phe)Thr-Leu-Thr-Ile-Ser-Arg/
Ser-Cys-Arg/ - - - - - - - - / - -Phe-Ser-Gly-Ser-Glu-Ser-Gly-Thr-Asp-Phe-Thr-Leu-Thr(Ile,Ser)Arg/

     80             85             90                   95            100
Leu-Glu-Pro-Glu-Asp-Phe-Ala-Val-Tyr-Phe(Cys,Gln,Gln,Tyr)Gly-Gly-Ser-Pro-Gln-Pro-Phe-Gly-Gln-

Leu-Glu-Pro-Glu-Asp-Phe-Ala-Val-Tyr-Tyr-Cys-Gln-Gln-Tyr-Glu-Thr-Ser-Pro-Thr-Thr-Phe.Gly-Gln-

Leu-Glx-Pro-Glx-Asx-Phe.Ala-Val-Tyr.Tyr-Cys-Gln-Gln-Tyr.Gly-Ser-Ser-Pro-Phe.Thr-Phe.Gly-Gln-

     105
Gly-Thr-Lys/Leu-Glu-Ile-Lys
Gly-Thr-Arg/Leu-Asp-Ile-Lys
Gly-Ser-Lys/Leu-Glu-Ile-Lys
```

with such a proposal. Table 1 shows the almost complete amino acid sequence of the N-terminal half of protein Bel, which is very similar to the sequence of other KI proteins, and Table 2 shows the partial sequence of Bence-Jones proteins Rad, Fr 4 and B6. These three sequences are not complete but they seem to define most of the N-terminal variable part of the third basic sequence of κ chains. Using these and other data (for list of references of proteins included in our comparisons see Table 3) the three basic sequences of type K Bence-Jones proteins can be defined reasonably well in some sections of the molecule (Tables 3, 4 and 5) but not all along. This is due to the presence of variants within each basic sequence. In order to start to define a basic sequence in a given stretch the sequence of the stretch must be known in at least two proteins, and preferably more. Each individual protein has a number of variants of the basic sequence scattered along the chain in a fairly random fashion, in most cases involving one base substitution. A repeat of a given residue along the sequence in at least two proteins is the minimum requirement indicating the provisional assignment of a residue in the basic sequence. When two proteins differ in a given position more data are necessary to judge the frequency of each variant. Very often variants occur only in isolated instances (like position 2 of protein BJ), but in other cases certain substitutions occur repeatedly, like Arg at position 24 of KI chains (Table 3). These repeated substitutions are of special interest to me and I will discuss this point further on. The variants are often incompatible with a mechanism invoking somatic crossing over between the basic sequences. See for instance BJ, position 2; Car, 20; Nig, 1; Gra, 12; Ag, 67 and 77; Bel, 81 etc.

The collected information on full sequences and on restricted sections of many Bence-Jones proteins has thus proved of special value and the definition of three basic sequences in the first 27 residues as shown in Table 3 rests on a reasonably solid base.

Another section which appears reasonably well defined goes from residue 59 to 90 and is shown in Table 4. It is very interesting to note that all the proteins that were defined in the N-terminal section as from a given basic sequence have characteristic stretches which differ from the homologous stretch in the proteins previously classified as from a different basic sequence. This is particularly striking in the stretch between residues 77 and 85 with three or more light chains represented in each subtype.

In other words, we can confidently say that up to residue 90 the proteins do not as a general rule "change tracks", as one would expect if random somatic recombination between basic sequences was operative. Residue 90 is only 15 residues removed from the beginning of the invariable section. Between residues 27 (end of Table 3) and 59 (beginning of Table 4) there are 30 residues which so far I have been unable to define with a good degree of confidence for the three basic sequences. More data are required, and we are looking forward to our own results (which we are collecting at the moment) and the results from other

Table 3. Three basic sequences in the N-terminal section of κ chains.

		5	10	15	20	25
Common residues	I	T Q S P	L	G	C	S Q
I	D	Q M	S S	S A S V	D R V T	I T	Q A
II	D	V M	L S	P V T P	E P A S	I S	R S
III	E	V L	G T	S L S P	E R A T	L S	R A

I

Roy	[27]	———————————————————————(———)
Ag	[28]	——————————————————————————
Ker	[29]	—(—)(————)———————I———
BJ	[29]	—(V—)——(————)(———)———
Bel		———L———————————————————
Eu	[30]	—————————T——————————R—
Car	[31]	————(———)T——————A———R—

I I

Cu	[27]	E————————T——————(———)-(—)
Mil	[32]	————L———————————————————
Man	[21]	—(—————————)———————————

I I I

Fr 4		—(———)———————————————
Rad		————————————————D————
Nig	[33]	K——————————————————————
Cas	[33]	——————————————————————
Smi	[33]	—————A————————————————
Gra	[33]	—M—M——————A————M————D————
B6		(———————————————————)

The conventions used are as follows:

Each basic sequence is constructed at the top of the table by assigning an amino acid residue (using the one letter code) at each position. When the assigned residue is identical in the three basic sequences the residue is put in the first line as "common residue", i.e. identical in the three basic sequences. At positions where the assigned residues are not identical, these are displayed in the three following lines. The myeloma κ chains are then matched against each basic sequence and listed in one of the three groups below (I, II, III).

When the individual protein has a stretch identical to the basic sequence this is indicated by a line. The line is interrupted when a difference occurs and the variant residue is included. For instance, at position 24 basic sequence I contains glutamine (Q), but basic sequences II and III Arg. Thus all proteins from the first group (I) with a line at that position have been reported as Glutamine (Eu and Car are exceptions, containing Arginine instead). In the second and third groups of proteins (II and III) the line indicates that Arginine has been found in that position in the indicated protein.

The brackets indicate that the evidence for the enclosed stretch derives from amino acid composition only. Often when the amide groups of specific proteins are unknown, assignment was made to minimize differences. The one letter amino acid code is as used by R. V. Eck and M. O. Dayhoff in the Atlas of Protein Sequence.

One letter Amino Acid Code

Gly	Ala	Val	Leu	Ile	Ser	Thr	Pro	Cys	Met	His
G	A	V	L	I	S	T	P	C	M	H

Lys	Arg	Asp	Glu	Asn	Gln	Asx	Glx	Tyr	Phe	Trp
K	R	D	E	N	Q	B	Z	Y	F	W

Table 4. Three basic sequences in κ chains between residues 59 and 90.

Common	60			65			70			75			80		85			9
residues	P	R F S G	S G S G T D	F T		I S			E D			Y Y C					
I	S				F T		S L Q P		I A T									Q
II	B				L K		R V Z A		V G V									
III	(B)				L T		R L E P		F A V									Q

I

Roy	————T					
Ag	——F—		—G—			
Eu	—I—	—Z—L—•		—F—		
Bel	—E—H;	—/—L—	—?—	—A—F—		

I I

Cu	—Z–B	
Mil	—Z–B	
Man	—Z–B——I—	

I I I

Fr 4		—F(——
Rad	—E—	
B6		

The conventions used are as follows:

Each basic sequence is constructed at the top of the table by assigning an amino acid residue (using the one letter code) at each position. When the assigned residue is identical in the three basic sequences the residue is put in the first line as "common residue", i.e. identical in the three basic sequences. At positions where the assigned residues are not identical, these are displayed in the three following lines. The myeloma κ chains are then matched against each basic sequence and listed in one of the three groups below (I, II, III).

When the individual protein has a stretch identical to the basic sequence this is indicated by a line. The line is interrupted when a difference occurs and the variant residue is included. For instance, at position 24 basic sequence I contains glutamine (Q), but basic sequences II and III Arg. Thus all proteins from the first group (I) with a line at that position have been reported as Glutamine (Eu and Car are exceptions, containing Arginine instead). In the second and third groups of proteins (II and III) the line indicates that Arginine has been found in that position in the indicated protein.

The brackets indicate that the evidence for the enclosed stretch derives from amino acid composition only. Often when the amide groups of specific proteins are unknown, assignment was made to minimize differences. The one letter amino acid code is as used by R. V. Eck and M. O. Dayhoff in the Atlas of Protein Sequence.

One letter Amino Acid Code

Gly	Ala	Val	Leu	Ile	Ser	Thr	Pro	Cys	Met	His
G	A	V	L	I	S	T	P	C	M	H

Lys	Arg	Asp	Glu	Asn	Gln	Asx	Glx	Tyr	Phe	Trp
K	R	D	E	N	Q	B	Z	Y	F	W

Table 5. "Hot Spots" in κ chains. Sequence around residues 91-107 in several proteins.

		95	100	105	Residue
Common residues	Y	P	T F G Q G T K	V D / L E	I K	191

I	D ? L	?
II	L ? ?	?
III	G ? S	?

I

Roy	F——N————L————G————V D F——	L
Ag	——T————R————————L E——	V
Ker	——D————P————————P————V D L——	L
BJ	—E N————Y————L E——	L
Eu	—— S B S K M————————V Z V——	V
Bel	—B H F——L ————————G————Z V Z V——	V

II

Cu	R——E I——Y————————L E——R	V
Mil	A——Q T——L————————G————N V E——	V
Man	V E——	V

III

Rad	—E T————T————————R L D——	V
Fr 4	——G————Q P————————L E——	L
B6	——S————F————————S——L E——	V

The conventions used are as follows:

Each basic sequence is constructed at the top of the table by assigning an amino acid residue (using the one letter code) at each position. When the assigned residue is identical in the three basic sequences the residue is put in the first line as "common residue", i.e. identical in the three basic sequences. At positions where the assigned residues are not identical, these are displayed in the three following lines. The myeloma κ chains are then matched against each basic sequence and listed in one of the three groups below (I, II, III).

When the individual protein has a stretch identical to the basic sequence this is indicated by a line. The line is interrupted when a difference occurs and the variant residue is included. For instance, at position 24 basic sequence I contains glutamine (Q), but basic sequences II and III Arg. Thus all proteins from the first group (I) with a line at that position have been reported as Glutamine (Eu and Car are exceptions, containing Arginine instead). In the second and third groups of proteins (II and III) the line indicates that Arginine has been found in that position in the indicated protein.

The brackets indicate that the evidence for the enclosed stretch derives from amino acid composition only. Often when the amide groups of specific proteins are unknown, assignment was made to minimize differences. The one letter amino acid code is as used by R. V. Eck and M. O. Dayhoff in the Atlas of Protein Sequence.

One letter Amino Acid Code

Gly	Ala	Val	Leu	Ile	Ser	Thr	Pro	Cys	Met	His
G	A	V	L	I	S	T	P	C	M	H

Lys	Arg	Asp	Glu	Asn	Gln	Asx	Glx	Tyr	Phe	Trp
K	R	D	E	N	Q	B	Z	Y	F	W

laboratories to fill the gap. I expect that these will confirm the general conclusions I have drawn from the present results.

After residue 90 the picture starts to change. At positions 92 and 94 the three basic sequences are still largely distinguishable (Table 5) but positions 93 and 96 are so variable that so far I have not been able to assign, with any degree of confidence, characteristic residues to any of the three basic sequences. Position 96 in Kl chains (studied in six proteins) includes five variants. In all the proteins listed in Table 5 (eleven specimens) eight different residues are found at positions 93 and 96. If any position in the light chain is involved in the active centre of antibodies, these two are certainly excellent candidates. To add an element of complication, between the highly variable positions 94 and 96 a conservative Pro at position 95 has been consistently found in all Bence-Jones proteins except one.

After position 96 no clear distinction between the three basic sequences is apparent. Residues 104 and 105 are found as either valine or leucine and aspartic or glutamic acid, respectively, in all basic sequences; in basic sequence II, however, only glutamic acid at 105 was found in the three proteins listed, but this should remain open until more data are available.

These results raise many different questions and I would like to conclude with some results relevant to three of these—namely, (1) can these three basic sequences be recognized in normal light chains; (2) is any of them an allelic form of another; and (3) are the basic sequences the expression of three or more structural genes? In order to investigate these problems I studied the occurrence in normal light chains of a selected peptide which I could easily recognize as originating from a given basic sequence.

The sequence around the cysteine 23 was an obvious choice. This can be easily labelled and thus radioactive techniques applied. Furthermore, as shown in Table 6, a very characteristic tryptic peptide derived from basic sequence III can be prepared in reasonable yields. In addition, a variant of sequence I has a substitution of Gln for Arg, giving a second peptide equal in size but differing by three residues.

Both peptides were in fact found in normal pooled light chains. Their compositions and N-terminal residues were determined after purification (Table 7) and found to be in close agreement with equivalent peptides isolated from pathological light chains. Furthermore, enough peptide TN2 could be prepared and its sequence established as—

Val-Thr-Ile-Thr-Ccm-Arg

which is identical to the variant of basic sequence I including the Arg substitution in residue 24.

This result indicates therefore that representative peptides of the basic sequences are indeed present in normal light chains and they provide further support to the idea that myeloma proteins are representative examples of the normal immunoglobulin population.

Peptide TN2 (a variant of basic sequence I) was present in fairly good yields when compared with the yields of TN1, but this was the only variant of the basic sequences which could be confidently detected. If crossing over between basic sequences was a common occurrence I should have expected to identify certain

Table 6. Sequence around Cys 23 of κ chains. (The arrows show the position of tryptic cleavage).

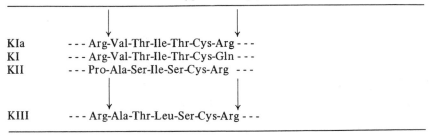

KIa   - - - Arg-Val-Thr-Ile-Thr-Cys-Arg - - -
KI   - - - Arg-Val-Thr-Ile-Thr-Cys-Gln - - -
KII   - - - Pro-Ala-Ser-Ile-Ser-Cys-Arg - - -

KIII   - - - Arg-Ala-Thr-Leu-Ser-Cys-Arg - - -

Table 7. Amino acid composition and N-terminal residues of two peptides isolated from normal pooled human light chains. (Compare with sequences in Table 6).

Amino Acid	TN1	TN2
Arginine	1·0	1·0
CMCys	0·61	0·68
Threonine	0·99	1·75
Serine	0·97	< 0·1
Glycine	< 0·1	< 0·1
Alanine	1·02	
Valine		1·02
Leucine	0·97	0·15
Isoleucine		1·02
N-terminus	Ala	Val

variant peptides. For example, a variant of TN1 containing isoleucine instead of leucine should not separate from TN1 and should have given a certain amount of isoleucine in the analysis, but this was not observed (see Table 7). In fact the analyses were reasonably clean and the small amount of residues, other than those accounted for by the sequences, are commonly observed impurities at the low levels of peptide analysed.

The fact that the Arg 24 version of KI was present in such good yields prompted us to investigate the possibility of its being an allelic form of basic sequence I.

Through the kindness of Dr. Darnborough of the Blood Transfusion Centre, Cambridge (who provided the sera), I isolated the light chains from seventeen individual normal sera and proceeded to establish the presence of TN1 and TN2 by a fingerprint procedure. Both peptides were in fact present in the light chains of the seventeen normal donors. Furthermore, I cut out each spot and estimated their relative yields with respect to the amount of one of the peptides derived from the invariable section of κ chains (Table 8). The results shown in Table 8 are from a single experiment and they may be subject to considerable error.

Table 8. Relative amounts of peptide TN1 and TN2 (see Table 7) obtained from the light chains of 17 normal donors. The numbers indicate the relative amount of each peptide in individual samples. The amount of a reference peptide (tryptic peptide including Cys 194) was arbitrarily taken as 1 in each sample.

Donor	TN1	TN2	Donor	TN1	TN2
735	0·23	0·19	780	0·13	0·21
740	0·16	0·27	739	0·20	0·31
595	0·10	0·30	764	0·19	0·21
823	0·23	0·28	718	0·17	0·24
724	0·31	0·36	762	0·18	0·25
577	0·36	0·30	521	0·13	0·20
810	0·32	0·31	686	0·13	0·14
585	0·23	0·32	646	0·11	0·12
656	0·33	0·32			

They suggest, however, that together the two peptides may account for something between 30 and 50% of the total light chain population. Although the relative proportion of each of them appears to be subject to considerable individual variation, peptide TN2 (the arginine variant of KI) was never significantly lower than TN1 (the representative of KIII).

In conclusion then: The observations made so far suggest that the basic sequences are not the result of polymorphism and that no random recombination events seem to occur between them—except at the very end of the N-terminal half. If this is so, we should conclude that there are indeed several "half genes" coding for the N-terminal half of κ chains which become integrated with a single "half gene" coding for the C-terminal half. In this case one would expect that the Leu and Val at position 191 (the Inv allotypes) will not be linked to any of the basic sequences. This is shown in Table 5 to be so for basic sequences I and III. All three proteins belonging to basic sequence II have so far been of the Inv b type, but this may only reflect the fact that Inv b is far more frequent than Inv a. This is, to our minds, the strongest evidence obtained so far in support of a mechanism of chromosomal re-arrangement or insertion as part of the control of κ-chain synthesis. The nature of the variability at residues 104 and 105 is compatible with such a scheme. Such a mechanism has been proposed [23] as the only way of overcoming the structural difficulties imposed by the existence of a single C-terminal half and the very large number of N-terminal halves required by a germ line theory of variability. However, it is equally possible that the number of genes coding for the N-terminal half is much more restricted in the germ line and that further variability is achieved by somatic mutation operating on a restricted section of the genome [24, 25].

The frequency of a variant of a basic sequence, studied in normal individual donors by the presence of variant Arg 24 of KI, suggests that this is also unlikely to be the result of polymorphism. It is most likely that as more pathological κ chains are sequenced Arg 24 will appear to be associated with the KI basic sequence in many more cases. Is such a variant the expression of yet a different gene in the germ line? Although one could easily imagine good reasons to say that it could originate by polymorphism in the population or by somatic mutation and selection, I am inclined to think otherwise; namely that it is the expression of a different gene. Once we are forced to believe in the presence of at least three "half genes" to code for the N-terminal half, I find it not very difficult to accept a few more. The real question is how many more?

REFERENCES

1. Cohen, S. and Milstein, C., *Adv. Immun.* **7** (1967) 1.
2. Milstein, C., *J. molec. Biol.* **9** (1964) 836.
3. Hilschmann, N. and Craig, L. C., *Proc. natn. Acad. Sci. U.S.A.* **53** (1965) 1403.
4. Titani, K., Whitley, Jr., E. J., Avogadro, L. and Putnam, F. W., *Science, N.Y.* **149** (1965) 1091.
5. Milstein, C., *Proc. R. Soc.* Ser. B, **166** (1966) 138.
6. Wikler, M., Titani, K., Shinoda, T. and Putnam, F. W., *J. biol. Chem.* **242** (1967) 1668.
7. Milstein, C., Clegg, J. B. and Jarvis, J. M., *Nature, Lond.* **214** (1967) 270.
8. Hill, R. L., Lebovitz, H. E., Fellows, R. E. and Delaney, R., *in* "Gamma Globulins", Nobel Symposium 3 (edited by J. Killander), Almqvist and Wiksell, Stockholm, 1967, p. 109.
9. Pink, J. R. L. and Milstein, C., this volume, p. 177.
10. Pink, J. R. L. and Milstein, C., *Nature, Lond.* **214** (1967) 92.
11. Frangione, B. and Milstein, C., *Nature, Lond.* **216** (1967) 939.
12. Pink, J. R. L. and Milstein, C., *Nature, Lond.* **216** (1967) 941.
13. Cebra, J. J., *Cold Spring Harb. Symp. quant. Biol.* **32** (1967) 65.
14. Press, E. M. and Piggot, P. J., *Cold Spring Harb. Symp. quant. Biol.* **32** (1967) 45.
15. Steiner, L. A. and Porter, R. R., *Biochemistry, N.Y.* **6** (1967) 3957.
16. Frangione, B. and Milstein, C., *J. molec. Biol.* **33** (1968) 893.

17. Feinstein, A. and Rowe, A. J., *Nature, Lond.* **205** (1965) 147.
18. Valentine, R. C. and Green, N. M., *J. molec. Biol.* **27** (1967) 615.
19. Hood, L., Gray, W. R., Sanders, B. G. and Dreyer, W. J., *Cold Spring Harb. Symp. quant. Biol.* **32** (1967) 133.
20. Smithies, O., *Science, N.Y.* **157** (1967) 267.
21. Milstein, C., *Nature, Lond.* **209** (1966) 370.
22. Milstein, C., *Nature, Lond.* **216** (1967) 330.
23. Dreyer, W. J. and Bennett, J. C., *Proc. natn. Acad. Sci. U.S.A.* **54** (1965) 864.
24. Brenner, S. and Milstein, C., *Nature, Lond.* **211** (1966) 242.
25. Cohn, M., *in* "Rutgers Symposium on Nucleic Acids in Immunology", (edited by O. J. Plescia and W. Braun), Springer-Verlag, New York, 1968.
26. Waxdal, M. J., Konigsberg, W. H. and Edelman, G. M., *Cold Spring Harb. Symp. quant. Biol.* **32** (1967) 53.
27. Hilschmann, N., *Hoppe-Seyler's Z. physiol. Chem.* **348** (1967) 1077.
28. Titani, K., Whitley, Jr., E. J., and Putnam, F. W., *Science, N.Y.* **152** (1966) 1515.
29. Milstein, C., *Biochem. J.* **101** (1966) 352.
30. Cunningham, B. A., Gottlieb, P. D., Konigsberg, W. H. and Edelman, G. M., *Biochemistry, N.Y.* **7** (1968) 1983.
31. Milstein, C. P., unpublished results.
32. Dreyer, W. J., Gray, W. R. and Hood, L., *Cold Spring Harb. Symp. quant. Biol.* **32** (1967) 353.
33. Niall, H. D. and Edman, P., *Nature, Lond.* **216** (1967) 262.
34. Frangione, B., Milstein, C. and Franklin, E. C., *Biochem. J.* **106** (1968) 15.

FEBS Symposium, Volume 15, 1969, pp. 57-74

Structural Studies on Immunoglobulins and their Genetic Implications for Antibody Formation

N. HILSCHMANN, H. U. BARNIKOL, M. HESS, B. LANGER, H. PONSTINGL,
M. STEINMETZ-KAYNE, L. SUTER and S. WATANABE

Max-Planck-Institut für experimentelle Medizin, Göttingen, Germany

Antibodies are multichain structures, consisting of two identical light (L) and heavy (H) chains which are linked by disulfide bridges and noncovalent bonds [1, 2]. Analogous to enzymes, their specificity is determined by the sequence of the constituent chains, different antibody molecules having different primary structures [3-5].

Sequence studies on the immunoglobulin chains are greatly hampered by the fact that they are extremely complex mixtures of different, but very similar, proteins. Several types of heterogeneity within a single species can be distinguished [6]: *Isotypic variants* which are present in every individual and are identical with the chain types (κ, λ, γ, μ, α) which constitute different immunoglobulin classes (IgG, IgM, IgA), *allotpyic variants* which are inheritable characteristics not found in every individual, and *idiotypic variants* which are an expression of the individual specificity of every single γ-globulin molecule, independent of chain type and genetic constitution. These idiotypic differences determine antibody specificity. All these variants are present in γ-globulin preparations and also in most so-called pure antibodies, even when prepared against single haptens. Chemical homogeneity with one idiotypic specificity can only be observed with myeloma proteins or Waldenström's macroglobulins because these proteins are derived from one single unipotent cell-clone.

In order to obtain an insight into immunoglobulin structure and the genetic mechanism which determines antibody specificity, sequence studies were performed mainly with these monoclonal proteins. These investigations were facilitated by the use of Bence-Jones proteins which are identical to L chains of the corresponding myeloma protein [7] and are easily available and differ from patient to patient. For comparative sequence studies, proteins of the same isotypic and allotypic specificity, but different idiotypy, are used. Thus, differences between the structures are solely attributable to these idiotypic

3 57

differences and cannot be caused by evolution or allotypes, factors not necessarily connected with antibody specificity.

These studies demonstrated that L chains are composed of two parts of equal length, the C-terminal half being identical in different L chains of the same type (constant (C) part), the N-terminal part being different in length and sequence, but homologous (variable (V) part). This observation was first made with two human Bence-Jones proteins of the κ type [8-10], but was soon shown to be of general validity. It has been observed for human [11, 12] and murine [13] κ-type proteins, for human λ-type proteins [14-17], and L chain preparations from whole γ-globulin mixtures [18]. A genetic factor (inv), which is an allele, inherited codominantly in a simple Mendelian manner, was found to be localized in position 191 of the constant part of human κ-type L chains, inv a^+ having leucine and inv b^+ having valine in this position [8, 19-21]. This factor was absent in mouse κ-type proteins [13]. The foregoing observation was made with the use of only the partial formulas of these proteins, but important conclusions concerning the genetic control could immediately be deduced from these data.

The allotypes, localized on the constant part of these molecules, indicated that this part of the molecule must be controlled by one single gene, while several genes had to be assumed for the variable part, in accordance with the one gene one polypeptide chain dogma. This excluded the possibility that the structural differences in the variable part, which closely resembled differences found in proteins which are phylogenetically related like the hemoglobins, could be caused by an evolutionary process restricted to one half in the whole L-chain gene. In this case, the inv factors could not have segregated in a simple Mendelian manner, and also these allotypes, which are not present in mouse proteins, would have had to be introduced in a great number of genes at exactly the same position. All these arguments point out that L-chain genes cannot be inseparably inherited, but that a special mechanism has to be assumed to explain the variability of the N-terminal part.

Several hypotheses have been proposed to explain the variability of the V genes, some involving a somatic hypermutation process of one [22] or a limited number of genes [23-26], others postulating separate genes in the germ line [27]. There were many arguments for and against all these hypotheses [28-31]. It was impossible to prove or disprove these possibilities in the absence of additional data on different Bence-Jones proteins.

LIGHT CHAIN STRUCTURE

We therefore extended our studies from the κ type of proteins Roy and Cum, where the original observations of the variable and constant part had been made, to other selected L chains; two λ-type (New and Kern) and one κ-type (Ti) protein. The V and C parts [15, 16] of the two λ-chain proteins were completely sequenced, while sequence work on the κ-type protein was limited to the V part [32].

Figure 1 shows all the variable parts of the λ-type proteins thus far determined. To simplify the presentation, the proteins New [16] and Kern [15] have been included and will be discussed together with the other proteins.

As with κ-type proteins, the variable parts of the λ-type proteins represent one half of the molecule and extend to position 109. The switch to the constant part occurs at a position exactly homologous to that in κ chains.

On the basis of the chemical homology which exists between the different variants, at least four groups or subgroups can be distinguished. Members of one subgroup have certain common basic sequences which are replaced by other sequences in other subgroups. For example, group I has valine in position 3, group II alanine, group III glutamic acid, and group IV has no definite amino acid at this position but does have a tyrosine in position 2. These group-specific differences are randomly distributed all over the variable part and are marked by light boxes in Fig. 1. They are mostly paralleled by a characteristic number of sequence gaps in positions 1, 28, and 95/96. Members of groups I and II have as the N-terminal amino acid always a blocked glutamic acid, most likely α-pyrrolidone carbonic acid; in groups III and IV this position is not occupied by any residue. A gap of three amino acid residues in position 28 is characteristic for groups III and IV. This gap is filled with three residues in group II and two or three residues in group I. A particularly interesting gap is the one in position 95/96 in group IV. This gap makes λ chains of group IV exactly as long as κ chains in this region. This means that, when κ and λ chains are compared in this area, an insertion of two amino acids has to be assumed for λ chains of groups I to III (Fig. 2).

These group-specific sequences are superimposed by single amino acid exchanges characteristic for one individual chain within one group. Where these individual sequences differ from the basic group-specific sequences, the exchanges have been marked by dark boxes in Fig. 1. While group-specific sequences amount to about 40–50% of the variable part, individual-specific differences within one group do not exceed 25%, but seem to be randomly distributed all over the chain.

Certainly one or the other of the sequences marked as group-specific will prove to be individual-specific when more comparable data are available. This holds particularly true for groups II and III. For the same reasons the assumption of four groups is only a preliminary figure.

It should be noted that, contrary to the κ chains, the constant part of the λ chains does not appear to be entirely constant. In protein Kern a serine-glycine exchange has been observed in position 154 [37], an arginine-lysine exchange in Oz+ proteins [38, 39] in position 191, and a double exchange in position 145 and 173 for the Mz [40] protein (Fig. 3). It is still an open question as to

I

			1										10									20							28	28a		30		

New   Glp Ser Val Leu Thr Gln Pro Pro Ser Val Ser Ala Ala Pro Gly Gln Lys Val Thr Ile Ser Cys Ser Gly Ser Ser Thr Asn Ile - Gly Asn Asn Tyr Val Ser
Ha   Glp Ser Val Leu Thr Gln Pro Pro Ser Val Ser Gly Ala Pro Gly Gln Arg Val Thr Ile Ser Cys Ser Gly Ser Ser Ser Asn Ile Gly Thr Asn Asn Tyr Val Ser
HBJ 7
HBJ 98 Glp/Ser Val Thr/Glx Pro Pro Ala/Asp Val/Gln Ala/Val Thr /Ile Ser/Cys
HBJ 11
Mz   Glp Ser Val Thr Gln Pro Pro Ser Val Ser Ala Ala Pro Gly Gln Lys Ile Ala Ile Ile Ser Cys Ser Gly Ser Ser Ser Asn Ala Met

II

Bo   Glp Ser Ala Leu Thr Glx Pro Ala Ser Val Ser Gly Ser Pro Gly Gln Ser Ile Thr Ile Ser Cys Thr Gly Thr Ser Ser Asp Val Gly Ala Asp Asn Lys Tyr Ser
HBJ 2 Glp Ser Ala Leu Thr Gln Pro Ala Ser Val Ser Gly Ser Pro Gly Gln Ser Val Thr Ile Ser Cys Thr Gly Thr Ser Val
HBJ 8 Glp Ser Ala Leu Ala Gln Pro Ala Ser Val Ser Gly Ser Pro Gly Gln Ser Ile Thr Thr
HBJ 15 Glp Ser Ala Leu Thr Gln Pro Ala Ser Val Ser Gly Ser Pro Gly Gln Thr Ile Thr

III

Sh   - Glu Leu Thr Gln Pro Ala Ser Val Ser Val Ala Leu Gly Gln Thr Val Arg Ile Thr Cys Gln Gly Asp Ser Leu Arg - - - Gly Tyr Asp Ala Ala

IV

Kern   - Tyr Ala Leu Thr Gln Pro Pro Ser Val Ser Val Ser Pro Gly Gln Thr Ala Ser Ile Thr Cys Ser Gly Asp Asn Leu Glu - - - Lys Thr Phe Val Ser
X   - Tyr Asp Leu Thr Gln Pro Pro Ser Val Ser Val Ser Pro Gly Gln Thr Ala Arg Ile Thr Cys Ser Gly Asp Lys Leu Gly - - - Asp
1 1 1
Mil   - Tyr Glu Leu Thr Gln Pro Pro

	40										50										60							70			

I

New   Trp His Gln Leu Pro Gly Thr Ala Pro Lys Leu Leu Ile Tyr Glu Asp Asn Lys Arg Pro Ser Gly Ile Pro Asp Arg Ile Ser Gly Thr Ser Ala Thr Gly Leu Arg
Ha   Trp Tyr Gln Gln Leu Pro Gly Thr Ala Pro Lys Leu Leu Ile Tyr Glu Arg Lys Lys Arg Pro Ser Gly Val Pro Asp Arg Phe Ser Gly Ser Lys Ser Gly Thr Ser Ala Ser Leu Ala Leu Leu Arg

II

Bo   Trp Tyr Gln Gln His Pro Gly Arg Ala Pro Lys Val Leu Ile Phe Glu Val Ser Asn Arg Pro Ser Gly Val Pro Asp Arg Phe Ser Gly Ser Lys Ser Gly Asn Thr Ala Ser Leu Thr Val Ser Gly Leu Arg

III

Sh   Trp Tyr Gln Gln Lys Pro Gly Gln Ala Pro Val Leu Val Ile Tyr Gly Lys Asn Asn Arg Pro Ser Gly Ile Pro Asp Arg Phe Ser Gly Ser Ser Ser Gly His Thr Ala Ser Leu Thr Ile Thr Gly Ala Gln

IV

Kern   Trp Phe Gln Gln Arg Pro Gly Gln Ser Pro Leu Leu Val Ile Tyr His Glu Asp Arg Pro Ser Gly Ile Pro Glu Arg Phe Ser Gly Thr Ser Ser Gly Thr Thr Ala Thr Leu Thr Ile Ser Gly Ala Gln

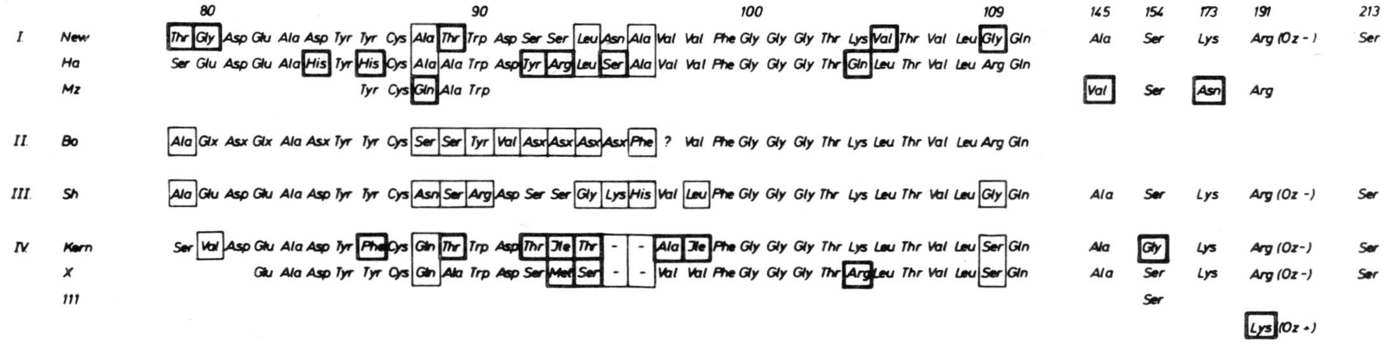

Figure 1. Comparison of the variable parts of λ-type Bence-Jones proteins Kern [15], New [16], Sh, Ha, Bo [14], X, Mil, Mz[33, 34], HBJ 2, HBJ 7, HBJ 11, HBJ 15 [35], and HBJ 98 [36]. On the basis of their chemical homology the proteins are divided into groups (I-IV).

Group-specific exchanges against a hypothetical basic sequence (identical residues in at least two groups) are marked by light boxes, individual-specific exchanges by dark boxes, deletions by –. Residues within brackets mean that this sequence is not yet determined. Exchanged amino acids in the constant part are shown for the Kern [37], the Oz + [38, 39] and the Mz [40] protein.

In comparison to [15] the sequence of Kern has been reversed in positions 30/31.

whether these exchanges are allotypes or an expression of a beginning subgroup following gene duplication of the C gene, since no genetic analysis has established allotypy. All attempts to link one of these exchanges to one of the subgroups in the variable part have failed; for example, protein X [33] and protein 111 [15, 42], which have an N-terminal tyrosine, do not have glycine, like protein Kern [15], in the corresponding position of the constant part.

Figure 4 shows a comparison of the variable parts of all κ chains whose structures are known, including Roy, Cum, and the Ti protein, whose sequence has just recently been determined in our laboratory [32].

			90										100									110	
Kern(λ)	Cys	Gln	Thr	Try	Asp	Thr	Ile	Thr	–	–	Ala	Ile	Phe	Gly	Gly	Gly	Thr	Lys	Leu	Thr	Val	Leu	Ser	Gln
X (λ)	Cys	Gln	Ala	Try	Asp	Ser	Met	Ser	–	–	Val	Val	Phe	Gly	Gly	Gly	Thr	Arg	Leu	Thr	Val	Leu	Ser	Gln
New(λ)	Cys	Ala	Thr	Try	Asp	Ser	Ser	Leu	Asn	Ala	Val	Val	Phe	Gly	Gly	Gly	Thr	Lys	Val	Thr	Val	Leu	Gly	Gln
Roy (κ)	Cys	Gln	Gln	Phe	Asp	Asn	Leu	Pro	–	–	Leu	Thr	Phe	Gly	Gly	Gly	Thr	Lys	Val	–	Asp	Phe	Lys	Arg

Figure 2. Unequal chain length in position 95/96 of λ-type L chains. In comparison to λ-type L chains of groups I-III. λ-type proteins of group IV have a deletion of two amino acids in position 95/96, rendering them equally long as κ chains in this region. It should be noted that deletions in L chains always occur in positions adjacent to Cysteine residues which are connected by disulfide bonds [33]. For references see Figs. 1 and 4. The arrow marks the beginning of the constant part.

As shown earlier, three different subgroups can be distinguished in κ chains on the basis of sequence homology in the variable part. While Roy and Cum are members of subgroups I and II, the Ti protein represents subgroup III, where less complete data were available so far. These three subgroups can be most clearly recognized in the N-terminal 20 residues of the variable part. Thus in position 13, group I has alanine, group II valine, and group III leucine in a corresponding position. Superimposed on these group-specific differences are single amino acid exchanges on the individual chains, again indicated by dark boxes. Most of the exchanges within one group can be explained by single point mutations. The rate of exchanges within one group is much lower (10–25%) than between groups (40–50%). Moreover the chain length seems to be consistent with the sub-grouping. The members of group I have a gap of six amino acids in position 29, when compared to Cum. Whether all proteins of group II will have the same length in this area must be confirmed, but group III seems to have a group-specific gap of five amino acids.

The overall picture is the same for κ and λ chains, except that, at the end of the variable part of the κ chains (position 90 to 107), the number of individual exchanges within one group is increased; in this area, group-specific sequences can hardly be recognized. The sequence of the constant parts of the κ chains are

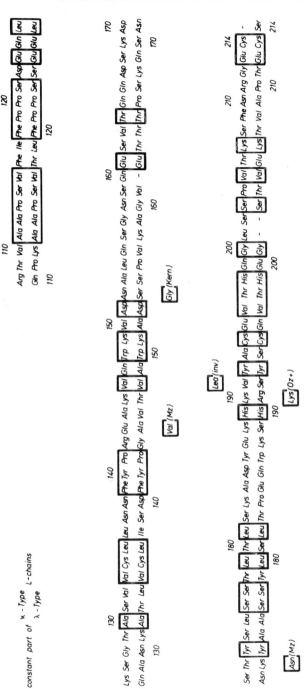

Figure 3. Comparison of the constant parts of κ and λ chains [9, 11, 15-17, 41]. Homologous positions between the two chain-types are marked by boxes. Also indicated are amino acid exchanges in the constant parts of both chains. For λ chains exchanges have been found in the Oz + [38, 39], the Kern [37], and the Mz [40] protein. In κ chains only the Val-Leu exchange in position 191 was shown to be an allotypic variant [8, 19-21].

N. HILSCHMANN, *et al.*

Figure 4a.

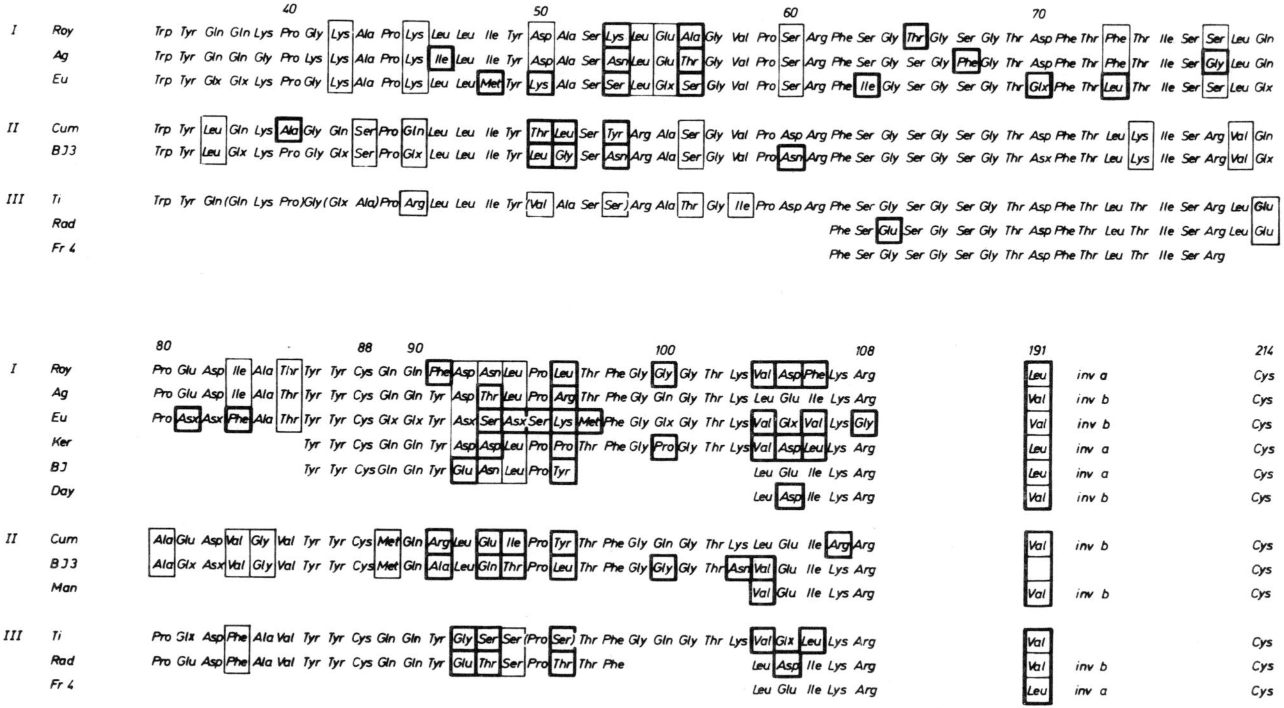

Figure 4b.

Figures 4a and 4b. Comparison of the variable parts of κ-type Bence-Jones proteins of Roy [9], Cum [10, 65], Ti [32], Ag [11], Eu [43], Ker, BJ, Day, Man, Rad, Fr 4 [44, 45], HBJ 1, HBJ 10, HBJ 4, HBJ 5, HS 4 [35], HBJ 3 (Mil) [47], Cra, Pap, Lux, Mon, Con, Fra, Nig, Win, Gra, Cas, Smi, and Pool [46].
On the basis of their chemical homology the proteins are divided into groups I–III. For symbols used see legend to Fig. 1.
In comparison to [9] the sequence of Roy has been extended for positions 25–28 and 31, 32, and reversed for positions 39 and 41.

identical, except for the valine-leucine exchange at position 191, which is caused by an allotype (Fig. 3). There seems to be no correlation between these allotypes and any particular group- or individual-specific sequence within one group.

HYPOTHESES OF ANTIBODY DIVERSITY

Several hypotheses have been proposed in order to explain the variability observed in the N-terminal part of the immunoglobulin chains. In general, two categories of hypotheses can be distinguished; models, involving one or a limited number of genes, and the multiple germ line hypothesis. Both types of hypotheses (except those involving just one gene) imply that the variable and the constant parts are under separate genetic control, i.e. one gene for the constant part and a greater number of genes for the variable part. Both categories also imply that the outer limits of variability are determined by the V genes which are separated in the germ line and whose structural differences have been acquired by an accumulation of point mutations during evolution. However, while the multiple germ line models assume that these evolutionary differences are solely responsible for the structural diversity in the variable part, and that therefore as many V genes as V parts have to be inherited, somatic mutation models explain structural diversity by a somatic recombination process between only a small number of genes, thus minimizing the number of genes which have to be carried in the germ line. This situation is schematically shown in Fig. 5.

As has already been pointed out, varying chemical homologies between the variable parts of different L chains of one antigenic type closely resemble structural variations in other homologous proteins. Chemical and phylogenetical relationships have been intensively investigated for the haemoglobins [48] and the cytochromes [49], and summarized in well established evolutionary trees. The V parts of the κ and λ chains also can be ordered in a similar fashion, the subgroups being the main branches, the individual chains the terminal ramifications of such an evolutionary tree. A comparison with the haemoglobins is of particular interest, because the κ as well as the λ chains seem to mimic haemoglobin evolution not only qualitatively but also quantitatively.

The α and β chains of human haemoglobin are homologous proteins which differ in multiple amino acid exchanges and some deletions. The number of exchanges amounts to 57%, when 148 residues are compared (deletions treated as exchanges). When two Bence-Jones proteins of the same chain type, but of different subgroupings, are compared, i.e. Roy (I) and Cum (II), the exchange rate of the variable part is 51% (in general 40—50%) (Fig. 6). From the varying degree of homology between the different haemoglobin chains, it has been concluded that the haemoglobin genes are derived from one primordial gene which underwent several subsequent gene duplications, followed by an accumulation of point mutations on these duplicated and dislocated genes. The first gene duplication seems to have occurred 400 million years ago [50]. This evolutionary tree fits well with the finding that primitive fishes, like the lampreys, still have only one haemoglobin chain with a molecular weight of 16,000 [51].

Assuming the same phylogenetic relationship and also the same mutation rate for the V genes of immunoglobulins, we should expect for the lower vertebrates

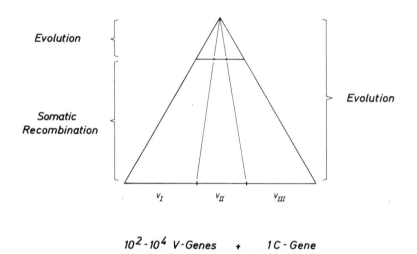

Figure 5. Alternative hypotheses of antibody diversity. The triangle demonstrates the differentiation of V genes from one precursor gene to a definitive number of V genes coding for different V parts. $V_I - V_{III}$ indicates the groups. Multiple germ line models limit this diversification process to evolution, which acts on genes separated in the germ line. Somatic hypermutation models explain antibody diversity partly by evolution, partly by recombination, between a small number of phylogenetically-related genes.

N-terminal parts which are no longer variable but possess one amino acid sequence. If the immune response depends on differences in structures, these animals should have no antibody activity. The lampreys, which have been examined in this respect [52], still have antibodies which show, as they should, differences in structure. But in hagfish, their somewhat lower relatives, no antibody activity could be detected and no γ-globulin band was present in serum electrophoresis [53]. It should, however, be noted that lower vertebrates which can produce antibodies, like the leopard shark and the paddle fish, already show diversities in the structures of the L chains, similar to that found in the different subgroups of human and murine L chains. Each H chain, however, has one unique structure for the N-terminal five residues [54, 55].

An additional insight into whether the variability of the N-terminal parts of the immunoglobulin chains is caused by a hypermutation process or evolution might be gained by a comparison of certain characteristics in κ and λ chains. The question is whether multiple V genes were already present in the primordial gene

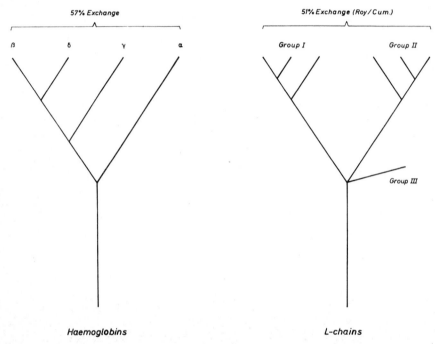

Figure 6. Schematic phylogenetic trees for human haemoglobin and immunoglobulin L chains. The exchange rate of amino acids between α and β chains of haemoglobin and between group-specific sequences of one antigenic type (κ) is compared.

of the κ chains and λ chains before they separated in evolution (Fig. 7a) or if they were produced afterwards (Fig. 7b). One very characteristic feature in both κ and λ chains are the sequence gaps or deletions. Although the size of these sequence gaps seems to be specific for each subgroup, they occur in κ as well as λ chains in positions 29 and 28 respectively, which are homologous positions in both proteins.

The homologous positions of these deletions in both the κ and λ chains could more plausibly be explained on the assumption that they have already been present in the precursor genes of the κ and λ genes than by an introduction in exactly homologous positions of the already separated κ- and λ-chain genes. This assumption is supported by a comparison of complete κ- and λ-type chains. The homology of these chains is expressed in 40% identity of the amino acid sequences in both chains. The equal distribution of these identities between the V and C parts in both types indicates equal phylogenetic distance from a common precursor. A comparison of the C-terminal parts of κ and λ chains is shown in Fig. 3.

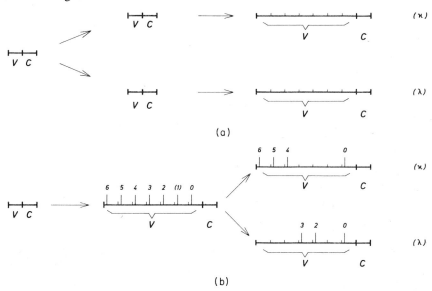

(a)

(b)

Figure 7. Two possibilities for generation of diversity in κ- and λ-chain genes.
(a) Variability, indicated by several V genes, was introduced after duplication and independent evolution of κ- and λ-type genes.
(b) Variability was already present in the precursor gene of κ- and λ-type genes. Numbers indicate the differences in length in the homologous positions 29 or 28 of κ or λ chains respectively.

One argument against multiple germ line has always been the enormous number of genes which would have to be carried in the germ line in order to code for all the different variable parts of the immunoglobulin chains. There is no reasonable estimation of the maximum number of different V genes, but an estimation can be made for the minimal number of genes involved from data already present. There are data for at least twenty-five different L chains of one antigenic type, most of them only fragmentary, but sufficient to show that none of these proteins is identical in structure. According to a calculation made by Cohen and Milstein [34], based on fingerprint data, which can now be replaced by sequence data, the number of the variants in the κ chains, for instance, is at least 250. Since this calculation would already be valid for variants which differ in only one amino acid, the number of variants might even be much higher, considering the number of exchanges present among different proteins even of one subgroup.

The question arises whether so many genes can be carried in the germ line. According to its DNA content, one human sperm cell has 4×10^9 nucleotides [56], or 0.67×10^9 triplets, per single DNA strand. Assuming that the variable parts of L and H chains contain 110 amino acid residues (which is not yet sure for the H chain), one would still arrive at 6×10^3 different variable parts when only 0.1% of the DNA content is engaged in antibody synthesis. Provided that L and H chains can combine unrestrictedly (which they cannot [57]), 10^7 different antibody molecules would result, a number which would suffice to explain the observed variety in antibody specificity.

So far no serious arguments speak against multiple germ line. There is, however, one argument which seems to be incompatible with multiple genes separated in the germ line. It is the observation that species-specific differences in invariable positions of the variable part have been maintained during evolution. This argument has been raised by Doolittle [58] and is demonstrated in Fig. 8 which shows the N-terminal five residues of human, mouse and rabbit κ chains. Position 2, which is invariable within every species, is isoleucine in man and mouse, and valine in the rabbit. Multiple germ lines would imply multiple point mutations at exactly the same positions in all genes carried in the germ line, which seems to be unlikely. There could be selection for a protein-carrying valine in position 2, but this could be more readily and plausibly explained with only a few genes in the germ line. In a recent investigation the N-terminal ten amino acids of mouse λ chain have been determined [59]. This sequence is very similar to the one proposed for the rabbit κ chains, but has also some correspondence to rabbit λ chains [60].

Somatic recombination models try to minimize the number of genes which have to be carried in the germ line. They take advantage of evolutionary differences between two or more basic genes inherited in the germ line. One of these models implies somatic interallelic recombination between a limited number of serially repeated homologous V genes, the C gene being excluded from this recombination process because of the low homology between V and C genes. Simultaneously, the V genes in the germ line are shortened to their definitive length by controlled deletions. This model has been discussed in detail elsewhere [23].

There are, however, still unsolved problems with all recombination models. Minimum models [24], which assume only two basic genes, have difficulties in explaining the three or four basic sequences which have already been found in κ or λ chains respectively. But even if one extends these minimum models to three or four basic genes, one has to consider that the observed variability is very difficult to explain by recombination between these three or four basic genes.

As sequence studies on κ and λ chains have shown, the basic sequence within one group is remarkably constant. This argument holds true for the group-specific sequences as well as for the number of deleted amino acid residues, which also seem to be constant within one group, both in κ and λ chains. A crossing over between these basic genes would lead to a structure which might have group-specific sequences derived from one group in one part and group-specific sequences from another group in another part of the molecule. The same should be found for the deletions. It is difficult to conceive of recombination between genes of unequal length. The deleted sections are therefore likely to be excluded from recombination, and sequences in the neighbourhood of these deletions should thus be rather constant within one group; this is, however, not observed.

	1	2	3	4	5	6
Mouse and Human κ	Asp Glu	Ile	Val Gln	Val Leu Met	Thr	Gln
Rabbit Pool	Ala	Val	Val Leu	Val	Gln	Gln
	(Ile) (Asp) (Glu)	(Leu)	(Gln) (Glu)	(Gln) (Glu)		(Thr) (Ala)

Figure 8. Invariable positions in the variable part of L chains in different species [58].

Furthermore, individual-specific exchanges in one group are difficult to explain by the crossing over between genes coding for different groups. Thus, for example, the valine-alanine exchange in position 13 of κ-type protein Pap (Fig. 4) can hardly be explained by crossing over with the basic gene of group II, which has valine in this position. When crossing over occurs, it would be expected that the neighbouring proline and threonine residues should also be exchanged. The most plausible explanation for the valine in position 13 of Pap is a point mutation caused by a one base exchange. The same is true for the methionine-leucine exchange at position 4 of the κ chains. Most of the single amino acid exchanges within one subgroup can be explained by a one base exchange. So far no blocks of exchanged amino acids have been observed in the N-terminal section of the variable part of the κ and λ chains although sufficient data are available for the N-terminal part of these molecules.

However, this does not exclude the possibility that recombination might have occurred in other parts of the molecule, where less data are available. The question is what should be expected from the structures in this case. It always has to be kept in mind that, in any recombination model, the analyzed sequences are not reprints of the basic genes, but are already their recombination products. What should be observed, no matter what the basic genes look like, and how often crossing over occurs between them, is an increased disturbance of the group-specific sequences when one proceeds from the N- to the C-terminal end of the variable part. This implies that a subgrouping based on sequence homologies of the N-terminal parts should not be valid for the C-terminal end of the variable part. With the symbols used in Figs. 1 and 4, this would mean that individual-specific exchanges, as a deviation from specific exchanges marked by dark boxes, should increase towards the C-terminal end of the variable part. This is, as Fig. 4 shows, the case only for positions 90–107 of κ-type proteins. These structural peculiarities were observed very early [8], and were so far the only indications in the L chain structure that a hybridization process might have occurred. But then these accumulated exchanges should not be limited only to that part of the molecule where both the recombination and the multiple germ line hypotheses claim fusion between V and C genes.

Furthermore, accumulated individual-specific exchanges have not been observed in the λ chains; these exchanges are equally distributed along the chain. The group-specific sequences on the λ chains can be recognized throughout the variable part; no linkage groups can be detected indicating crossover between the groups. This is particularly true for the proteins Kern and X of group IV, which have several distinct markers; the N-terminal tyrosine, deletions in positions 28 and 95/96, and a serine at position 109, immediately adjacent to the constant part.

This almost completely excludes models which postulate recombination between two or three basic genes. More complex models, assuming recombination between a larger number of basic genes, cannot be discarded from the present data. The recombination processes should then be limited to genes of one subgroup. This makes the number of V genes or V-gene pairs involved, at least as large as the number of subgroups in one chain type [16]. The number of genes will increase whenever a new subgroup becomes apparent from new sequence data. Arguments against multiple germ line could be equally applied to recombination models with a large number of genes. Structurally they would be indistinguishable.

So sequence studies with monoclonal proteins have shed some light on the genetic mechanism which determines antibody specificity. Although many questions are still open, the fusion of the V and C genes being only one, these studies have lent support to the idea that many homologous V genes, randomly generated as in evolution, must take part in the control of immunoglobulin synthesis. This concept is certainly not easy to reconcile with the "one gene one protein" dogma, although it is not in direct opposition to it. It is completely in agreement with another more recent finding that, for example, the γ chain of human foetal haemoglobin must be controlled by several structural genes [61]. Serial repetitions of genes in organisms belonging to the chromosomal kingdom seem to be no exception and have been discussed recently [62, 63]. The more serious problem will be to understand how so many serially repeated genes can be maintained during evolutionary and individual development, and not deleted, as might be surmised from viral and bacterial genetics [64].

REFERENCES

1. Fleischman, J. B., Porter, R. R. and Press, E. M., *Biochem. J.* **88** (1963) 220.
2. Edelman, G. M. and Gally, J. A., *Proc. natn. Acad. Sci. U.S.A.* **51** (1964) 846.
3. Whitney, P. L. and Tanford, C., *Proc. natn. Acad. Sci. U.S.A.* **53** (1965) 524.
4. Haber, E., *Proc. natn. Acad. Sci. U.S.A.* **52** (1964) 1099.
5. Koshland, M. E. and Englberger, F. M., *Proc. natn. Acad. Sci. U.S.A.* **50** (1963) 61.
6. Oudin, J., *J. exp. Med.* **112** (1960) 125.
7. Edelman, G. M. and Gally, J. A., *J. exp. Med.* **116** (1962) 207.
8. Hilschmann, N. and Craig, L. C., *Proc. natn. Acad. Sci. U.S.A.* **53** (1965) 1403.
9. Hilschmann, N., *Hoppe-Seyler's Z. physiol. Chem.* **348** (1967) 1077.
10. Hilschmann, N., *Hoppe-Seyler's Z. physiol. Chem.* **348** (1967) 1718.
11. Titani, K., Whitley, E. J., and Putnam, F. W., *Science, N.Y.* **152** (1966) 1513.
12. Milstein, C., *Proc. R. Soc.* Ser. B, **166** (1966) 138.
13. Gray, W. R., Dreyer, W. J. and Hood, L., *Science, N.Y.* **155** (1967) 465.
14. Putnam, F. W., Shinoda, T., Titani, K. and Wikler, M., *Science, N.Y.* **157** (1967) 1050.
15. Ponstingl, H., Hess, M. and Hilschmann, N., *Hoppe-Seyler's Z. physiol. Chem.* **349** (1968) 867.
16. Langer, B., Steinmetz-Kayne, M. and Hilschmann, N., *Hoppe-Seyler's Z. physiol. Chem.* **349** (1968) 945.
17. Milstein, C., Clegg, J. B. and Jarvis, J. M., *Nature, Lond.* **214** (1967) 270.
18. Milstein, C., *Nature, Lond.* **205** (1965) 1172.
19. Milstein, C., *Nature, Lond.* **209** (1966) 370.
20. Baglioni, C., Alescio-Zonta, L., Cioli, D. and Carbonara, A., *Science, N.Y.* **152** (1966) 1519.
21. Hilschmann, N., *Proc. 11th Int. Congr. Blood Transf.* Sydney, 1966, and *Biblthca. haemat.* No. 29, Part 2, p. 501. Karger, Basel/New York, 1968.
22. Brenner, S. and Milstein, C., *Nature, Lond.* **211** (1966) 242.
23. Hilschmann, N., *Hoppe-Seyler's Z. physiol. Chem.* **348** (1967) 1291.
24. Smithies, O., *Science, N.Y.* **157** (1967) 267.
25. Edelman, G. M. and Gally, J. A., *Proc. natn. Acad. Sci. U.S.A.* **57** (1967) 353.
26. Whitehouse, H. L. K., *Nature, Lond.* **215** (1967) 371.
27. Dreyer, W. J. and Bennett, J. C., *Proc. natn. Acad. Sci. U.S.A.* **54** (1965) 864.
28. Cohn, M., *in* "Gamma Globulins", Nobel Symposium 3 (edited by J. Killander), Almqvist and Wiksell, Stockholm, 1967, p. 615.
29. Discussion, in *Cold Spring Harb. Symp. quant. Biol.* **32** (1967) 169.
30. Lennox, E. S. and Cohn, M., *A. Rev. Biochem.* **36** (1967) 365.
31. Cohn, M., *in* "Rutgers Symposium on Nucleic Acids in Immunology", (edited by O. J. Plescia and W. Braun), Springer-Verlag, New York, 1968, p. 671.

32. Suter, L., Barnikol, H. U., Watanabe, S. and Hilschmann, N., *Hoppe-Seyler's Z. physiol. Chem.* **350** (1969) 275.
33. Milstein, C., *Cold Spring Harb. Symp. quant. Biol.* **32** (1967) 31.
34. Cohen, S. and Milstein, C., *Adv. Immun.* **7** (1967) 1.
35. Hood, L., Gray, W. R., Sanders, B. G. and Dreyer, W. J., *Cold Spring Harb. Symp. quant. Biol.* **32** (1967) 133.
36. Baglioni, C., *Biochem. biophys. Res. Commun.* **26** (1967) 82.
37. Ponstingl, H., Hess, M., Langer, B., Steinmetz-Kayne, M. and Hilschmann, N., *Hoppe-Seyler's Z. physiol. Chem.* **348** (1967) 1213.
38. Ein, D. and Fahey, J. L., *Science, N.Y.* **156** (1967) 947.
39. Appella, E. and Ein, D., *Proc. natn. Acad. Sci. U.S.A.* **57** (1967) 1449.
40. Milstein, C., *Biochem. J.* **104** (1967) 28C.
41. Wikler, M., Titani, K., Shinoda, T. and Putnam, F. W., *J. biol. Chem.* **242** (1967) 1668.
42. van Eijk, H. G. and Monfoort, C. H., *Biochim. biophys. Acta* **86** (1964) 410.
43. Cunningham, B. A., Gottlieb, P. D., Konigsberg, W. H. and Edelman, G. M., *Biochemistry, N.Y.* **7** (1968) 1983.
44. Milstein, C., *Nature, Lond.* **216** (1967) 330.
45. Milstein, C., *Biochem. J.* **101** (1966) 352.
46. Niall, H. D. and Edman, P., *Nature, Lond.* **216** (1967) 262.
47. Dreyer, W. J., Gray, W. R. and Hood, L., *Cold Spring Harb. Symp. quant. Biol.* **32** (1967) 353.
48. Braunitzer, G., Hilse, K., Rudloff, V. and Hilschmann, N., *Adv. Protein Chem.* **19** (1964) 1.
49. Margoliash, E. and Schejter, A., *Adv. Protein Chem.* **21** (1966) 113.
50. Braunitzer, G., *Naturwissenschaften* **54** (1967) 407.
51. Rudloff, V. and Zelenik, M., *Hoppe-Seyler's Z. physiol. Chem.* **344** (1966) 289.
52. Marchalonis, J. J. and Edelman, G. M., *J. exp. Med.* **127** (1968) 891.
53. Good, R. A. and Papermaster, B. W., *Adv. Immun.* **4** (1964) 1.
54. Suran, A. A. and Papermaster, B. W., *Proc. natn. Acad. Sci. U.S.A.* **58** (1967) 1619.
55. Pollara, B., Suran, A., Finstad, G. and Good, R. A., *Proc. natn. Acad. Sci. U.S.A.* **59** (1968) 1307.
56. Müller, H. J., *Bull. Am. math. Soc.* **64** (1958) 137.
57. Mannik, M., *Biochemistry, N.Y.* **6** (1967) 134.
58. Doolittle, R. F., *Proc. natn. Acad. Sci. U.S.A.* **55** (1966) 1195.
59. Appella, E. and Perham, R. N., *J. molec. Biol.* **33** (1968) 963.
60. Rüde, E. and Givol, D., *Biochem. J.* **107** (1968) 449.
61. Schroeder, W. A., Huisman, T. H. J., Shelton, J. R., Shelton, J. B., Kleihauer, E. F., Dozy, A. M. and Robberson, B., *Proc. natn. Acad. Sci. U.S.A.* **60** (1968) 537.
62. Callan, H. G., *J. cell. Sci.* **2** (1967) 1.
63. Whitehouse, H. L. K., *J. cell. Sci.* **2** (1967) 9.
64. Thomas, C. A., *in* "Progress in Nucleic Acid Research and Molecular Biology", Vol. 5, (edited by J. N. Davidson and W. E. Cohn), Academic Press, New York and London, 1966, p. 315.
65. Hilschmann, N., *Naturwissenschaften*, in press.

FEBS Symposium, Volume 15, 1969, pp. 75-81

Variable Structures in Pig Immunoglobulin λ Chains

F. FRANĚK, B. KEIL and F. ŠORM

Department of Protein Chemistry,
Institute of Organic Chemistry and Biochemistry,
Czechoslovak Academy of Science,
Prague, Czechoslovakia.

When we isolate the light chains from normal immunoglobulin and investigate their physical and chemical characteristics, we find that possibly the only property which they share in common is their approximately identical chain length. The population of light chains can be divided into subpopulations which differ from each other both in amino acid composition and end groups, and also in antigenic properties. There exist subpopulations which do not show any feature in common when they are examined by the fingerprint technique [1]. An almost equal heterogeneity is displayed by light chains isolated from specifically purified antibodies, even though these antibodies have a narrow specificity, for example, to a synthetic hapten [2, 3]. As to the finding of highly restricted heterogeneity in antibody light chains of certain animal species, it has been shown that this phenomenon is the exception rather than the rule [4].

The unusual heterogeneity of the light chains finds its physical manifestation in multiple banding which occurs when normal or antibody light chains are subjected to gel electrophoresis at neutral or slightly alkaline pH [5]. The phenomenon of banding itself does not indicate whether the components represented by the individual bands are really homogeneous polypeptide chains or not. Neither does the electrophoretic pattern show whether the components are in some way related. Far more information in this respect is offered by peptide maps. These maps always include several peptide spots which are intense and a number of other, weaker spots. At the same time the total number of spots exceeds several times the number of peptides which could be expected to arise in theory, having regard to the specificity of the enzyme used.

As concerns pig immunoglobulin, which we have studied, we were able to achieve a very efficient fractionation of its light chains. The resulting light chain subpopulations showed entirely different sets of intensive peptide spots [1]. As we found later, these subpopulations differed also in their antigenic properties and we were therefore fully justified in considering them as light chain types [3]. The pig immunoglobulin light chains were subsequently resolved into electrophoretically-homogeneous components [6]. Even these components were found to represent subpopulations, each consisting of many variants differing in amino acid sequence.

Summarizing the information which we have obtained in our studies on subpopulations of pig immunoglobulin light chains, we can conclude that the population of normal immunoglobulin light chains consists of two or more types. Variants which belong to the same type possess a considerable portion of their polypeptide chain in common. There exist, however, sections of the polypeptide chain which are extremely variable. These sections are the source of all physical and chemical differences found between individual variants. The number of existing variants is hardly to be estimated [7]. All that has been said about normal pig immunoglobulin light chains complies with the concept that these chains represent a mixture of polypeptide chains of the same character as the Bence-Jones proteins of man and mouse whose primary structures are in several cases completely known. To our expectation our first data on the amino acid sequence of pig immunoglobulin—sequences around the cystine bridges of the λ chains—have confirmed the existence of a high degree of similarity between λ chains of normal pig immunoglobulin and human type L Bence-Jones proteins [7, 8].

When determining the amino acid sequence of the variable portion of the immunoglobulin chains, we have to face problems not encountered in studies on the primary structure of homogeneous proteins. The fragmentation of polypeptide chains possessing sections with a mixed sequence gives rise to a jumble of peptides, notwithstanding that the fragmentation procedure was highly specific. With some of the resulting peptides it is impossible to decide whether they are derived from different variant chains or from the same polypeptide chain in which they were originally linked together. This difficulty can be circumvented by a fragmentation strategy which respects several reference points, i.e. amino residues, the position of which may be considered as invariant in the particular subpopulation of light chains. We have made an effort to employ as such reference points, in the variable portion of the λ chains, the half-cystine residues of which form a disulfide bond. We started with the tryptic digest and made a search for such tryptic peptides, the amino acid pattern of which would show the presence of half-cystine residues and in which the sum of lysine and arginine residues would equal two. Only these features guarantee that the peptides under consideration have been liberated by specific tryptic cleavage and that their C-terminal lysines or arginines may serve as additional auxiliary reference points. The tryptic digest of the λ chains with intact intrachain disulfide bonds was fractionated first on Sephadex G-50 in order to separate the fraction of large peptides from the fraction of small peptides. Individual

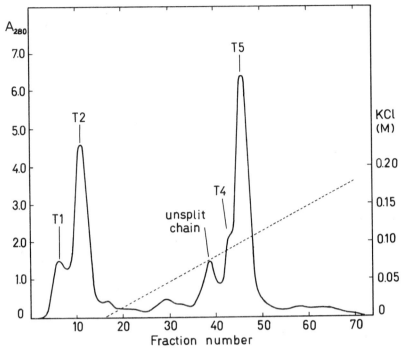

Figure 1. Ion-exchange chromatography on SE-Sephadex of large peptides from the tryptic hydrolyzate of pig immunoglobulin λ chains. The column (6 x 40 cm) was equilibrated with a buffer containing 0·005 M potassium formate and 8 M urea; the pH was adjusted with formic acid to 3. After applying the sample (5 g) the column was eluted with a linear gradient of potassium chloride in the buffer. Fraction volume is 100 ml. Solid curve—absorbance at 280 nm. Dotted line—molarity of potassium chloride in the eluate.

Table 1. Amino acid composition of peptide T2.

Lys	0·9	Ala	7·3
His	—	1/2Cys	2·0
Arg	1·0	Val	4·3
Asp	3·7	Met	1·0
Thr	9·4	Ile	2·2
Ser	7·1	Leu	4·0
Glu	9·3	Tyr	2·9
Pro	5·9	Phe	2·9
Gly	6·5	Trp	1·0

Number of residues of individual amino acids are given. The values shown represent extrapolated values from two analyses (20 h and 70 h hydrolysis). The half-cystine content was determined as cysteic acid from the analysis of a performic acid oxidized aliquot.

components of the fraction of large peptides were then resolved by chromatography on SE-Sephadex in formate buffer at pH 3, 8 M in urea (Fig. 1). As can be seen from the amino acid composition (Table 1), our requirements are fulfilled for peptide T2. It contains one disulfide group, 1 arginine, and 1 lysine. The total number of amino acid residues in peptide T2 is 70 or 71. This number represents possibly an average value, since the individual variants may differ in the length of their chain by several residues.

When chromatographed on SE-Sephadex, peptide T2 appears to emerge as a homogeneous peak. This is not surprising since at pH 3 only the positive electric

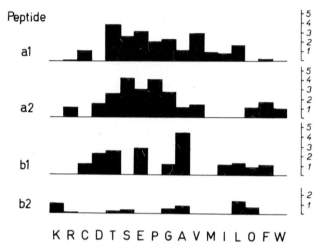

Figure 2. Amino acid composition of peptides derived from peptide T2. The numbers of residues are represented as heights of the columns. Scales for number of residues are on the right side. The amino acids are designated by one-letter symbols [10] placed beneath the columns.

charge of basic amino acids plays a role and, in fact, all variants of this peptide have the same content of basic amino acids. The amino acid composition indicates convincingly that most of the amino acids are not present as integral multiples of residues. Peptide T2 does not contain histidine. This provides additional evidence that peptide T2 originates from variable part, since the analogous peptide from the invariant part of the chain contains two histidine residues in the close vicinity of a half-cystine residue. The strongly acidic character of peptide T2 suggests that this peptide might involve the N-terminal end of the chain whose amino group is blocked. The ultimate proof of this statement will emerge from data to be presented below.

For the subsequent fragmentation of peptide T2 the two reference points—the cysteine residues—were utilized. The disulfide bond was reduced by dithiothreitol in 6 M guanidine hydrochloride and the cysteine residues were converted into aminoethylcysteine residues. Peptide T2 yields two fragments, peptides T2a and T2b which were separated from each other on SE-Sephadex under conditions analogous to those used for the separation of the hydrolyzate. Each of these two peptides was then digested with trypsin. The products were resolved either by gel filtration or by ion-exchange chromatography and characterized by amino acid analysis (Fig. 2). The composition of these peptides shows certain characteristic features which permit their alignment. Two of the peptides each contain one aminoethylcysteine residue, one peptide contains one lysine residue and the last one contains arginine residue. The terminal amino acid of peptide a1 cannot be determined. This peptide contains 22 or 23 residues. When we compare this data with the known structures of λ chains of human immunoglobulin [9] it becomes apparent that peptide a1 represents most likely

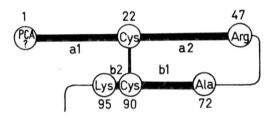

Figure 3. Tentative alignment of peptides a1, a2, b1, and b3. Numbers show the positions of individual residues in the pig immunoglobulin λ chains. N-terminal residue is numbered 1. The section of the chain covered by peptides a1, a2, b1, b2 is represented by a thick line. S-S bridge is illustrated as a double line. PCA stands for pyrrolidone carboxylic acid.

the N-terminal peptide. The half-cystine residue in this peptide occupies position 22 (or 23); the corresponding position of this half-cystine residue in human λ chains is position 22. The position of the half-cystine residue in peptide b1 was designated as 90 in analogy to human λ chains. The tentative arrangement of peptides a1, a2, b1, and b2 into the primary structure of the λ chains is demonstrated in Fig. 3.

By now we have determined the amino acid sequence of peptide b2 and partly of peptide b1. The mixture of peptides b2, most of which are tetra-peptides, was resolved by a combination of ion-exchange chromatography on Dowex 1 with paper techniques. The structures determined so far are presented in Table 2. The amounts of individual peptides present in the mixture widely differ. Most, but not all positions in the region which has been sequenced so far proved to be variable.

Information on the primary structure of normal immunoglobulin polypeptide chains is very incomplete so that no general conclusions can be drawn. It would appear that the overall concept of the light chain as consisting of the variable N-terminal portion and of the invariant type-specific C-terminal portion will be confirmed also for normal immunoglobulin light chains. On the other hand, the increasing amount of information on the primary structure of pathologic light chains of man and mouse [10] raises doubts as to whether the concept of the variable and invariant half of the light chain does not oversimplify the situation. From initial data on amino acid sequence of Bence-Jones proteins the conclusion was drawn that amino acid replacements are predominantly localized in the N-terminal half of the chain [11]. Until a fairly large number of individual Bence-Jones proteins was sequenced, it was impossible to estimate which positions in the N-terminal half have variable character and which are possibly invariant. Summarizing of recent data [10] leads to the conclusion that most likely there exist positions in the N-terminal half which are invariant with respect to different variant chains belonging to the same type. A few of these

Table 2. Amino acid sequence of peptides b1 and b2.

Peptide b2 variants:
Ala-Leu-Tyr-Lys
Ala-Leu-Leu-Tyr-Lys
Ala-Leu-Gly-Lys
Ser-Leu-Tyr-Lys
Thr-Leu-Tyr-Lys
Gly-Leu-Tyr-Lys
Ala-Leu-Gly-Arg
N-terminal sequence of peptide b1:
Ala-Ala-Leu-Leu-
Thr   Gly
          Thr

residues have such a conservative character that they are invariant even with respect to light chains of different animal species. In addition to the invariant residues or stretches, sections characteristic for a subtype were, in a number of cases, established [12-14].

The investigation of the primary structure of normal light chains is at least to some extent equivalent to a simultaneous investigation of primary structures of a great number of different Bence-Jones proteins or myeloma light chains. Therefore, possible invariant positions in the variable half of the chain are expected to be established without difficulties. The amino acid sequence reported in this paper may serve as a modest proof of this assumption. Finally the variable structures of the light chains participate in forming the antibody-combining site. No matter whether their role is direct or indirect, it is evident that one or more sections of variable character must be responsible for this function.

Our considerations present the problems of the structure of normal immuno-globulin light chains in a form which by no means negates the immense complexity of this field. It might even appear that such a presentation of the problems could discourage investigators who intend to undertake studies on the structure of normal and antibody immunoglobulins. It is, however, our sincere belief that the initial results of sequence studies presented in this paper will be followed by other data which will establish convincing evidence permitting us to consider the studies on variable structures of immunoglobulins and antibodies as being without methodical problems in the near future.

REFERENCES

1. Franěk, F. and Zorina, O. M., *Colln. Czech. chem. Commun.* **32** (1967) 3229.
2. Choules, L. and Singer, S. J., *Immunochemistry* **3** (1966) 21.
3. Yamashita, T., Franěk, F., Škvařil, F. and Simek, L., *Eur. J. Biochem.* **6** (1968) 34.
4. Brenneman, L. and Singer, S. J., *Proc. natn. Acad. Sci. U.S.A.* **60** (1968) 258.
5. Cohen, S. and Porter, R. R., *Biochem. J.* **90** (1964) 278.
6. Franěk, F., Pačes, V., Keil, B. and Šorm, F., *Colln. Czech. chem. Commun.* **32** (1967) 3242.
7. Franěk, F., *in* "Gamma Globulins", Nobel Symposium 3 (edited by J. Killander), Almqvist and Wiksell, Stockholm, 1967, p. 221.
8. Franěk, F., Keil, B., Novotný, J. and Šorm, F., *Eur. J. Biochem.* **3** (1968) 422.
9. Putnam, F. W., *in* "Gamma Globulins", Nobel Symposium 3 (edited by J. Killander), Almqvist and Wiksell, Stockholm, 1967, p. 45.
10. Dayhoff, M. O. and Eck, R. V., "Atlas of Protein Sequence and Structure 1967-68". National Biomedical Research Foundation, Silver Spring, 1968.
11. Hilschmann, N. and Craig, L. C., *Proc. natn. Acad. Sci. U.S.A.* **53** (1965) 1403.
12. Niall, H. D. and Edman, P., *Nature, Lond.* **216** (1967) 262.
13. Milstein, C., *Nature, Lond.* **216** (1967) 330.
14. Hilschmann, N., Barnikol, H. U., Hess, M., Langer, B., Ponstingl, H., Steinmetz-Kayne, M., Suter, L. and Watanabe, S., this volume, p. 57.

FEBS Symposium, Volume 15, 1969, pp. 83-91

Electron Microscopic Studies of some Immunoglobulin Components

S. HÖGLUND

Institute of Biochemistry, University of Uppsala, Uppsala, Sweden

INTRODUCTION

There exist structural relationships between the major classes of human immunoglobulins [1], each possessing a multichain structure of two heavy and two light polypeptide chains. The light chains are of two antigenic types, K and L. The IgM molecule, with a molecular weight of about 900,000, probably comprises five 7S subunits [2]. In IgM the weak noncovalent subunit interaction and the unusually high frictional ratio indicate some degree of rotational freedom about the inter-subunit disulphide bonds [2]. This conclusion is also supported by fluorescence depolarization studies [3]. IgG, having a molecular weight of about 150,000, is split by papain into three fragments of about 50,000 molecular weight [4]. Two of these fragments, F_{ab}, are identical and possess an antigen-combining site, while the third fragment, F_c, is chemically and biologically different. The biological activities associated with the F_{ab} and F_c fragments are unaffected by papain digestion, which indicates that their configuration is unaltered by the cleavage [1]. Sedimentation and viscosity studies indicate that the three fragments of IgG are compact globular proteins, and in a likely IgG model the fragments should be joined in a flexible manner [5]. Further evidence in support of this was provided by fluorescence depolarization studies [1]. Sixty per cent of IgG of normal human serum contains light chains of type K and 30% possesses light chains of type L, but myeloma proteins and Bence-Jones proteins from one individual contain only one of these types [1].

A new immunoglobulin class has been described which is called IgND (IgE) [6]. This immunoglobulin was isolated as a myeloma protein, but it has been obtained also from healthy individuals and patients with certain allergic diseases. IgND has a sedimentation constant of 8S and a molecular weight of 200,000 [6].

Bence-Jones proteins are obtained in urine or plasma from patients with multiple myeloma [7]. These proteins are antigenically and chemically related to immunoglobulins [8]. Most Bence-Jones proteins have a sedimentation constant of 3·5S, and occur both as disulphide-linked and non-covalently linked dimers of free light chains with a molecular weight of about 40,000 [8].

MATERIALS AND METHODS

Electron microscopy was used to show the general shape of some immuno-globulin components of IgM and IgC; the latter was compared to IgND, and the dimer of a Bence-Jones protein of type L. In addition IgG interaction with particulate antigens was studied. Each sample of immunoglobulin, particulate antigen, or immunological complex, was carefully purified before preparation for electron microscopy by a combination of fractionation steps including electrophoresis, chromatography, centrifugation and distribution in polymer two-phase systems. A detailed description of these purification procedures is given elsewhere [9-11]. Highly purified IgND was prepared by Johansson and Bennich [6] and homogenous solutions of disulphide-linked dimers of a urinary Bence-Jones protein of type L were obtained by Berggård and Pettersson [7].

Biological macromolecules do not scatter electrons easily in the electron microscope and specimen contrast must be enhanced by introducing heavy atoms. Three contrast methods are now in use, namely shadow casting, negative, and positive contrasting. As the specimen is exposed to high vacuum in the electron microscope, it is seen in a dry state. This drying of the sample might damage especially flexible protein molecules, such as IgM. Protein molecules also have a great tendency to aggregate during drying. We have minimized this aggregation by the use of a high pressure spray gun for the application of the molecules on the specimen grid [9, 11]. We have prepared series of parallel specimens of the protein sample using different contrast methods, which are described in detail elsewhere [9-11].

RESULTS AND DISCUSSION

Studies of IgM

The IgM molecules were easily penetrated by the negative contrast agent employed. The shape of IgM was ovoid or round with a distinctly rough periphery on the negatively contrasted specimens. Their average dimensions were about 200 Å × 300 Å [10]. Occasionally, elongated subunits of IgM were detected (Fig. 1). By the use of the Markham stroboscopy technique [12] it was possible to show that IgM could comprise five elongated, morphological subunits (Fig. 1). A few projections extending from negatively contrasted IgM molecules have sometimes been observed, and spider-like structures were shown by a representative number of Waldenström macroglobulins [13]. Our electron micrographs suggest a swollen, flexible IgM structure, which is compatible with observations by other physico-chemical methods [2]. However, it is difficult to establish whether the projections of the IgM molecules were produced during the preparation of the electron microscopy specimen. It has also been shown that

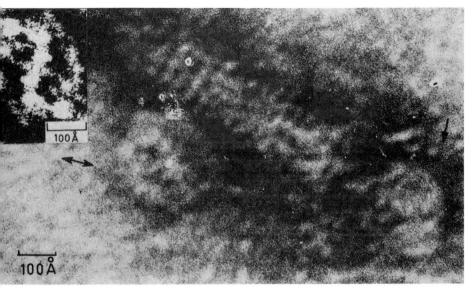

Figure 1. Two IgM antibody molecules (indicated by arrows) connected to the tail of a T2 phage. The IgM molecule to the left clearly shows elongated subunits by stroboscopy with two-fold rotation (insert).

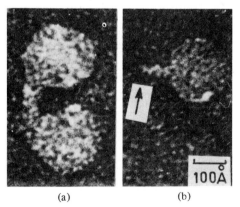

(a)   (b)

Figure 2. (a) Adjacent TNV satellite particles, probably bridged by two or more parallel IgG antibody molecules.
(b) An IgG antibody molecule is connected by one of its ends to a TNV satellite, thus projecting from the virus surface (indicated by the arrow).

myeloma IgM molecules possess linear subunits or extending projections (Beale, D., personal communication).

Studies of IgG

Rabbit IgG antibodies were produced against TNV satellite, which is the smallest virus known to date. Small virus antibody complexes were formed, usually at slight antigen excess, and the complexes were freed from non-specific IgG by particle sieve chromatography [11]. With the microscope, individual IgG molecules were seen within complexes comprised by a few virus particles joined by irregular antibody bridges [11]. The IgG molecules had a length of 100–150 Å and a breadth of about 30–40 Å. Sometimes an antibody bridge about 60 Å broad was detected between two virus particles, probably comprised of two or more parallel antibody molecules (Fig. 2a). IgG molecules linked by one end to single TNV satellite particles were also observed (Fig. 2b) [11].

The interaction of specific IgG with poliovirus

Rabbit IgG was prepared against poliovirus type 1 [14]. Some of this was labelled with I^{131} [15], and tracer amounts of labelled IgG were added back to the unlabelled pool for the detection of virus antibody complexes. Labelled IgG preparations and purified poliovirus type 1 were mixed at equivalence for 12 h at 4°C. The virus-antibody complexes were separated from non-specific IgG by CsCl-gradient centrifugation, and the isolated complexes were dialyzed overnight against 0·5 M ammonium acetate [16]. The complexes appeared in different sizes in the electron microscope. The virus-antibody complexes were dissociated by diluting the material from the CsCl gradient ten-fold in 2·2 M NaI buffered with 0·05 M Tris at pH 7·5 [17] and incubating for 30 min at room temperature. Specific antibodies were then separated by an additional centrifugation on a preformed CsCl gradient. The neutralizing activity of the isolated specific antibodies amounted to 5–20% of the activity of the original IgG preparation, but this varied considerably in different experiments [16]. The specific IgG antibodies were mixed with purified poliovirus at equivalence, incubated overnight at 4°C, and samples were withdrawn for electron microscopic analyses. Very small complexes of a few virus particles joined by IgG, and occasionally IgG combined to isolated virus particles, were detected (Fig.3). Most of the IgG molecules had a rounded shape which differed from the elongated structure of IgG in the TNV satellite antibody complexes (Fig. 2) [11]. This rounded configuration of the specific IgG molecules could be due to a partial denaturation due to the treatment with NaI.

IgG from normal human serum

The IgG molecules were well separated on the electron microscopic specimen when applied with the aid of the high pressure spray gun (Fig. 4a). The IgG

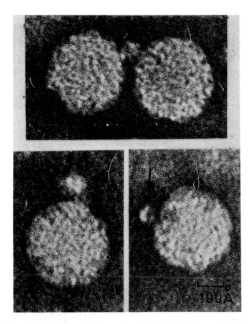

Figure 3. Specific IgG against poliovirus occasionally linking adjacent poliovirus particles (above) or combined with separate viruses (below).

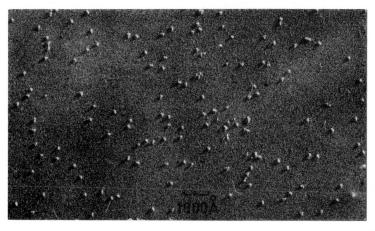

Figure 4a. Shadow cast IgG molecules from normal human serum, distributed with the aid of the high pressure spray gun.

molecules have different configurations [18] comprised of three globular, morphological subunits. These seem to be arranged in a triangular configuration or to be more elongated (Fig. 4b). Occasionally the IgG molecule appears to be curved, or one of its units is placed on the other two (Fig. 4b). For comparison, three-unit models were constructed with globular subunits which were illuminated by a spot light at the same angle as the shadow casting angle for IgG

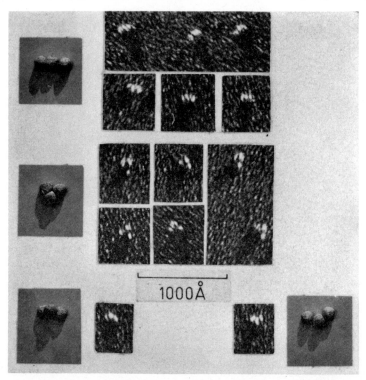

Figure 4b. Selected electron micrographs of shadow cast IgG having different configurations comprised of three morphological subunits. Three different models composed of three globular subunits and illuminated by a spot light at the angle used for the shadow casting of IgG are seen to the left, and one such model is seen to the right. These models appear to have the same appearance as the selected electron micrographs of IgG.

and photographed. The appearance of the shadow cast IgG molecules fits the three-unit models presented in Fig. 4b.

In an important investigation Valentine and Green [19] showed rabbit IgG to be Y-shaped comprised of two F_{ab} and one F_c fragment, by linking anti-dinitrophenyl (DNP) antibodies with a specially synthesized divalent DNP hapten. The three globular subunits seen in Fig. 4 may represent the F_{ab} and F_c fragments. This view seems to agree with the flexible three-unit model of Noelken *et al.*

[5]. Alternatively, the different configurations of IgG may represent different types of rather rigid structures, although the samples appeared homogeneous by the physico-chemical analyses performed in this study. The structural heterogeneity of IgG could also account for the great difficulty in preparing ordered crystals for X-ray crystallographic studies. The average width and height of IgG were 113 Å and 41 Å respectively, and the diameter of the subunits of IgG was approximately 40–50 Å [11]. Valentine [20] calculated a maximum stretch of rabbit IgG to be 120 Å with the F_{ab} fragment 60 Å × 35 Å and the F_c fragment 40 Å × 45 Å.

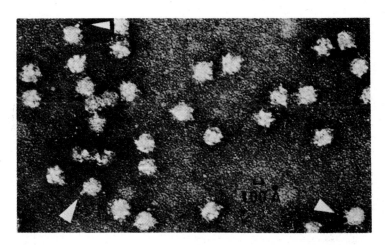

Figure 5. TNV satellite particles with combined F_{ab} fragments on their surface (indicated by arrows).

IgND is separated from IgG by gel filtration [6]. Comparison of IgND and IgG shows that they have different shapes. IgND appears as a rather compact molecule with a rounded, flattened shape in the electron microscope. The average dimensions are 110–120 Å across with a height of about 40 Å.

F_{ab} fragment of IgG

Rabbit IgG against TNV satellite was split by papain [4]. The fragments of IgG were then mixed with purified TNV satellite particles and incubated overnight at 4°C. Precipitation tests in capillary tubes by mixing intact virus (standard solution), or virus treated with IgG fragments and IgG antibody, showed the degree of combination of F_{ab} fragments to the virus. Virus with combined F_{ab} fragments was purified from other IgG fragments by chromatography [21], and was prepared for electron microscopy. Short, rod-shaped F_{ab} fragments were found projecting from the surface of the virus (Fig. 5).

4

Studies of Bence-Jones protein

The disulphide-linked dimer of a Bence-Jones protein of type L was separated
from monomer and polymers by gel filtration on Sephadex G-100 [7] and
shortly thereafter was prepared for electron microscopic examination. The
protein molecules appeared as small light areas of approximately 60 Å × 40 Å
(Fig. 6). Occasionally a substructure of the molecules was detected having the

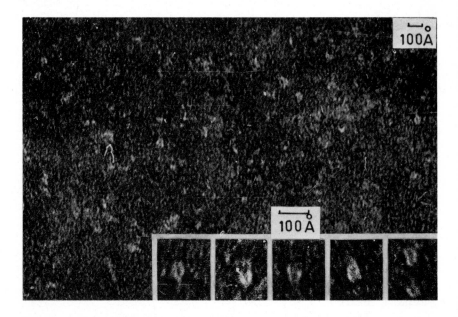

Figure 6. Disulphide-linked dimers of a Bence-Jones protein of type L, showing small,
light areas. A substructure comprised of two chain units is indicated for selected molecules
(insert).

appearance of two parallel units, about 20 Å thick, joined lengthwise (Fig. 6,
insert). This result was verified by taking electron micrographs in through-focal
series [9]. Assuming that each of these subunits represents a monomer (light
chain) [22, 23], then the height of the whole molecule should be approximately
20 Å, the same as the diameter of one chain unit. Using these outer dimensions
and a partial specific volume of 0·73 [24], the molecular weight is calculated to
be just below 40,000, which is in accord with other calculations [8, 22, 24]. The
average major particle axes of Bence-Jones protein are 21·0 Å × 48·3 Å × 74·8
Å as estimated from small-angle X-ray scattering studies [24].

REFERENCES

1. Stanworth, D. R. and Pardoe, G. I., *in* "Handbook of Experimental Immunology" (edited by D. M. Weir), Blackwell Scientific Publications, Oxford and Edinburgh, 1967, p. 134.
2. Miller, F. and Metzger, H., *J. biol. Chem.* **240** (1965) 3325.
3. Metzger, H., Perlman, R. L. and Edelhoch, H., *J. biol. Chem.* **241** (1966) 1741.
4. Porter, R. R., *Biochem. J.* **73** (1959) 119.
5. Noelken, M. E., Nelson, C. A., Buckley, C. E. and Tanford, C., *J. biol. Chem.* **240** (1965) 218.
6. Johansson, S. G. O. and Bennich, H., *Immunology* **13** (1967) 381.
7. Berggård, I., and Pettersson, P., *in* "Gamma Globulins", Nobel Symposium 3 (edited by J. Killander), Almqvist and Wiksell, Stockholm, 1967, p. 71.
8. Bernier, G. M. and Putnam, F. W., *Nature, Lond.* **200** (1963) 223.
9. Höglund, S., *Ark. Kemi* **28** (1968) 505.
10. Höglund, S., *Virology* **32** (1967) 662.
11. Höglund, S., *J. Gen. Virol.* **2** (1968) 427.
12. Markham, R., Frey, S. and Hills, G. J., *Virology* **20** (1963) 88.
13. Svehag, S. E., Chesebro, B. and Bloth, B., *Science, N.Y.,* **158** (1967) 933.
14. Philipson, L. and Bennich, H., *Virology* **29** (1966) 330.
15. Hunter, W. M. and Greenwood, F. C., *Nature, Lond.* **194** (1962) 495.
16. Philipson, L. and Höglund, S., (in preparation).
17. Avrameas, S. and Ternynck, T., *Biochem. J.* **102** (1967) 37C.
18. Höglund, S., *in* "Proceedings of the 6th International Conference on Electron Microscopy", II (edited by R. Uyeda), Maruzen Co., Tokio, 1966, p. 123.
19. Valentine, R. C. and Green, N. M., *J. molec. Biol.* **27** (1967) 615.
20. Valentine, R. C., *in* "Gamma Globulins", Nobel Symposium 3, (edited by J. Killander), Almqvist and Wiksell, Stockholm, 1967, p. 251.
21. Johansson, A. and Höglund, S., (in preparation).
22. Putnam, F. W., *in* "The Proteins" (edited by H. Neurath), Academic Press, New York, 1965, p. 153.
23. Edelman, G. M. and Gally, J. A., *Proc. natn. Acad. Sci. U.S.A.,* **51** (1964) 846.
24. Holasek, A., Kratky, O., Mittelbach, P. and Wawra, H., *J. molec. Biol.* **7** (1963) 321.

FEBS Symposium, Volume 15, 1969, pp. 93-104

Initiation and Assembly of the Immunoglobulin Peptide Chains

C. BAGLIONI

Department of Biology,
Massachusetts Institute of Technology,
Cambridge, Massachusetts, U.S.A.

The synthesis of immunoglobulins (Ig) has been investigated in intact lymphoid cells and in cell-free systems derived from these cells. The general progress in the field of protein synthesis has allowed a rapid advance in our understanding of the biosynthesis of Ig. Methods devised for the study of other cell types have thus been applied to the study of Ig synthesis by lymphoid cells. However, the peculiar heterogeneity and molecular structure of the Ig have presented the investigator with a number of problems.

The biological activity of antibodies, i.e. the binding of a specific antigen, depends upon the combination in each Ig molecule of a specific heavy (H) and light (L) chain [1]. Attempts to synthesize active antibodies in a cell-free system with free polyribosomes have thus often failed because of the random combination of H and L chains. Antibodies directed against an identical antigen are heterogeneous [2] and the lymphoid cells engaged in the synthesis of these antibodies, which are used as the source of the cell-free system, synthesize a heterogeneous collection of L and H chains. Random combination of these chains would cause the formation of hybrid molecules with two different L and/or H chains and moreover, if several different chains are synthesized, the proper combination of a specific L chain with a specific H chain would be extremely unlikely.

These problems do not apply to intact lymphoid cells. Each cell synthesizes one species of L and H chain only and the complete assembly of the Ig molecule takes place within the lymphoid cell.

CELL-FREE SYNTHESIS OF ANTIBODIES

The synthesis of protein for excretion is carried out by the membrane-bound polyribosomes of the endoplasmic reticulum (ER). Undifferentiated lymphoid cells have very little ER, while plasma cells active in the synthesis of Ig are extremely rich in ER. Studies on the synthesis of Ig by lymphoid cells have shown a characteristic delay of approximately 30 min in the excretion of Ig, which is caused by the passage of the newly synthesized Ig through the spaces of the ER [3, 4]. The biosynthesis of the peptide chains of Ig takes place on polyribosomes of different size [5-7]. The pattern of polyribosomes in plasma cells shows a characteristic biphasic distribution, with two major clusters containing 7–8 and 16–20 ribosomes respectively [5-7]. L chains are synthesized on the small polyribosomes, whereas H chains are synthesized on the large polyribosomes [5, 6]. The fact that H and L chains are synthesized on separate polyribosomes is in agreement with the notion that the structural genes for the H and L chains are not linked [8].

Polyribosomes are prepared from lymphoid cells by the use of detergents [5]. These solubilize the membranes of the ER and leave free the polyribosomes that can be analyzed by centrifugation or used in a cell-free system for the synthesis of Ig with the necessary supernatant factors and an energy-generating system. The cell-free system in which free polyribosomes are used has the disadvantage which has been outlined in the introduction, the random assembly of H and L chains. Since the normal process of assembly takes place in intact cells in the vesicles of the ER, it seemed a logical step to use polyribosomes bound to microsomal vesicles for the cell-free synthesis of Ig [9].

The microsomal vesicles of the ER, to which the polyribosomes active in the synthesis of Ig remain bound, are easily obtained by homogenization of the lymphoid cells in a medium containing 0·88 M sucrose [9]. High concentrations of sucrose stabilize the lysosomes, preventing liberation of lysosomal nucleases which inactivate the cell-free system [9]. Moreover, the rough ER, which is rich in polyribosomes, can be separated by differential centrifugation from the smooth ER and from free polyribosomes, which are probably active in the synthesis of endogenous proteins [9, 10]. The microsomal fraction is thus enriched for polyribosomes active in the synthesis of Ig and the assembly of corresponding H and L chains can take place within the microsomal vesicles in a normal way [9, 10]. Polyribosomes active in the synthesis of H and L chains are presumably contiguous on the membrane of a microsomal vesicle and the correct assembly of Ig takes place after the passage of the newly synthesized chains into the vesicles. The products of this cell-free synthesis are not released in the supernatant at the end of the incubation, but it is necessary to disrupt the microsomal vesicles with detergent to obtain a soluble product [10]. The newly synthesized protein can then be characterized for its biological activity.

Identification of antibody activity in the product of cell-free synthesis has been carried out by a co-precipitation [11] assay or by the use of a specific immunoadsorbent [10]. This last method has given the most reliable results. Vassalli *et al.* [10] have characterized the synthesis of an anti-DNP antibody in this way and have made the following observations:

1. Less than 10% of the immunoglobulin synthesized by a cell-free system

prepared from lymphonodes of animals immunized with DNP-bovine immunoglobulin and *H. pertussis* has anti-DNP antibody activity.

2. 50% or more of the immunoglobulin synthesized appears to be of small molecular weight, possibly L chains.

3. At least some Ig molecules are assembled from L and H chains, the synthesis of which is completed during the cell-free incubation. Assembly of Ig molecules can thus proceed in the microsomal vesicles under the conditions of the cell-free incubation.

4. Liver enzymes and tRNA can be utilized by the lymphonode cell-free system in the synthesis of active antibody. This last observation, which is confirmed by studies of Mach *et al.* [12] on a mouse myeloma cell-free system, seems to rule out any translational theory on the variability of the amino acid sequence of Ig. This theory postulates that a special vocabulary of tRNA's is present in antibody-producing cells [13]. If polyribosomes of these cells can utilize the tRNA and activating enzymes of liver for synthesis of active antibody, it follows that no special tRNA needs to be involved in the synthesis of antibodies. Since most, if not all, Ig chains synthesized in a cell-free system are chains which have been completed *in vitro*, whereas no new chains are initiated, it is possible that the variable part of Ig chains, which is restricted to the N-terminal half, is not synthesized in the cell-free system. The fact that no new chains are initiated in the cell-free system may lead one to think that chain initiation of Ig requires some specific factors which are not present in this system. The failure to initiate new chains is, however, observed in all mammalian cell-free systems, with the exception of reticulocytes [14]. Cell-free systems prepared from rabbit reticulocytes display a limited amount of chain initiation and ribosome recycling [14]. The reasons for this peculiar property of the reticulocyte cell-free system are not known.

INITIATION OF THE PEPTIDE CHAIN OF IMMUNOGLOBULINS

The amino acid which is used for peptide chain initiation in *E. coli* is *N*-formyl-methionine [15], which has a blocked amino group. After this observation was made in *E. coli,* a search for initiating amino acids with blocked amino groups was carried out in higher organisms. Candidates for a role in chain initiation were the *N*-acetyl-amino acids, which are found at the N-terminus of many proteins, and pyrrolidone-carboxylic acid (PCA), which is found at the N-terminus of most H chains and of some L chains.

The role of *N*-acetyl-amino acids in chain initiation was ruled out after it had been shown that acetylation of the free NH_2-terminal group occurs after completion of peptide chain synthesis in some proteins [16]. It thus remained of interest to establish whether PCA could serve a unique role in the initiation of the peptide chains of Ig.

Experiments on charging of PCA on tRNA obtained from lymphoid cells have been reported [17]. These experiments were, however, somewhat inconclusive. I have thus attempted to analyze directly the terminal residue of growing H chains to establish whether a free NH_2-terminal is present in these chains.

A mouse myeloma line was used in these studies. This myeloma (ADPG-9, obtained from Dr. Paul Knopf of the Salk Institute, San Diego, Calif.) synthesizes an Ig, whose H chains have N-terminal PCA. Suspension of myeloma cells obtained as described by Lennox *et al.* [18] were used for all the incubations.

It was first attempted to establish whether PCA could be utilized by these cells and incorporated into Ig. However, no measurable uptake of PCA by lymphoid cells was observed. Also, the uptake of glutamic acid was rather slow and it was thus decided to use [^{14}C] glutamine in these experiments. The incubation was thus carried out in minimal Eagle medium [19], without added glutamine. Under these conditions of incubation all the labelled glutamine is taken up by the plasma cells within a few minutes. The lack of glutamine, however, prevents these cells from carrying out sustained protein synthesis. When incubations have to be carried out for hours in order to obtain a uniformly-labelled product, the addition of cold glutamine is necessary.

The pathway of Ig synthesis shows a continuous flow of newly made protein from polyribosomes, to the content of the microsomal vesicles and then to the extracellular medium [4]. It is thus possible to analyze the newly made Ig obtained from these different compartments. A short incubation—2 to 3 min—is necessary to obtain maximum labelling of the polyribosome-bound protein, whereas a prolonged incubation is necessary to obtain maximum yield of labelled protein from the content of the microsomal vesicles.

After a short incubation with [^{14}C] glutamine the plasma cells were rapidly chilled and homogenized in a medium containing 0·88 M sucrose, following the same procedure used for the preparation of the microsomal fraction used in experiments on cell-free synthesis of Ig [9]. The polyribosomes were then prepared by homogenizing the microsomal pellett in medium containing 0·5% deoxycholate. In several 2 min incubations approximately 50% of the labelled protein remained in the polyribosome pellett, which was separated from the protein of the microsomal vesicles by centrifugation through a layer of 1·3 M sucrose. Several attempts have been made to release the peptidyl-tRNA from these polyribosomes, by treating them with sodium dodecyl sulphate or with EDTA, which are known to release specifically the peptidyl-tRNA in other systems [20, 21]. It was however impossible to release all the peptidyl-tRNA of deoxycholate-treated polyribosomes. This may be caused by some alteration of the polyribosomes during the treatment with detergent. It was thus necessary to analyze the growing peptide chains while still attached to the polyribosomes through the tRNA.

Conditions were devised, in which the presence of the polyribosomes did not interfere with the chemical analysis. The polyribosome pellett was resuspended in 8 M urea and reacted with fluoro-dinitro-benzene (FDNB) according to the procedure suggested by Fraenkel-Conrat et al. [22].

At the end of the reaction the excess FDNB was reacted with ammonia and the protein was precipitated with trichloroacetic acid; after a one hour incubation at 37°C the protein was filtered on a Whatmann GF/2 glass filter, washed with 5% trichloroacetic acid, alcohol/ether (1/1) and ether, dried and hydrolyzed in 6 N HCl.

The ether extract of the hydrolyzate was mixed with carrier dinitrophenyl-amino acids and analyzed by thin layer chromatography [23]. The spots were cut and counted in a liquid scintillation counter.

It was thus found that approximately 0·6% of the c.p.m. incorporated into the growing peptide chains chromatographed with carrier DNP-Glu. This indicates that the NH_2-terminal amino acid of some ribosome-bound peptide chains is free to react with FDNB and that it is either glutamic acid or glutamine. These data, although preliminary, support the idea that no special initiator codon for PCA exists, and that PCA is formed by cyclization of glutamine, when this amino acid occupies the N-terminal position in a peptide chain. These experiments will be reported in detail elsewhere.

ASSEMBLY OF IMMUNOGLOBULINS

Proteins made up of two different peptide chains have to be assembled in the correct quaternary structure after chain synthesis has been completed. The problem of assembly has been particularly studied in the case of hemoglobin [24, 25] and of immunoglobulins [26-29]. It was initially discovered that a pool of free L chains exists in lymphoid cells synthesizing normal or pathological Ig [5, 6, 23, 24]. It was thus concluded that newly made L chains are released from ribosomes and enter a pool of free L chains. It was also observed [5] that complete L chains are present on large polyribosomes which are active in the synthesis of H chains. A model of Ig assembly was thus proposed [5] in which L chains from the pool of free L chains became associated with nascent or incomplete polyribosome-bound H chains.

This model received support from an investigation on the relative specific activity of L and H chains after pulse labelling or uniform labelling of human myeloma cells [28]. The H chains isolated from Ig assembled after pulse labelling had higher specific activity than the L chains [28]. After uniform labelling, L and H chains had the same specific activity.

The failure to observe myelomas in which excess H chains are produced and

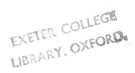

the absence of free monomeric H chains in lymphoid cells, suggested that H
chains are not released from polyribosomes unless they are associated with L
chains [5]. In the model of Ig assembly proposed [5] the association between L
and H chains at the polyribosome level may be an obligatory intermediary step
in the assembly process. In this model the HL half molecule is released from
polyribosomes either upon completion of H chains synthesis, if L chains
associate with incomplete H chains, or after a complete H chain becomes
associated with an L chain.

A search for intermediates in the assembly process was thus begun. Scharff
[26] presented evidence for the existence of the HL intermediate, whereas
Askonas and Williamson [27] found by a different method of analysis evidence
for the existence of an H_2 dimer. This last result is somewhat difficult to
reconcile with the observations made by others [26, 29]. Schubert [29] has
recently investigated the assembly of Ig in another mouse myeloma line and
has obtained results which are substantially in agreement with the model proposed by Shapiro et al. [5]. In this investigation [29] light and heavy polyribosomes have been analyzed. It has been found that the L chain is covalently
bound with an H chain of heavy polyribosomes [29]. This polyribosome-
bound HL intermediate can only be separated into its constituents in reducing
and dissociating solvents. This observation provides evidence that the formation
of the covalent disulphide bond between H and L chains occurs when these
chains first become associated [29]. It cannot be excluded that disulphide
bonds are formed during the isolation of polyribosomes, however. The HL half
molecule combines then with another half molecule either at the polyribosome
level or after being released; inconclusive evidence for the existence of free HL
intermediate was obtained [29].

This model of assembly of Ig is formally similar to that of hemoglobin
assembly [24, 25]. A small pool of free α chains exists in reticulocytes [25].
Complete α chains become bound to polyribosomes that presumably synthesize β
chain (the polyribosomes that synthesize the two chains of hemoglobin cannot
be distinguished, since they have identical size). The $\alpha\beta$ half molecule is then
released from polyribosomes and appears as an intermediate, which can be easily
distinguished, since it does not yet contain heme [25]. The final step in the
assembly process is the combination of heme with globin and the dimerization
of the $\alpha\beta$ intermediate to form hemoglobin.

The combination of α chain with β chain of hemoglobin at the polysome level
is thought to have a regulatory role in the biosynthesis of these chains [24]. In
reticulocytes the two chains of hemoglobin are synthesized at an identical rate
[24]; it follows that some mechanism is operating to equilibriate the rate of
synthesis of one chain to that of the other. If the combination of α with β chain
at the polysome level facilitates the release of the β chain from polysomes, a
simple and efficient mechanism is operating. In this case the rate of synthesis of β

chain should potentially exceed that of the α chain to have a complete feedback control of the rate of synthesis of both chains. In individuals carrying mutations of the hemoglobin genes (thalassemias) which decrease the rate of synthesis of hemoglobin chains, overproduction of either hemoglobin chain is observed. The α chain produced in excess precipitates [30] within the red cell precursors, whereas the β chain produced in excess aggregates to form abnormal β_4 tetramers. This indicates that the control of the release of β chain from polyribosomes by the α chain is not stringent.

The assembly of H and L chains of Ig on polyribosomes may be thought to serve a similar purpose, that of equilibriating the rate of synthesis of the two component chains of Ig. For this reason the rate of synthesis of H and L chains has been studied in several human and mouse myelomas [5, 6, 26-29] and in normal lymphoid cells [31-33]. In most myelomas excess synthesis of L chains has been observed [24-26], in agreement with the notion that in a high proportion of myelomas, L chain dimers (Bence-Jones proteins) are excreted in the urine. Excess L chain synthesis has also been observed in lymph nodes of immunized animals [31]. These observations have suggested that the synthesis of the peptide chains of Ig is unbalanced and that L chains are normally produced in excess over H chains.

In a few myelomas [24, 26] and in normal lymphoid cells [32], however, the peptide chains of Ig appear to be synthesized at an equal rate. It thus seems possible that normally the synthesis of Ig chains is balanced and that the polyribosomal assembly of Ig has a regulatory control on the rate of synthesis of Ig chains. This control is quite stringent since no excess H chains are produced, or, if they are synthesized in excess, they are not secreted by plasma cells. The problem of the balanced synthesis of Ig chains is complicated by the finding that some myelomas [28, 29] synthesize L chains in excess over H chains, but do not secrete the excess L chains. These chains could possibly be degraded or in any event removed from the pool of free L chains which participate in the assembly of Ig.

The formation of L_2 dimers is in some respects analogous to the polymerization of the β chains of hemoglobin, when they are produced in excess over α chains. The L_2 dimers are the normal secretory form of L chain; monomeric L chains excreted in the urine may have formed by disulphide interchange of dimers with cystine [34]. L chains may be synthesized in excess and not secreted if they are unable to dimerize; alternatively, only some species of L_2 dimers may be secreted by plasma cells, while others are unable to pass into the vesicles of the ER. Cioli and Baglioni [28] have suggested that the L_2 dimers do not participate in the assembly of Ig and that only free monomeric L chains associate with polyribosome-bound H chains. This suggestion was based on the observation that the relative rate of labelling of L and H chains is not appreciably different between myeloma cells that synthesize L chains in excess but do not secrete them, and myeloma cells that show a balanced synthesis of L and H chains [28].

CONCLUSIONS

Much has been learnt about the biosynthesis of immunoglobulins, but some of the more fundamental problems remain unsolved. The origin of the peculiar structure of the Ig chains, made up of a variable N-terminal part and of a constant C-terminal part, is the major unresolved problem in this field. An apparently unlimited number of different amino acid sequences is found in the N-terminal half of human Bence-Jones proteins. In a study of 100 Bence-Jones proteins obtained from different patients with myeloma, no two identical proteins have been found [35]. It has thus been calculated that at least 5000 different amino acid sequences exist in humans for the variable half of the L chain. This impressive number of different amino acid sequences corresponds to an identical number of structural genes. It has not been established whether these genes exist in the genome of each cell (germ line theory) or whether different genes are formed by somatic differentiation of a few genes coding for the variable half of L chains (somatic differentiation theory). In the first case each cell has several genes for variable sequences of Ig, whereas in the other case each cell has only a few genes; in any case only a few genes coding for the constant part of Ig chains exist [2].

If the germ line theory were correct it seems possible that the variable and constant parts of Ig chains would be synthesized separately and then joined together by a special *ad hoc* mechanism. To explore this possibility several investigators have attempted to determine whether the variable and constant parts of Ig chains are synthesized separately or whether they are synthesized in a single sequence. Two recent reports indicate that the L chain synthesized by a mouse myeloma and the H chain of IgG synthesized by rabbit lymph node are synthesized in a single sequence [36, 37]. These experiments seem to indicate that the messenger RNA for the variable and constant regions of Ig chains is a single polynucleotide sequence, in agreement with the size of this RNA estimated from the dimension of the polyribosomes coding for the L and H chains [5-7].

Studies on the amino acid sequence of human L chains have recently shown that the two L chain types (κ and λ) recognized in man can be subdivided into a few subtypes, which have in common the same constant C-terminal half, but have distinctly different sequences in the N-terminal half [38, 39]. Three subtypes for κ and four subtypes for λ chains have so far been distinguished [38, 39], but it seems likely that more subtypes will be discovered as more sequences become available. Since each subtype differs from the other subtypes considerably in amino acid sequences and in many cases in chain length, it seems likely that at least one structural gene for each subtype is present in each cell.

Thus, separate genes which code for the variable and constant parts of the Ig chains exist and the problem of the fusion of the products of translation or transcription of these genes remain unresolved. As an alternative, it has been suggested that variable region genes can be fused to a constant region gene by a specific mechanism of excision, translocation, and insertion [40]. This ingenious theory receives some support from the observation that in cells heterozygous for an allotypic marker of the constant region of Ig chains, only one allele is utilized for the synthesis of Ig [41]. If the constant region were translated or transcribed as a separate unit, one does not see why both alleles, which are equivalent, should not be utilized. If, on the other hand, a specific variable gene is translocated and fused to one of the two allelic genes, one can see why only that allele is utilized for the synthesis of that given variable sequence.

The problem of the existence of many genes in each cell, or of a few genes which undergo somatic differentiation, is still one of the major unresolved problems of molecular genetics and immunology. Some recent studies on the amino acid sequence of the α chain of human haptoglobin have pointed out an extremely interesting homology in amino acid sequence between this haptoglobin chain and the variable region of L chains [42]. The α chain of haptoglobin is somewhat shorter than the variable region of L chains (83 vs. $\sim$ 107 amino acids), but it seems possible that this has been formed in the course of human evolution by duplication and evolutionary changes of an ancestral immunoglobin gene coding for a chain approximately half as long as present-day L chains. The existence of such an ancestral gene has been suggested to account for the homology in sequence between variable and constant regions of immunoglobulin chains [43].

A new insight into the origin of immunoglobulin genes and their evolutionary divergence is provided by the discovery of their homology in amino acid sequence with the α chain of haptoglobin. This finding demonstrated that duplications of immunoglobulin genes and evolutionary specialization of the duplicated genes has repeatedly taken place. It may be supposed that other secretory proteins with specialized and extremely specific binding activity (e.g. thyroglobulin) have a common evolutionary origin with immunoglobulins. If the structural genes coding for these proteins have been formed by processes of duplication and independent evolution, one does not see why all the genes coding for the variable part of Ig chains should not have originated by the same mechanism. Genes that were duplicated early in the evolution of vertebrates diverged more and provided the genetic material for the evolution of secretory proteins related to immunoglobulins; other duplicated genes formed the variable and constant regions of L and H chains of different classes of immunoglobulins [43]; recently duplicated genes formed the numerous variants of each subtype of L and possibly H chains.

A consequence of the evolutionary scheme proposed is a relatively limited number and a considerable uniformity of the immunoglobin genes coding for variable regions in different individuals of the same species. Antibody response in individuals of the same species should then be relatively homogeneous in the molecular species of antibodies synthesized, whereas any mechanism which produces somatic random variability in amino acid sequences of Ig chain will give a rather heterogeneous population of antibody molecules in different individuals. Studies on antibody heterogeneity have so far been limited by the lack of physico-chemical techniques which allow separation of complex mixtures of antibody molecules. One analytical technique, which has been recently introduced, isoelectric focusing, seems to be adequate to resolve antibody molecules into distinct electrophoretic components [44]. It is quite striking that antibodies synthesized in response to the same antigen by different animals, show a remarkably similar banding pattern [44].

This survey of immunoglobulin synthesis is necessarily restricted to those areas of research which are more close to the interests of the author. No attempt has been made to cover this field of investigation comprehensively. The main intent of the author has been that of presenting some of the most interesting developments of recent research work, with special emphasis on those aspects which appear to be particularly promising in relation to the fundamental problems of molecular immunology.

ACKNOWLEDGEMENT

This investigation has been supported by grant RO1 A108116 of the National Institute of Health and grant GB-7226 of the National Science Foundation.

REFERENCES

1. Fleischman, J. B., A. Rev. Biochem. 35 (1966) 835.
2. Cohen, S. and Milstein, C., Adv. Immun. 7 (1967) 1.
3. Kern, M. and Swenson, R. M., Cold Spring Harb. Symp. quant. Biol. 32 (1967) 265.
4. Swenson, R. M. and Kern, M., Proc. natn. Acad. Sci. U.S.A. 57 (1967) 4177.
5. Shapiro, A. L., Scharff, M. D., Maizel, J. V. and Uhr, J. W., Proc. natn. Acad. Sci. U.S.A. 56 (1966) 216.
6. Williamson, A. R. and Askonas, B. A., J. molec. Biol. 23 (1967) 201.
7. Becker, M. J. and Rich, A., Nature, Lond. 212 (1966) 142.
8. Oudin, J., Proc. R. Soc. Ser. B, 166 (1966) 207.
9. Vassalli, P., Proc. natn. Acad. Sci. U.S.A. 58 (1967) 2117.

10. Vassalli, P., Lisowska-Bernstein, B., Lamm, M. E. and Benacerraf, B., *Proc. natn. Acad. Sci. U.S.A.* **58** (1967) 2422.
11. Gusdon, J. P., Jr., Stavitsky, A. B. and Armentrout, S. A., *Proc. natn. Acad. Sci. U.S.A.* **58** (1967) 1189.
12. Mach, B., Koblet, H. and Gros, D., *Proc. natn. Acad. Sci. U.S.A.* **59** (1968) 445.
13. Potter, M., Appella, E. and Geisser, S., *J. molec. Biol.* **24** (1965) 361.
14. Williamson, A. R. and Schweet, R., *J. molec. Biol.* **11** (1965) 358.
15. Marcker, K., Clark, B. F. C. and Anderson, J. S., *Cold Spring Harb. Symp. quant. Biol.* **32** (1966) 279.
16. Marchis-Mouren, G. and Lipmann, F., *Proc. natn. Acad. Sci. U.S.A.* **53** (1965) 1147.
17. Moau, B. and Harris, T. N., *Biochem. biophys. Res. Commun.* **29** (1967) 773.
18. Lennox, E. S., Knopf, P. M., Munro, A. J. and Parkhouse, R. M. E., *Cold Spring Harb. Symp. quant. Biol.* **32** (1967) 249.
19. Eagle, H., *Science, N.Y.* **130** (1959) 432.
20. Gilbert, W., *J. molec. Biol.* **6** (1963) 389.
21. Penman, S., Vesco, C. and Penman, M., *J. molec. Biol.* **34** (1968) 49.
22. Fraenkel-Conrat, H., Harris, J. I. and Levy, A. L., in "Methods in Biochemical Analysis, Vol. 2" (edited by D. Glick), Interscience Publishers, New York, 1955, p.359.
23. Wang, K. T., Huang, J. M. K. and Wang, I. S. Y., *J. Chromat.* **22** (1966) 362.
24. Colombo, B. and Baglioni, C., *J. molec. Biol.* **16** (1966) 51.
25. Baglioni, C. and Campana, T., *Eur. J. Biochem.* **2** (1967) 480.
26. Scharff, M. D., in "Gamma Globulins", Nobel Symposium 3 (edited by J. Killander), Almqvist and Wiksell, Stockholm, 1967, p. 385.
27. Askonas, B. A. and Williamson, A. R., in "Gamma Globulins", Nobel Symposium 3 (edited by J. Killander), Almqvist and Wiksell, Stockholm, 1967, p. 369.
28. Cioli, D. and Baglioni, C., in "Gamma Globulins", Nobel Symposium 3 (edited by J. Killander), Almqvist and Wiksell, Stockholm, 1967, p. 401.
29. Schubert, D., *Proc. natn. Acad. Sci. U.S.A.* **60** (1968) 683.
30. Fessas, P., Stoamatoyannopoulos, G. and Karaklis, A., *Blood* **19** (1962) 1.
31. Shapiro, A. L., Scharff, M. D., Maizel, J. V. and Uhr, J. W., *Nature, Lond.* **211** (1966) 243.
32. Askonas, B. A. and Williamson, A. R., *Nature, Lond.* **211** (1966) 369.
33. Williamson, A. R. and Askonas, B. A., *Archs Biochem. Biophys.* **125** (1968) 401.
34. Milstein, C., *Nature, Lond.* **205** (1965) 1171.
35. Baglioni, C., Cioli, D., Quatrocchi, R. and Alescio-Zonta, L., in "Abstracts 5th Meeting Europ. Biochem. Soc.", Prague 1968, p. 176.
36. Knopf, P. M., Parkhouse, R. M. E. and Lennox, E. S., *Proc. natn. Acad. Sci. U.S.A.* **58** (1967) 2288.
37. Fleischman, J. B., *Cold Spring Harb. Symp. quant. Biol.* **32** (1967) 233.
38. Hood, L., Gray, W. R., Sanders, B. G. and Dreyer, W. J., *Cold Spring Harb. Symp. quant. Biol.* **32** (1967) 133.
39. Milstein, C., *Nature, Lond.* **216** (1967) 330.
40. Dreyer, W. J., Gray, W. R. and Hood, L., *Cold Spring Harb. Symp. quant. Biol.* **32** (1967) 353.

41. Pernis, B., *Cold Spring Harb. Symp. quant. Biol.* **32** (1967) 333.
42. Black, J. A. and Dixon, G. H., *Nature, Lond.* **218** (1968) 736.
43. Singer, S. J. and Doolittle, R. F., *in* "Structural Chemistry and Molecular Biology" (edited by A. Rich and N. Davidson), Freeman, San Francisco, 1967, p. 173.
44. Awdeh, Z. L., Williamson, A. R. and Askonas, B. A., *Nature, Lond.* **219** (1968) 66.

FEBS Symposium, Volume 15, 1969, pp. 105-116

Control of Immunoglobulin Formation

B. A. ASKONAS, A. R. WILLIAMSON and Z. L. AWDEH*

National Institute for Medical Research, London, England

GENE EXPRESSION IN SINGLE CELLS

The number of structural genes coding for immunoglobulins carried in the germ line is at present unclear; however, each cell must carry a gene for each of the several classes and subclasses of heavy chains and each of the types of light chains. It is most probable that the antibody specificities associated with the different classes in a given cell would be different so the precursor cell could be expected to be multi-potential for immunoglobulin production. At the level of the differentiated immunoglobulin-forming cell the products of single plasma cells have been analysed by a number of workers [1-5] and certain general restrictions have been found to apply. The immunoglobulin product has been found to have a single antibody specificity and belong to a single class or subclass of Ig and to have a single type of light chain. It should be added that exceptions to these restrictions have in fact been observed but these now are attributed generally to methodological difficulties. However, these phenotypic restrictions defined for individual cells leave considerable scope for hetero-geneity of the immunoglobulin product at a molecular level. Plasma cell tumours derived from single cell clones provide the only immunoglobulin-forming cell clones whose products can be readily analysed at a molecular level. Originally, examination of the myeloma proteins found in serum of animals bearing these tumours, or in patients with myeloma, showed that the heterogeneity of the product at a molecular level was clearly very restricted. However, a number of protein bands were observed by starch gel electrophoresis at alkaline pH and the heterogeneity was reflected in heterogeneous light and heavy chains (see review by Fahey [6]). This left open the possibility that these differentiated cells were expressing a number of structural genes for closely related heavy and light chains. The protein product of murine plasma cell tumour 5563 is a good example of the type of heterogeneity mentioned above. We have made extensive use of this particular tumour in our biosynthetic studies and recently we have endeavoured to characterize the biochemical nature of the original product of

*Present address: American University, Beirut.

this tumour. Comparison of freshly synthesized ^{14}C-labelled myeloma protein with that found in the sera of tumour, bearing animals showed that the former is much more homogeneous on electrophoresis or chromatography [7]. Application of the high resolution technique of isoelectric focusing in thin layers of polyacrylamide gels [8], followed by autoradiography, showed that originally only a single molecular species of myeloma protein is synthesized by the tumour cell (Awdeh, to be published); this product is subsequently converted into the multiple molecular species found in serum.

The differentiated plasma cell therefore appears to express structural genes for a single heavy chain and for a single light chain. Modification of the assembled single immunoglobulin molecule then occurs after synthesis to give the limited heterogeneity of G-myeloma protein in serum in murine or human plasmacytomas. The molecular basis for these changes is not known as yet; however, by analogy with other heterogeneous proteins the properties of the myeloma protein components found in serum suggest that the loss of labile amide groups may be occurring.

CONTROL OF LIGHT AND HEAVY CHAIN SYNTHESIS

At the translational level present evidence would indicate that both light and heavy chains are synthesized as single and separate polypeptide chains. Evidence for this comes from the characterization of the size of polyribosomes bearing nascent light and heavy chains and from pulse-labelling studies designed to measure the number of growing points in light and heavy chains [9-12]. This evidence at the level of protein synthesis, however, does not exclude the possibility that two structural genes are required to code for each of the chains. All three classes of rabbit immunoglobulin (IgG, IgA and IgM) carry identical markers on the Fab fragments, i.e. the Fd part of the rabbit heavy chain [13, 14]. This observation, together with the sequence data on κ light chains from myeloma proteins [15], has led to the suggestion that the variable and constant regions of both light and heavy chains could be controlled by different cistrons with gene fusion preceding transcription. On the other hand, there is genetic evidence that at least a large part of the heavy chain is controlled by a single structural gene. In the human, genetic markers located on different parts of the γ_1 heavy chain (for example Gm(z) on Fd and Gm(a) on Fc fragments) are inherited as a single gene in a given population [16]. In addition, in rabbits, allotype-related amino acid sequence variation has been found to occur near the N-terminal end of the heavy chain and also near the N-terminal end of the Fc fragment [17]. Thus, a mechanism comprising the linkage of two equally sized cistrons coding for the Fd and Fc regions of the heavy chain, or the variable and constant regions of the light chain, seems incompatible with the data. More complicated models of gene fusion, particularly those involving interpolation of a piece of genetic material, seem implausible.

The structural genes for heavy and light chains are inherited separately and thus referred to as unlinked (see review by Mårtensson [18]). Our studies [19, 20] indicated that in lymph nodes from normal and immunized mice, gene expression is controlled in such a way that there is an overall balanced synthesis of equal numbers of light and heavy chains so that the only immunoglobulin product secreted from the cells are the final immunoglobulin molecules, and no subunits are secreted. However, in rabbits, excess light chain production has been reported in lymph nodes from immune animals [21], and in normal rabbit spleen, but not in spleen at the height of a secondary response [22]. In plasmacytomas, defects in this synchrony of chain production occur frequently as discussed previously in detail [23].

ASSEMBLY OF IgG MOLECULE

Pool of free light chains

A number of steps in the assembly of the completed heavy and light polypeptide chains into IgG can now be defined. Our previous findings in plasma cell tumour 5563 [24] and mouse lymph nodes [20] have shown that completed light chains are autonomously released from polyribosomes into an intracellular pool of free light chains. This pool is small, relative to the intracellular pool of IgG (molar ratio approximately 1:4). Free light chains in the pool turn over rapidly as intermediates in IgG assembly, thus maintaining the pool at a constant size. Evidence for the intermediate role of free light chains comes from the time course of labelling of free light chains and of light chains in assembled IgG [25], as well as from "pulse chase" experiments. In the latter experiments, lymph node or tumour plasma cells are incubated for brief periods (5-10 min) with radioactive amino acids and then during subsequent incubation with non-radioactive amino acids the radioactivity in the free light chain pool is "chased", i.e. decreases with concomitant increase in radioactivity of IgG. The existence of this small light chain pool does not conflict with the evidence for balanced synthesis of heavy and light chains [19] mentioned in the last section. A potential role for free light chains in controlling assembly will be discussed below.

Disulphide bond formation

In studying the assembly of immunoglobulin G we need to distinguish between covalent and non-covalent assembly of the molecules. Covalent assembly, that is the formation of the interchain disulphide bonds, is the easiest process to follow experimentally since the intermediate stages are identifiable. We will describe our search for covalently-linked intermediates and then later discuss non-covalent assembly in the light of these results.

Our experimental design in searching for covalently-linked intermediates has been to expose 5563 ascitic tumour cells to brief pulses of labelled amino acids, to disrupt the cells in the presence of alkylating agents to prevent further disulphide bond formation, and to purify the pulse-labelled myeloma protein determinants from the cells under conditions of chromatography which do not dissociate non-covalently linked subunits. Subsequent analysis by poly-acrylamide gel electrophoresis under dissociating conditions was followed by autoradiography or identification of protein components by precipitation with specific antisera [26]. A polyacrylamide gel analysis of myeloma protein determinants labelled during a four minute pulse is shown in Fig. 1. Alignment of the autoradiograph with the stained gel by means of the spots of radio-active ink shows that radioactivity is present in myeloma protein, heavy chain dimer (H-H), and heavy chain dimer with one light chain attached (H-H-L). The positions of these components in this electrophoretic system has been previously characterized [28]. Further evidence for the identity of the radioactive protein components was obtained by cutting up the polyacrylamide gel, eluting the radioactive protein and precipitating with antisera specific for heavy chain determinants or light chain determinants. Radioactivity in all three components was found to be precipitable with antisera to heavy chain determinants, while only radioactivity in myeloma protein and H-H-L was precipitable with antisera to light chain determinants [26]. The relative labelling of these components as a function of the time of pulse labelling suggested that they are intermediates in IgG assembly [26]. A number of trace components were found to be labelled on autoradiographs; the positions of these components varied from one preparation to another and they have not been identified. In particular, no radioactivity was found in the position corresponding to half molecules (H-L) (Fig. 1).

We conclude from these findings that in this tumour which forms mouse G_{2a}-myeloma protein, formation of interchain disulphide bonds takes place in the stepwise fashion thus: H + H $\rightarrow$ H $-$ H $\xrightarrow{+L}$ H $-$ H $-$ L $\xrightarrow{+L}$ L $-$ H $-$ H $-$ L, with the formation of the disulphide bond between two heavy chains pre-ceding the formation of the inter L $-$ H disulphide bonds.

This raises the possibility that intrapolyribosomal interaction between the heavy chains and formation of the heavy chain dimer could occur before release of heavy chains from the polyribosomes. Figure 2 shows a schematic drawing of the possible interaction between immunoglobulin chains, while completed or nearly completed heavy chains are still attached to the polyribosomes. Such nascent chains may already have adopted their ultimate secondary and tertiary configuration, or chain–chain interaction may well play a role in this process. It needs to be stressed that the order of interchain disulphide bond formation does not necessarily reflect the sequence of non-covalent interaction between the immunoglobulin chains. Particularly in the presence of excess light chains one might expect non-covalent interaction between light chains and heavy chains to

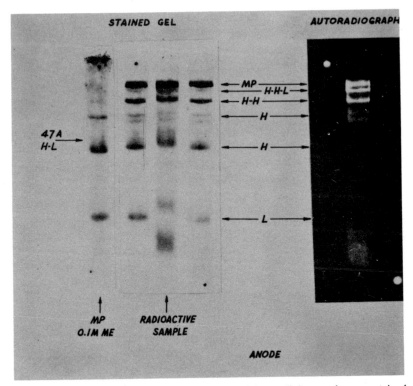

Figure 1. Autoradiographic analysis of alkylated intracellular myeloma protein determinants.

Plasma cells (5563 tumour line) were incubated for 4 min with a [^{14}C]amino acid mixture, and the cells disrupted in the presence of 0·15 M iodoacetamide. The purified myeloma protein determinants were analysed by polyacrylamide gel electrophoresis in SDS-urea-phosphate pH 7·2 followed by autoradiography [26]. Stained gels, left to right (1-4). Arrow on left indicates position of half-molecules (H-L) excreted by tumour line 47A [27]. (1) 5563 myeloma protein (M.P.) reduced with 0·1 M 2-mercaptoethanol (ME); (2), (4) M.P. protein plus its partial reduction mixture (0·01 M ME); (3) Radioactive sample plus carrier proteins as in (2). Radioactive ink spots facilitated alignment of autoradiograph of gels (2), (3) and (4) and stained gels.

take place. There have been two reports on the presence of half molecules (H-L) in tumours producing excess light chains, suggesting that in these tumours the light-heavy chain disulphide bond precedes formation of the inter-heavy chain bond. In a plasmacytoma-producing γ_1-myeloma protein (MOPC 21), half molecules (H-L) were extracted from polyribosomes with urea and sodium dodecyl sulphate [10], but were not detected in the cell sap and there is no kinetic evidence that these are intermediates; MPC-11 (G_{2b}-myeloma protein producer) was found to contain and secrete half molecules which did not show a precursor-product relationship to the four chain myeloma proteins [29].

It may be too early to give a general scheme of assembly. Since immunoglobulins are very heterogeneous and show a range of structural stabilities to low concentrations of reducing agents [28]–there is no reason why one assembly order should apply to all immunoglobulins. It is possible that, following non-covalent interaction between the chains, the actual disulphide bond formation may depend on the reducing conditions within the cisternae of the endoplasmic reticulum, where assembly takes place. In elucidating the order of assembly it is most important to show that any partially assembled structures are in fact intermediates and not aberrant end-products of the tumour cell or

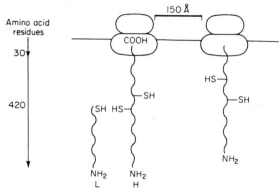

Figure 2. Schematic presentation of the possible interactions which could occur between heavy polypeptide chains or light and heavy chains on polyribosomes forming heavy chains. H = heavy chains, L = light chains.

artefacts of isolation. Moreover, while the study of imbalanced synthesis in tumour cells is very useful, caution must be used in interpreting the results in terms of normal balanced synthesis.

The possible interaction of light chains with nascent heavy chains; further studies

The two different approaches to the study of assembly of IgG, i.e. study of the kinetics of assembly on the one hand and the study of disulphide bond formation on the other, lead to rather conflicting ideas. The presence of a rapidly turning over light chain pool which is maintained in size within the cell by donating light chains for the assembly of IgG molecules, suggested that this pool might well play a role in controlling the assembly process. The lag in the appearance of label in heavy chains of assembled IgG [25] suggested that this role might be a mediation of heavy chain release from the site of synthesis by attachment of light chains. One attraction of this idea is that the presence of light chains would stabilize the conformation of heavy chains since we know that the isolated heavy chains, and especially the Fd portion of the heavy chains, have a tendency to aggregate and to lose their stable configuration. This sort of assembly procedure might suggest that half molecules, L-H, would be intermediates. However, the studies on the order of interchain disulphide bond formation during assembly of G_{2a}-myeloma protein 5563 described above do not provide evidence to support this proposal.

The evidence for the presence or absence of light chains on heavy-chain-synthesizing polyribosomes is rather conflicting. In our experiments on the characterization of heavy-chain-synthesizing polyribosomes by precipitation of radioactively labelled nascent chains with antisera specific for heavy chains, it was also observed that very little radioactivity on the heavy-chain-synthesizing polyribosome was precipitable with antisera against light chains [9]. On the other hand, Shapiro and his colleagues [30] have reported the presence of radioactive light chains on heavy polyribosomes; nascent chains released from polyribosomes with ribonuclease, and treated with 1% sodium dodecyl sulphate, 0·5 M urea and 0·13 M mercaptoethanol were distributed across the polyacrylamide gel after electrophoresis and all radioactivity found in the same position as light chains was taken to represent light chains. Since this separation procedure fractionates molecules mainly on the basis of their size, further characterization of radioactive components as light chain would be required. The tumour studied by these authors synthesizes a large excess of free light chains, and since light chains released from their site of synthesis are randomly mixed with the intracellular free light chain pool [25], the specific activity of free light chains from this pool would be expected to be low after a short pulse (1·5 min) and chase (30 s).

Recent studies by Schubert [10] using plasmacytoma MOPC 21 have suggested covalent binding of light chains to heavy chain polyribosomes. These tumour cells form a γ_1-Ig and are reported to produce, but not to secrete, excess light chains, whose fate is enigmatic. In this study polyribosomes were examined after a 10 min pulse. With a pulse of this duration a further problem arises, i.e. the intracellular myeloma protein is also extensively labelled and any non-specific binding of myeloma protein to ribosomes would complicate detection of specific attachment of radioactive light chains to nascent heavy chains. A series of time points would be useful in clarifying this finding.

In our own attempts along these lines we have tried to increase the sensitivity of detection of light chains by labelling non-alkylated light chains of myeloma protein 5563 with ^{131}I and permitting these to interact in vitro with polyribosomes. These experiments, although avoiding some difficulties mentioned above, could not be expected to reveal the pathway of assembly and were intended only to test for the possible interaction of light chains with nascent heavy chains. The results described below show clearly the low levels of light chains involved in such interaction and the difficulties of detection in pulse-labelling experiments.

Polyribosomes were isolated by treatment of post-mitochondrial supernatant with deoxycholate [31]. ^{131}I-labelled light chains were obtained by iodination of purified G-myeloma protein 5563 by the chloramine-T method [32] to a specific radioactivity of about 800 μc/mg protein, followed by reduction with 0·2M mercaptoethanol and separation of light and heavy chains on Sephadex

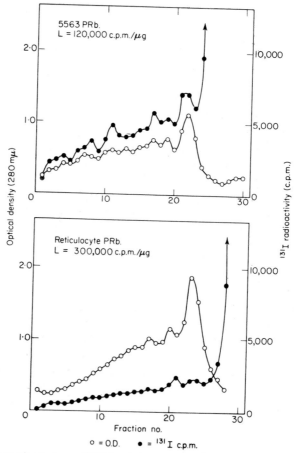

Figure 3. Interaction between ^{131}I-light chains and polyribosomes *in vitro*.
^{131}I-light chains (prepared from 5563 myeloma protein) were incubated with poly-ribosomes for 10 min at 20° C in the absence of an energy source. The incubation mixtures were layered on 10–47% (w/v) linear sucrose gradients and centrifuged for 3 h at 24,000 r.p.m. in a Spinco SW 25 rotor. Top figure: polyribosomes prepared from the 5563 plasmacytoma; lower figure: reticulocyte polyribosomes. ○–optical density of poly-ribosomes at 280 mμ, ●–radioactivity due to ^{131}I-labelled light chains.

G-100 in 1 N acetic acid [33]. The acid was removed on a G-25 Sephadex column equilibrated with 0·1 M tris pH 7·5 and the radioactive light chains immediately incubated with the polyribosomes and the mixture fractionated on a linear sucrose gradient (Fig. 3). Radioactive light chains are seen to be distributed across the polyribosome profile. Since in the upper portion of the gradient, separation from the large excess of soluble ^{131}I-light chains was not complete, fractions from three regions of the gradient corresponding to large polyribosomes, medium sized polyribosomes and single ribosomes were pooled and pelleted by centrifugation for 90 min at 100,000 g. The amount of radioactive light chain remaining bound to the pelleted ribosomes was then measured and is shown in Table 1. Over 70% of the ^{131}I-light chain radioactivity remained bound to the heavy ribosomes. The extent to which ^{131}I-light chain remains bound to ribosomes is expressed in Table 2 as a function of the number of 80S ribosome monomers required to bind one light chain; considered together with the size of polyribosomes in the three pools, this calculation reveals that very few single ribosomes, and less than 10% of medium sized polyribosomes, bind light chains, while there is one light chain bound to almost every large polyribosome.

Since non-specific sticking of protein to ribosome can occur, two types of control were performed: (1) the binding of ^{131}I-myeloma globulin (5563) to 5563 plasmacytoma polyribosomes was measured; and (2) the binding of ^{131}I-light chain (5563) to rabbit reticulocyte polyribosomes was measured (Fig. 3, lower figure). These controls were carried out as described above, incubating the labelled protein with the ribosomes and then spreading out the polyribosomes on linear sucrose gradients. Ribosomes were *not* pelleted from the gradient fractions and the total amount of labelled protein associated with polyribosomes in the various regions of the reticulocyte polyribosome gradient are shown in Table 3, expressed as before. Free light chain is found associated with reticulocyte polyribosomes of all sizes but the extent of this binding, even in the absence of a second pelleting, is very low. The amount of light chain associated with reticulocyte polyribosomes in the lower third of the gradient (Table 3) is about 8-fold less than that associated with 5563 plasmacytoma ribosomes in the same region (Table 2). The extent of binding of 5563 myeloma protein to heavy 5563 polyribosomes (Table 2) is 10-fold less than the extent of light chain binding.

These experiments show that there is some specificity of interaction of light chains with heavy-chain-synthesizing polyribosomes and suggest that free light chains can associate with nascent heavy chains. The extent of light chain attachment is small, but it approaches the theoretical value calculated on the assumption that only one heavy chain (completed or near completion) per heavy-chain-synthesizing polyribosome (14-18 ribosomes) is capable of receiving a light chain. Although the attachment of light chains to nascent heavy chains

Table 1. Binding of radioactive light chains to polyribosome fractions

Gradient tubes	% of ^{131}I-L-chain in gradient fractions bound by ribosomes
1-11	71
12-20	60
21-24	30

[131]I-light chains were incubated with isolated 5563 polyribosomes. Following fractionation of the polyribosomes on sucrose gradients (Fig. 3), pooled fractions were recentrifuged (90 min at 100,000 **g**) to pellet the ribosomes. The table gives the percentage of total ^{131}I-light chains in each pool bound to polyribosomes.

Table 2. Amount of ^{131}I-light chains bound to 5563-polyribosomes

Gradient tubes	$\mu\mu$ moles ^{131}I-L-chain bound	$\mu\mu$ moles ribosomes	No. of ribosomes/molecule L-chain bound
1-11[a]	4·5	100	22
12-20[a]	2·7	130	54
21-24[a]	0·5	80	160

	$\mu\mu$ moles ^{131}I-myeloma protein bound		No. of ribosomes/molecule of myeloma protein
4-11	0·42	100	238

[a]Ribosomes pelleted by centrifugation (90 min, 100,000 **g**).
Isolated 5563 polyribosomes were incubated with 17 μg ^{131}I-L-chain (2 × 10[6] c.p.m.) or 45 μg ^{131}I-myeloma protein (6 × 10[6] c.p.m.) and ^{131}I-protein binding by different-sized polyribosomes (Fig. 3, top) was determined.

Table 3. Amount of ^{131}I-light chain bound to reticulocyte polyribosomes.

Gradient tubes	$\mu\mu$ moles L/O.D. unit	$\mu\mu$ moles ribosomes	No. of ribosomes/molecule of L-chain
1-12	0·13	20·8	160
13-20	0·13	20	160
21-25	0·14	20·8	143

Reticulocyte polyribosomes were incubated with 3·3 μg ^{131}I-L-chain (1 × 10[6] c.p.m.) and the ^{131}I-L-chain associated with different-sized polyribosomes (Fig. 3, lower) was determined.

appears possible, there is no evidence to show that this pathway is necessary for, or even facilitates, heavy chain release.

The autonomous release of heavy chain has not been demonstrated but this is not surprising since even under normal conditons of balanced light and heavy chain synthesis there is a small free light chain pool and light-heavy chain interaction would occur rapidly. The identification of heavy chain dimers within the cell indicates that covalent light-heavy chain bonding is *not* necessary in heavy chain release. While excess light chain production has been frequently observed in tumour cells, synthesis of excess heavy chain may well have escaped detection because of the rapid denaturation of heavy chains.

CONCLUSIONS

1. Differentiated immunoglobulin-forming plasma cells express only structural genes for one variant of light and one variant of heavy chain.
2. Light and heavy chains are synthesized on separate polyribosomes.
3. Light chains are released into a small pool of free light chains, which turns over rapidly, from which light chains are incorporated into IgG.
4. ^{131}I-light chains appear to be able to interact with heavy γ chains while the latter are still on the polyribosomes; however, there is no evidence that this interaction is a necessary step in release of heavy chains.
5. The order of disulphide bond formation has been established for mouse IgG$_{2a}$ (plasmacytoma 5563). The disulphide bond between the two heavy chains precedes formation of the light-heavy interchain bonds; intra-polyribosomal association of heavy chains might be involved. It is not clear as yet whether the order of disulphide bond formation reflects the sequence of non-covalent chain interaction, or whether it depends on the local reducing conditions within the cell. If the latter is true, the order of covalent bonding may vary in different species or with different immuno-globulin classes, since inter-chain disulphide bonds vary in their suscepti-bility to reducing agents. In a mouse plasmacytoma-producing γ_1-myeloma protein and excess light chains, other workers suggest that disulphide bond formation between light and heavy chains may take place at the poly-ribosomal level.
6. Under normal conditions, in mouse lymphoid tissue, the production of light and heavy chains is balanced; this synchrony breaks down frequently in neoplastic plasma cells, leading to imbalance in the formation of the two types of chains.

REFERENCES

1. Mäkelä, O., *Cold Spring Harb. Symp. quant. Biol.* **32** (1967) 423.
2. Attardi, G., Cohn, M., Horibata, K. and Lennox, E. S., *Bact. Rev.* **23** (1959) 213.

116   B. A. ASKONAS, A. R. WILLIAMSON AND Z. L. AWDEH

3. Pernis, B., Chiappino, G., Kelus, A. S. and Gell, P. G. H., *J. exp. Med.* **122** (1965) 853.
4. Cebra, J. J., Colberg, J. E. and Dray, S., *J. exp. Med.* **123** (1966) 547.
5. Nossal, G. J. V. and Mäkelä, O., *J. Immun.* **88** (1962) 604.
6. Fahey, J. L., *Adv. Immun.* **2** (1962) 41.
7. Awdeh, Z. L., Askonas, B. A. and Williamson, A. R., *Biochem. J.* **102** (1967) 548.
8. Awdeh, Z. L., Williamson, A. R. and Askonas, B. A., *Nature, Lond.* **219** (1968) 66.
9. Williamson, A. R. and Askonas, B. A., *J. molec. Biol.* **23** (1967) 201.
10. Schubert, D., *Proc. natn. Acad. Sci. U.S.A.* **60** (1968) 683.
11. Fleischman, J. B., *Biochemistry, N.Y.* **6** (1967) 1311.
12. Lennox, E. S., Knopf, P. M., Munro, A. J. and Parkhouse, R. M. E., *Cold Spring Harb. Symp. quant. Biol.* **32** (1967) 66.
13. Oudin, J., *J. cell. comp. Physiol.* **67** (1966) 77.
14. Kelus, A. S. and Gell, P. G. H., *Prog. Allergy* **11** (1967) 141.
15. Milstein, C., *Nature, Lond.* **216** (1967) 330.
16. Litwin, S. D. and Kunkel, H. G., *J. exp. Med.* **125** (1967) 847.
17. Prahl, J. W. and Porter, R. R., *Biochem. J.* **107** (1968) 753.
18. Mårtensson, L., *Vox Sang.* **11** (1966) 521.
19. Askonas, B. A. and Williamson, A. R., *in* "Gamma Globulins", Nobel Symposium 3 (edited by J. Killander), Almqvist and Wiksell, Stockholm, 1967, p. 369.
20. Askonas, B. A. and Williamson, A. R., *Nature, Lond.* **216** (1967) 264.
21. Shapiro, A. L., Scharff, M. D., Maizel, J. V. Jr. and Uhr, J. W., *Nature, Lond.* **211** (1966) 243.
22. Skvortsov, V. T. and Gurvich, A. E., *Nature, Lond.* **218** (1968) 377.
23. Askonas, B. A. and Williamson, A. R., *Antibiotica Chemother* **15** (1968) 64, Karger, Basel/New York. Proceedings of Symposium "The Immune Respone and its Suppression".
24. Askonas, B. A. and Williamson, A. R., *Nature, Lond.* **211** (1966) 369.
25. Williamson, A. R. and Askonas, B. A., *Archs Biochem. Biophys.* **125** (1968) 401.
26. Askonas, B. A. and Williamson, A. R., *Biochem. J.* **109** (1968) 637.
27. Potter, M. and Kuff, E. L., *J. molec. Biol.* **9** (1964) 537.
28. Williamson, A. R. and Askonas, B. A., *Biochem. J.* **107** (1968) 823.
29. Scharff, M. D. *in* "Gamma Globulins", Nobel Symposium 3 (edited by J. Killander), Almqvist and Wiksell, Stockholm, 1967, p. 385.
30. Shapiro, A. L., Scharff, M. D., Maizel, J. V. Jr. and Uhr, J. W., *Proc. natn. Acad. Sci. U.S.A.* **56** (1966) 216.
31. Williamson, A. R., *Proc. Symp. Nucleic Acids in Immunology,* Rutgers Univ., 1967, p. 590.
32. Hunter W. M. and Greenwood, F. C., *Nature, Lond.* **194** (1962) 495.
33. Fleischman, J. B., Pain, R. H. and Porter, R. R., *Archs Biochem. Biophys.* **Suppl. 1** (1962) 174.

FEBS Symposium, Volume 15, 1969, pp. 117-131

Biosynthesis of γG Globulin and its Peptide Chains in a Cell-free System

R. S. NEZLIN and O. V. ROKHLIN

*Institute of Molecular Biology,
Academy of Science of the U.S.S.R.,
Moscow, U.S.S.R.*

Considerable advances in molecular biology are to a great extent accounted for by recent investigation of biological processes in more simple systems than the living cell. The first of these is the so-called cell-free system that reproduces the main steps of protein biosynthesis. These investigations have made it possible to elucidate the main processes leading to the formation of a specific protein molecule and to elucidate the genetic code.

However, attempts to use the cell-free systems for the study of antibody biosynthesis have not been numerous and up to now not very effective. Our efforts in this direction have concentrated on the study of the possibility of the formation of immunoglobulins and their peptide chains in cell-free microsomal systems.

There are data available according to which amino acids in cell-free systems of bacterial or animal origin can be incorporated into particular proteins synthesized by cells that were used to obtain microsomes and ribosomes. For instance, the microsomal fraction from rat liver can incorporate amino acids into proteins that are immunologically similar to albumin and a number of other proteins synthesized by the liver [1, 2], and ribosomes of reticulocytes can direct the formation of hemoglobin [3].

Recently, several laboratories have been dealing with the formation of antibodies or immunoglobulins in cell-free preparations from lymph nodes or spleen [4-15].

One of the difficulties experienced thereby is in the identification of protein synthesized in the cell-free system. Biological tests, such as neutralization of viruses [7], fail to give a clear answer to the question whether new peptide bonds are actually formed in the system. Direct proof for protein biosynthesis involves incorporation of radioactive amino acids into the peptide chains. The above investigations have shown that microsomes of lymphoid tissue are capable of incorporating labelled amino acids into proteins. Attempts to prove the presence of immunoglobulins or antibodies among the newly synthesized proteins are, however, rather complicated. The use of the corresponding antiserum for the precipitation of radioactive protein may be misleading, for the resulting precipitate may contain non-specific proteins in a small amount but with high radioactivity. Another reason for errors arising when using this precipitation procedure might be due to a high percentage of antibodies in the pH-5 fraction [9]. Radioimmunoelectrophoresis, used by some authors [8, 13], can give rise to artifacts of the same type and, besides, it is not a quantitative procedure.

It is well known that one of the optimum methods to determine both antibodies and antigens is immunoadsorption [16]. To characterize newly synthesized protein it is also possible to apply with advantage chemical methods as, for example, shown by Mach *et al.* [14].

In this work we have made use of the method of immunoadsorbents that is comparatively simple, strictly quantitative and, when combined with the isotope method, extremely sensitive. It is of great importance that, by means of immunoadsorbents, it is possible to identify not only the protein exhibiting the activity of an antibody but also that having the antigenic properties of immunoglobulins and even that with antigenic properties of different portions of immunoglobulin molecules. Thus, to detect the presence of the peptide chains of immunoglobulins, we have used these subunits in the fixed form.

Initial attempts to establish, with the aid of immunoadsorbents, biosynthesis of antibodies in cell-free systems of lymphoid tissue of rabbits and pigs, in Dr. Hrubešová's group (Institute of Microbiology, Prague) [9] and then in our laboratory [10], failed to show any unambiguous-specific adsorption on the fixed antigen. But, when experimenting with rat spleen microsomes, we succeeded in demonstrating and quantitatively characterizing the synthesis of γG globulin and its peptide chains. A preliminary report on these experiments has been published [12]. Recently Vassalli [15] has described successful experiments with fixed antigens used to detect antibodies synthesized by isolated microsomes.

The first part of this paper describes the experimental results of immunoadsorption, including the most rational use of immunoadsorbents for determination of radioactive antigens, the technique of counting the adsorbed protein, and the estimation of the activity of immunoglobulin subunits fixed on cellulose. The second part presents evidence for the formation, in the cell-free system from spleen, of proteins with antigenic properties of rat γG globulin. It is also shown that both heavy and light peptide chains of these proteins can be formed in this system.

IMMUNOADSORPTION TECHNIQUE

Optimum conditions for the determination of the protein bound to the immunoadsorbent

To prepare immunoadsorbents, proteins were conjugated to small cellulose particles through the diazogroups [17]. For the determination of antigens two types of immunoadsorbents were used. One of these consisted of a complex of the fixed antigen and the corresponding antibody (the "sandwich" technique) [18, 19], the other involved pure antibodies fixed on cellulose directly. First, the optimum conditions for the estimation of the protein that was being bound to the adsorbent were determined [20].

The immunoadsorbent* was mixed with the solution under investigation and washed 5-7 times with saline (pH 7) in centrifuge tubes. The bound proteins were eluted with concentrated formic acid (or 0·1 N HCl) and the amount of protein in the eluate was determined by Lowry's method or, in the case of labelled antigens and antibodies, in terms of radioactivity. In the latter case the eluate was applied on a disc of Whatman 3MM paper and allowed to dry. The radioactivity was counted in a liquid scintillation counter (efficiency about 70%). Another alternative consisted in smearing the washed sorbent without elution onto the disc, drying and then counting as above.

It will be seen from data in Table 1 that the second alternative leads to underestimated results (by 20-27%) due to the self-adsorption of the immuno-adsorbent. By repeated elution with concentrated formic acid it is possible to remove the whole protein bound to the adsorbent (96%). In other experiments it has been shown that 0·1 N HCl is somewhat less effective, leading to no more than 85-90% elution of the bound protein.

Pure antibodies fixed on cellulose

In a number of experiments [20] a comparison was made of the capacity for adsorption of antigen (rabbit γG globulin) by corresponding antibodies that had been made insoluble either by binding to the fixed rabbit globulin ("sandwich" technique) or by direct conjugation to cellulose. In the latter case, pure antibodies were used against rabbit γG globulin, isolated from donkey antiserum with fixed antigen. About 98% of the isolated protein could again be adsorbed by fixed antigen. Adsorbents with rat γG globulin were used as controls. In previously published studies [21, 22], fractions of immune globulins containing, together with antibodies, a considerable amount of non-specific proteins, were used for direct fixation.

It is seen from Table 2 that both types of adsorbents can react with antigen. Pure antibodies, directly fixed on cellulose, are 2-3 times as active. Non-specific

* The amount of adsorbent is expressed in terms of the quantity of dry cellulose used for preparation of a portion of adsorbent.

Table 1. Methods of determination of antigen and antibody bound to immunoadsorbents.

| Immunoadsorbent | Adsorbed [^{14}C] protein | Radioactivity, c.p.m. | | | | Radioactivity of discs with smeared adsorbent (without previous elution) | Underestimation of radioactivity values for discs with smeared adsorbents |
		1st eluate	2nd eluate	Residual on the adsorbent	Total	c.p.m.	%
Fixed HSA	anti-HSA	3347	498	147	3992	3164	20
Complex of fixed rabbit γG globulin and antibodies	rabbit γG globulin	563	111	25	710	514	27

[^{14}C] γG globulin (8750 c.p.m.) from rabbit immunized with human serum albumin (HSA) was added to 4 mg of immunoadsorbents. The elution was performed with conc. formic acid. Average from two determinations is given.

Table 2. Adsorption of antigen on complexes of fixed antigen and antibodies and on fixed pure antibodies.

Immunoadsorbents		Adsorbed radioactivity	Specifically-adsorbed antigen	
Fixed protein	Antibody bound to fixing antigen	Antibody on immunoadsorbent		
		μg	c.p.m.	c.p.m.	μg
Rat γG globulin	Rabbit anti-rat globulin	720	34	—	—
		720	69	—	—
Rabbit γG globulin	Donkey anti-rabbit globulin	700	572	520	74
		1000	379	327	47
Rat γG globulin	—	1000	67	—	—
		1000	67	—	—
Donkey anti-rabbit γG globulin	—	700	766	699	100
		1000	1415	1348	193

Rabbit [^{14}C] γG globulin (8750 c.p.m.) with specific activity 7000 c.p.m./mg was added to 4 mg of immunoadsorbents.

5

adsorption on fixed pure antibodies has been shown by special experiments to be very weak. The proportion between the amount of fixed pure antibodies and that of the adsorbed antigen amounted on the average to 5:1, ranging from 1:1 to 10:1, depending upon the amount of antibodies fixed on cellulose and upon the amount of antigen added to the fixed antibodies.

Hence, the optimum immunoadsorbents for isolation of antigen are pure antibodies fixed on cellulose. Apart from their high capacity, these antibodies can be stored and used not only for quantitative estimation but also for the isolation of antigens which cannot be achieved with complexes of fixed antigens and antibodies, excluding some particular cases such as the isolation of low-molecular proteins [16].

Fixed subunits of γG globulins

A number of our experiments were concerned with the possibility of fixing subunits of γG globulins (peptide chains and fragments) on cellulose [23]. If these subunits retained their activity after fixation, they could be used to prepare adsorbents that permit the biosynthesis of subunits to be recognized and quantitatively characterized in cell-free systems. Secondly, active fixed subunits would help to elucidate the immunogenicity of immunoglobulin peptide chains and fragments. And, thirdly, the fixed subunits might be useful to obtain monospecific sera and isolate pure antibodies to subunits.

It is conceivable that subunits, both free and fixed on cellulose, would not markedly change their spatial configuration as compared with the one they have when they form part of the whole molecule of γG globulin. This suggestion was, in particular, substantiated by experiments on free subunits of rabbit γG globulins by means of infrared spectroscopy and hydrogen-deuterium exchange. It was shown that the secondary structure of light chains and fragments of rabbit γG globulin resemble the secondary structure of whole molecules of these proteins [24].

This point of view is confirmed by Table 3. According to the data, subunits fixed on cellulose retain their capacity to react with antibodies, which is obviously possible only when the particular spatial structure of subunits remains unaffected.

The data listed in Table 3 lead to some quantitative conclusions regarding the immunogenicity of peptide chains and fragments. A considerable part of antigenic determinants (about 25%) of the whole molecule is on the light chains. The fixed peptic F(ab')$_2$-fragments adsorb somewhat more antibodies than do the papain Fab-fragments. This is readily explained by corresponding differences in their size. The sum of antibodies adsorbed by means of heavy and light chains is somewhat smaller than the amount of antibodies that has reacted with fixed γG globulin. This might possibly be due to the whole γG-globulin molecule-containing determinants composed of both light and heavy chains.

Such determinants have been described by a number of authors [16]. Another possibility might result from the disappearance of some of the antigenic determinants on isolation and fixation.

Summing up the data in Table 3, one may conclude that, in the cases under study, the proportion of antibodies to the particular subunit in all anti-γG-globulin antibodies is approximately equal to the weight per cent of the subunit in the whole molecule. For instance, about two-thirds of the molecule is accounted for by Fab-fragments and nearly the same amount of antibodies (73%) is sorbed on fixed Fab. The antigenic determinants of the investigated γG globulins appear to be rather uniformly distributed along the molecule. It is,

Table 3. Immunogenicity of γG globulin subunits.

| Fixed protein | Amount of antibodies adsorbed from 1 ml of antiserum[a] on fixed | | | |
| | rabbit proteins | | rat proteins | |
	μg	%	μg	%
γG globulin	1278	100	1522	100
Heavy peptide chains	733	57	978	64
Light peptide chains	334	26	321	21
F(ab')$_2$-fragments	968	76		
Fab-fragments	939	73		
Fab-fragments		74[b]		
Fc-fragments		48[b]		

[a]Donkey antiserum against rabbit globulins and rabbit antiserum against rat globulins were used.

[b]The average of two runs in another experiment.

however, not quite clear whether this regularity holds for other cases as well, e.g. when using antisera from animals of other species. A various degree of immunogenicity of papain fragments of rabbit γG globulin, when immunizing animals of various species, has been reported by Porter [25].

CELL-FREE SYSTEM FROM RAT SPLEEN

Materials and procedures

The main component of the cell-free system used, the microsomes, was isolated from spleen of rats (random bred or Wistar). In a number of experiments the rats were immunized with sheep red cells. The tissue was homogenized by 5-7 strokes of a loosely fitting spherical Teflon pestle in a medium of the following composition: 0·035 M Tris buffer (pH 7·8), 0·16 M sucrose, 0·07 M KCl, 0·01 M MgCl$_2$ and 0·006 M mercaptoethanol. The homogenate was centrifuged at

15,000 *g* for 20 min and at 105,000 *g* for 90 min. The sediment of microsomes was suspended in the medium of the same composition. The protein concentration was determined according to Lowry.

To the microsomes was added the pH-5 fraction from spleen or liver, the ATP-generating system, and ^{14}C-labelled amino acids (Soviet commercial preparations with specific activity about 10 mC/mM or those sold by NEN(USA) with specific activity from 116 to 248 mC/mM). The mixture was incubated for 25 min at 36·5°C, then puromycin (10^{-3} M) was added for the release of nascent

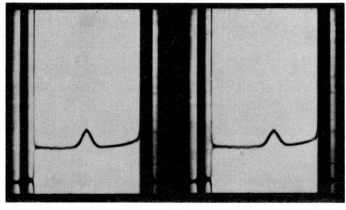

Figure 1. Photograph taken with Schlieren optics during ultracentrifugation of rat γG globulin in 0·1 M sodium acetate. Rotor speed 63,650 r.p.m. Exposures were taken at 55 min and 65 min. Calculated $S_{20w} = 6·3$.

polypeptide chains from polyribosomes and the incubation was continued for a further 5 min: The incorporation of [^{14}C] amino acids into proteins was determined in a liquid scintillation counter by means of the disc method [26]. After addition of deoxycholate (final concentration 0·5%) the mixture was centrifuged at 105,000 *g* for 90 min and the supernatant was analyzed for soluble proteins with antigenic properties of γG globulins or their peptide chains. The determination was carried out with complexes of fixed antigens and antibodies.

The interpretation of the results obtained is, of course, largely dependent on the purity of the antigen used for the preparation of immunoadsorbents. For fixation we have used rat γG globulin, isolated from pooled rat serum by precipitation with sodium sulphate two times at 18 and 14% saturation, followed by chromatography on DEAE-cellulose (Whatman, DE 50) in 0·0175 M phosphate buffer, pH 6·3. The preparation was found to be homogeneous in the analytical ultracentrifuge (Fig. 1) with a sedimentation constant of 6·3S. Immunoelectrophoretic investigation, using the rabbit antiserum against proteins of rat serum, revealed a strong precipitin band, similar to that of γ_2

globulin of other animal species, and a weak band for the protein with somewhat higher mobility. Further experiments are needed to show whether this protein is one of the subclasses of rat γG globulin (Fig. 2).

The complexes of fixed rabbit γG globulin with corresponding donkey antibodies were used as control adsorbents. Special experiments have shown that this control adsorbent, as well as specific adsorbents involving rat γG globulin or its peptide chains, adsorb non-specifically from solutions of $[^{14}C]$ amino acids a similar amount of the label.

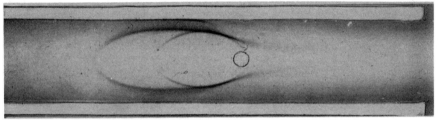

Figure 2. Immunoelectrophoretic patterns of rat γG globulin.

Amino acid incorporation into proteins by rat spleen or liver microsomes

Under conditions used, the spleen microsomes were capable of incorporating radioactive amino acids into proteins [12]. The data obtained with microsomes isolated from Wistar rats on the fifth day after a single intravenous immunization with sheep red cells are shown in Table 4. It will be seen from these data that, in the absence of the ATP-generating system, the label was not incorporated. Addition of puromycin also stopped almost entirely the protein synthesis. The extent of the incorporation of the label varied, depending on the amount of

Table 4. Incorporation of labelled amino acids into proteins by rat spleen and liver microsomes under different conditions.

Microsomes	Reaction mixture	Radioactivity incorporated into proteins
		c.p.m./mg microsome protein
Spleen	Complete	11,900
Spleen	+ puromycin(10^{-3}M)	870
Spleen	− ATP,GTP,PEP,PEP-kinase	50
Liver	Complete	15,540

Complete reaction mixture contained in a volume of 1 ml: 1 mg microsomes and 2·5 mg of pH-5 fraction from liver, 2 μmole ATP and 0·2 μmole GTP (Reanal, Hungary), 10 μmole phosphoenolpyruvate (Sigma, USA), 100 μg phosphoenolpyruvate kinase (Reanal), 1 μC of a mixture of ten ^{14}C-labelled amino acids (NEN, USA) with specific activity 116-248 μC/μM and 0·3 μmole of 10 other amino acids (non-labelled). The mixtures were incubated for 25 min at 36·5°C.

Table 5. Incorporation of radioactive amino acids into immunoglobulins and other proteins by rat spleen and liver microsomes.

Expt. No.	Micro-somes	pH-5 frac-tion	Radioactivity incorporated into proteins c.p.m./mg microsome protein	Total c.p.m. Soluble proteins	Sedimented proteins	Adsorption of the radioactive label from supernatants on non-specific adsorbent c.p.m.	on specific adsorbent c.p.m.	Soluble labelled proteins antigenically reacted as rat γG globulin c.p.m.
1.	Spleen	Spleen	1240	8000	12,780	540	484	no
2.	Liver	Spleen	1900	6800	7800	349	1000	651
3.	Liver	Liver	8640	—	—	—	—	—

The reaction mixture contained in a volume of 1 ml: microsomes (5·5 mg in Expt. 1 and 4 mg in Expt. 2), pH-5 fraction (25 mg in Expt. 1 and 11 mg in Expt. 2), 2 μmole ATP, 0·2 μmole GTP, 10 μmoles PEP, 100 μg PEP-kinase, 1 μC of mixture of ^{14}C-labelled amino acids (glutamic acid, alanine, arginine, serine and proline) with specific activity approx. 7 mC/mM and 0·3 μmole of other 15 amino acids (non-labelled). The mixtures were incubated for 25 min at 36·5°C, then puromycin was added (final concentration 10^{-3}M) and the incubation was continued for a further 5 min. After addition of deoxycholate (final concentration 0·5%) the mixtures were centrifuged for 90 min at 105,000 **g**.

added label, its specific activity, and on the source of the pH-5 fraction. This fraction from spleen was less active than that from liver. In most experiments we used the pH-5 fraction from liver. The liver microsomes were found in almost all experiments to possess a stronger ability to incorporate the label into proteins than did the spleen microsomes (Tables 4 and 5). The preparations of pH-5 fraction from liver were almost unable to effect this function.

Under the conditions of our experiments, sedimentation of particles left about 40-45% of radioactive proteins in the supernatant (Table 5). The remaining label was connected with the sediment obtained on centrifugation of the mixture during 90 min at 105,000 g.

Amino acid incorporation into γG globulins and its peptide chains

To detect labelled proteins possessing antigenic properties of γG globulins or their peptide chains, use was made of complexes of fixed antigens and antibodies. At first, to the incubation mixture treated with deoxycholate and freed from particles by centrifugation, was added the control adsorbent—a complex of fixed rabbit γG globulin and corresponding antibodies. The radio-activity of this adsorbent was taken as a measure of non-specific adsorption. When the adsorbent was removed a complex of rat γG globulin and correspond-ing antibodies was added. The difference between radioactivity adsorbed on this adsorbent and the control adsorbent was considered a measure of the amount of radioactive proteins with antigenic properties of rat γG globulins.

Table 5 lists the results of an experiment with liver and spleen microsomes of random bred rats that were twice immunized intraperitoneally and killed on the fifth day after the first injection of antigen. It will be seen that the first experiment with the pH-5 fraction from spleen revealed no specific adsorption. On the other hand, the second experiment with the pH-5 fraction from liver showed a considerable increase in radioactivity on the specific adsorbent, thus pointing to the synthesis of proteins with antigenic properties of rat γG globulins. From the data presented in Table 5 it can also be seen that the quantity of radioactivity accounted for by these proteins amounts to about 10% of soluble proteins and 5% of all radioactive proteins. Specific adsorption was, however, not revealed in all experiments or, rather, was found to be present in only half of them. In control experiments with liver microsomes, adsorption was found to be similar on both types of adsorbents.

It has been further studied whether proteins with antigenic properties of light and heavy polypeptide chains could be synthesized in a cell-free system. To this end complexes of fixed light and heavy peptide chains of rat γG globulins and corresponding antibodies were used. The chains were isolated according to Franěk [27]. As shown above, the peptide chains fixed on cellulose retain their ability to react with antibodies.

The results of an experiment concerned with the antigenic properties of proteins synthesized by microsomes from spleen of rats immunized intra-peritoneally are shown in Table 6. It will be seen that radioactive proteins are specifically bound to adsorbents with light and heavy peptide chains. The overall quantity of specifically-adsorbed protein amounted in this experiment to 9% of all radioactive proteins. It is evident that, in a cell-free system, proteins with antigenic properties of both light and heavy peptide chains can be synthesized. It is, however, difficult to estimate exactly in this case what kind of proteins, those

Table 6. Antigenic properties of proteins synthesized in a cell-free system from rat spleen.

Immunoadsorbent	Radioactivity adsorbed	Specifically adsorbed radioactivity
	c.p.m.	c.p.m.
1. Control adsorbent (complex of fixed rabbit γG globulin and corresponding antibodies)	239	–
2. Adsorbent-specific for light chains of rat γG globulins (complex of fixed light chains of rat γG globulins and corres-ponding antibodies)	530	291
3. Adsorbent-specific for heavy chains of rat γG globulin (complex of fixed heavy chains of rat γG globulins and corresponding antibodies)	534	295
4. Adsorbent-specific for γG globulins (complex of fixed rat γG globulin and corresponding antibodies)	251	12

To supernatant of the reaction mixture (as in Table 5) the immunoadsorbents were added one after another.

belonging to light or heavy chains, are predominantly synthesized because the adsorbent-binding light chains can also bind complexes of light and heavy chains. At the same time it is evident that radioactive free heavy chains are present in the incubation mixture. The possible admixture of light chains in the prepara-tion of heavy chains used for fixation should not affect the results obtained, because adsorbents with heavy chains were treated with antiserum which was completely freed of antibodies against light chains.

To estimate more precisely the relation between the light and heavy chains synthesized, the supernatant of the incubation mixture was divided into two equal parts, the former being treated as in the previous experiment and the latter undergoing a reverse order of treatment. Such a procedure makes it possible to estimate the amount of free chains and the amount of chains bound in the

Table 7. Synthesis of light and heavy chains of rat γG globulin in the cell-free system.

First part of supernatant		Second part of supernatant	
Immunoadsorbent specific for	Specifically-adsorbed radioactivity	Immunoadsorbent specific for	Specifically adsorbed radioactivity
	c.p.m.		c.p.m.
1. Light chains	318	1. Heavy chains	425
2. Heavy chains	179	2. Light chains	132
3. γG Globulins	0	3. γG Globulins	0
In all	497	In all	557

The reaction mixture contained in a volume of 1 ml: 1 mg of microsomes and 10 mg of pH-5 fraction from rat liver, 2 μC of mixture of [^{14}C] amino acids as in Table 5. Radioactivity incorporated into proteins was 6118 c.p.m./mg of microsome protein. At the end of incubation puromycin (10^{-3} M) was added.

complex. This procedure had been previously used to identify the microglobulin synthesized by rabbit spleen cells *in vitro* [23, 28].

Table 7 gives the results of this experiment (microsomes from random-bred non-immune rats being used). The overall quantity of proteins with properties of γG globulins amounted in this experiment to 1% of all radioactive proteins and about 3% of radioactive soluble proteins. As seen from Table 7, the proteins with antigenic properties of both light and heavy chains are partly involved in a complex, and partly exist in a free state.

In the described experiments (Tables 6 and 7) the radioactivity accounted for by free heavy chains formed in a cell-free system was in excess.

These experiments have thus shown that spleen microsomes can synthesize proteins with antigenic properties of light and heavy peptide chains of γG globulins. These were identified by means of fixed peptide chains. The fixed subunits of γG globulin are also likely to be useful for the study of the formation of N-terminal parts of chains in cell-free systems, i.e. those parts that display the primary function in the antibody activity of immunoglobulins.

ACKNOWLEDGEMENT

Some of the experiments were undertaken in collaboration with L. M. Kulpina and T. I. Vengerova. Some biochemicals used in this study were obtained through the Immunology Unit of the World Health Organization. Immuno-electrophoresis was performed in Dr. N. Kholchev's laboratory and analytical ultracentrifugation in Dr. V. Chernyak's laboratory. The authors would like to express their thanks to Mr. A. L. Pumpiansky for translation of the article.

REFERENCES

1. Campbell, P. N. and Kernot, B. A., *Biochem. J.* **82** (1962) 262.
2. Ganoza, M. C., Williams, C. R. and Lipmann, F., *Proc. natn. Acad. Sci. U.S.A.* **53** (1965) 619.
3. Bishop, J., Leahy, J. and Schweet, R., *Proc. natn. Acad. Sci. U.S.A.* **46** (1960) 1030.
4. Askonas, B. A., *in* "Protein Biosynthesis" (edited by R. J. C. Harris), Academic Press, London and New York, 1961, p. 363.
5. Ogata, K., Omori, S., Hirokana, R. and Takahashi, T., *in* "Proceedings of the 5th International Congress of Biochemistry", Symposium II, Publ. House Acad. Sci. U.S.S.R., 1962, Moscow, p. 194.
6. Eisen, H. N., Simms, E. S., Helmreich, E. and Kern, M., *Trans. Ass. Am. Physns* **74** (1961) 207.

7. Van der Meer, J. H. H. and Koningsberger, V. V., *Biochim. biophys. Acta* **103** (1965) 136.
8. Stenzel, K. H. and Rubin, A. L., *Science, N.Y.* **153** (1966) 537.
9. Hrubešová, M., *Folia microbiol., Praha* **11** (1966) 346.
10. Nezlin, R. S., *Biokhimiya* **31** (1966) 516.
11. Wust, C. J., *Archs Biochem. Biophys.* **118** (1967) 568.
12. Nezlin, R. S. and Kulpina L. M., *Biochim. biophys. Acta* **138** (1967) 654.
13. Gusdon, J. P., Stavitsky, A. B. and Armentrout, S. A., *Proc. natn. Acad. Sci. U.S.A.* **58** (1967) 1189.
14. Mach, B., Koblet, H. and Gros, D., *Cold Spring Harb. Symp. quant. Biol.* **32** (1968) 269.
15. Vassalli, P., Lisowska-Bernstein, B., Lamm, M. E. and Benacerraf, B., *Proc. natn. Acad. Sci. U.S.A.* **58** (1967) 2422.
16. Nezlin, R. S., *in* "Biochemistry of Antibodies", Nauka, Moscow, 1966 (Russian Edition); Plenum Publ. Co., New York, 1969 (English Edition).
17. Gurvich, A. E., *in* "Immunological Methods" (edited by J. F. Ackroyd), Blackwell, Oxford, 1964, p. 113.
18. Williams, R. R. and Stone, S. S., *Archs Biochem. Biophys.* **71** (1957) 377.
19. Gurvich, A. E. and Drizlikh, G. I., *Nature, Lond.* **203** (1964) 648.
20. Rokhlin, O. V. and Nezlin, R. S., *Vop. med. Khim.* in press.
21. Jagendorf, A. T., Patchornik, A. and Sela, M., *Biochim. biophys. Acta* **78** (1963) 516.
22. Gallop, R. G. C., Tozer, B. T., Stephen, J. and Smith, H., *Biochem. J.* **101** (1966) 711.
23. Nezlin, R. S. and Kulpina, L. M., *Immunochemistry* **4** (1967) 269.
24. Abaturov, L. V., Nezlin, R. S., Vengerova, T. I. and Varshavsky, Ya, M. *in* "Abstracts 5th FEBS Meeting (Prague)", 1968, p. 264.
25. Porter, R. R., *Biochem. J.* **73** (1959) 119.
26. Mans, R. J. and Novelli, G. D., *Archs Biochem. Biophys.* **94** (1961) 48.
27. Franěk, F. and Zikán, J., *Colln. Czech. chem. Commun.* **29** (1964) 1401.
28. Nezlin, R. S. and Kulpina, L. M., *Biokhimya* **31** (1966) 1257.

FEBS Symposium, Volume 15, 1969, pp. 133-168

Allotypic Specificity in Productive, Pre-Productive and Progenitor Cells

C.-T. CHOU, B. CINADER and S. DUBISKI

Departments of Medical Biophysics, Pathological Chemistry and Medicine, University of Toronto, Toronto, Canada

Antibody formation is preceded by differentiation from stem cells, by cell-cell interaction and by humoral factors which control certain stages of the cellular progression [1-12]. The point in this progression at which commitment to a particular antibody specificity occurs, is as uncertain as are the details of this process. It is clear, however, that productive-commitment involves not only the combining site of antibody for antigen, but also other structural features of the immunoglobulin. Whether commitment to all these facets of light and heavy chains occurs at the same, or at different stages, remains an intriguing problem. Individual productive cells, i.e. the final cellular stages, show a severe restriction of heterogeneity in their products. Concomitantly, individual cells are vastly different from one another in the combining sites of their immunoglobulins. This heterogeneity is less extensive with respect to certain structural features such as allotypic specificity, i.e. with respect to genetic markers which are not in the combining site of the antibody molecule. It is thus possible to carry out population studies of productive cells in terms of fairly large discrete subgroups of cells. It is also practicable to pursue the antecedents of productive cells in terms of the same genetic markers, which seem to be much more widely distributed than any combining capacity of antibody.

We propose to examine immunoglobulin production in terms of allotypic specificity. We shall first deal with population studies of cells in the productive state (i.e. manufacturing antibody), next with cells in the pre-productive state (i.e. cells which do not release immunoglobulin, but are affected by antibody directed against immunoglobulins) and, finally with progenitor cells which do not seem to have reached either of these stages, but generate the productive cell (i.e. cells which can transfer to an animal the ability to produce allotypic specificity). The first of these studies is based on the interaction between plaque-forming cells and anti-allotype antibody, the second deals with antibody-mediated phenotypic changes of newborn animals and the third is concerned with induction by cell-transfer of allotype-chimerism.

CELL IN THE PRODUCTIVE STATE

We have already referred to the relation between the extreme heterogeneity of circulating immunoglobulins on the one hand, and the homogeneity of immuno-globulins, produced by individual cells, on the other. We now know of some exceptions to the rule that all aspects of heterogeneity in the humoral antibodies can be attributed to heterogeneity of cell populations and we shall return to them in the discussion of "Pre-Committed Cells". In general, however, each productive cell releases antibody with a single genetic marker, even if the animal is heterozygous for this marker [13-15]. This is an intriguing phenomenon and in sharp contrast to production of other molecules, such as enzymes, by single somatic cells of heterozygous animals. In an attempt to understand this phenomenon, we are faced with two questions: Are individual homozygous cells indistinguishable from heterozygous cells? Are the two alleles from a hetero-zygous animal equally expressed, and, if not, is this due to different quantitative output by individual cells or is it due to different cell-numbers?

To answer these questions, we shall analyse cell populations from animals homozygous and heterozygous at the A_b locus.

The heterogeneity in hemolytic capacity of allotypically-defined plaque-forming cells. (Donors homozygous on A_b locus.)

The study of cell population requires a technique which can link the productive cell with well defined features of its soluble product. We shall therefore start with the analysis of the reactions which allow us to subdivide plaque-forming cells according to genetic markers on their light chains and according to their hemolytic capacity. We shall employ, for this purpose, antibody directed against allotypic specificity and we shall refer to it as "external" antibody. The effect of this "external" antibody on plaque formation by cells from homozygous animals shall form the first part of the experiments to be described. We shall then turn to some problems in this assay which become evident in the interaction of "external" antibodies with plaque-formation by cells from *heterozygous* animals and we shall, in particular, demonstrate an inhibiting effect of "normal" immunoglobulin.

Antibody against γ globulin ("external" antibody) can affect plaque formation in two ways; it may enhance plaque formation by promoting the hemolytic action of complement [16-20], and it may inhibit plaque formation by preventing antibody ("internal" antibody of the plaque-forming cells) from reaching the erythrocytes [1].

We first examined antibody-forming cells, obtained from rabbits which had been given one or two injections of sheep red cells and were sacrificed 6-8 days afterwards. Antibody against allotypic specificity ("external" antibody) A4 or A5 was incorporated into agar together with sheep erythrocytes and spleen cells of the immunized homozygous rabbits (A^4/A^4 or A^5/A^5).

The incorporation into agar of increasing amounts of "external" antibody (incorporation technique) resulted first in an increase of the observed plaque number, then in a decrease (Fig. 1). We were thus able to distinguish two types of plaque-forming cells; those which produced antibody capable of directly promoting complement-lysis (direct plaques due to antibody of high hemolytic capacity), and those which produced antibody that only promoted complement-lysis in the presence of "external" antibody (enhanceable plaques, due to

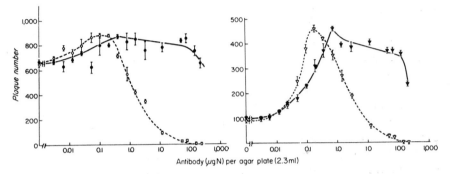

Antibody (μgN) per agar plate (2.3ml)

Figure 1. Early response. The effect on plaque formation of "external" (anti-allotype) antibody *during* and *after* the release by plaque-forming cells of "internal" antibody [23].

Rabbits received two i.v. injections of 6×10^9 sheep red blood corpuscles, one week apart, and were sacrificed six days after the second injection. Antibody directed against allotypic specificity of the light chains was either incorporated into the agar, together with spleen cells and erythrocytes (broken lines) or was allowed to enter the agar by diffusion, two hours after erythrocytes and spleen cells had been mixed with agar (full lines). For the incorporation technique, the quantity of antibody shown on the horizontal axis is the total quantity present in 2·3 ml of the agar cell mixture. For the overlay technique the quantity on the horizontal axis signifies the amount of "external" antibody in 2·3 ml of fluid layered above the agar cell mixture. The left-hand panel shows the interaction of antibody directed against A4 specificity with plaques from an A^4/A^4 rabbit. The right-hand panel shows the interaction between antibody to specificity A5 and plaque-forming cells from A^5/A^5 rabbits. Vertical bars signify one standard deviation. Plaque numbers are given for 10^6 spleen cells. Open symbols and broken lines show plaque numbers determined by the incorporation technique. Full symbols and full lines show plaque number determined by the overlay technique.

antibody of low hemolytic capacity). It is evident that the formation of both types of plaques could be inhibited by "external" antibody.

The increase in the number of plaque-forming cells in the presence of "external" antibody may be attributed to plaque-forming cells whose antibody could not promote hemolysis unless combined with "external" antibody [21].

Direct plaques, which are found in the absence of "external" antibody and are inhibitable by "external" antibody, may be largely due to γM "internal" antibodies; plaques which are only seen in the presence of "external" antibody may be largely due to γG "internal" antibodies. We shall see, in a later section, that this view gains support from experiments with mouse cells and antibody against the murine heavy chain-allotype MuA2. However, we have no compelling experimental evidence for this view and we shall, therefore, refer to direct plaques which are due to "internal" antibody of high hemolytic capacity, and to enhanceable plaques which are due to antibody of low hemolytic capacity, respectively.

It will be seen from the two curves shown in Fig. 1 that maximum enhancement of each of the sets of plaque-forming cells was brought about by well defined amounts of "external" antibody; we shall refer to these amounts as "optimal antibody".

The question arises whether the number of enhanceable plaque-forming cells may be deduced from the difference between the plaque number in the presence of optimal "external" antibody and the number of direct plaques. This difference will represent the number of enhanceable plaque-forming cells only if direct plaques are not inhibited by optimal antibody. We therefore asked the following operational question: Is "internal" antibody of high hemolytic capacity neutralized by optimal quantities of "external" antibody before it reaches the red cell? To answer this question, we allowed "external" antibody to enter the reaction *after* the "internal" antibody had combined with the sheep red cells (overlay technique). We examined spleen cells from animals which had been given one or two injections of 6×10^9 sheep erythrocytes and were sacrificed 8 or 13 days, respectively, after the initiating injection. In the overlay technique, as in the incorporation technique, the plaque number increased with increasing amounts of "external" antibody. The maximum number of plaque-forming cells was identical when "external" antibody was incorporated into agar (incorporation technique; broken lines, Fig. 1) and when it was added by diffusion after "internal" antibody had combined with the sheep erythrocytes (overlay technique; Fig. 1). In the former experimental arrangement, "internal" antibody could be neutralized by combination with the "external" antibody *before* it reached the red cells; in the latter experimental arrangement, none of the "internal" antibody was prevented from reacting with the erythrocytes. Since maximum enhancement was of the same magnitude whether optimal quantities of "external" antibody were present during or only after the release of "internal" antibody, it follows that the incorporation of optimal quantities of "external" antibody did not result in inhibition of plaque formation, which was due to "internal" antibody of high hemolytic capacity. It was therefore possible to obtain the total number of enhanceable plaque-forming cells from the results of the incorporation technique as the difference between the maximum number of plaques in the presence of "external" antibody and the number of direct plaques.

Thus in the *early* stages of the immune response, all enhanceable plaques were revealed before the direct plaques were inhibited. That this was *not* the case in the later stages of the immune response, could be seen by comparing the highest plaque number found by the incorporation technique and by the overlay technique. With cells obtained 18 days after an injection, the difference between the maximal plaque numbers obtained in overlay and incorporation techniques was about half the number of direct plaques; with cells obtained 28 days after the injection, the difference, obtained by overlay and incorporation techniques, was identical with the number of direct plaques. Thus, the incorporation of optimal quantities of "external" antibody resulted in inhibition of some plaques of high hemolytic capacity and simultaneous enhancement of plaques of low hemolytic capacity (Fig. 2).

We shall now turn to a consideration of the significance of the optimal quantity of "external" antibody. The curve relating direct plaques to varying quantities of "external" antibody will be sigmoid and the curve relating enhanceable plaque number to "external" antibody will be bell-shaped. The *experimentally*-observed relation (incorporation technique) between plaque number and "external" antibody may therefore be regarded as the summation of a sigmoid curve and of a bell-shaped curve. This is shown schematically in Fig. 3.

The amount of "external" antibody which corresponds to maximum plaque-number of the bell-shaped curve may be, (a) (in Fig. 3a) within the range of the horizontal portion of the sigmoid curve, or it may be (b) (in Fig. 3b) within the declining portion of the sigmoid curve, i.e. within the range in which the number of plaques of high hemolytic capacity (inhibitable plaques) begins to decrease as a function of the quantity of "external" antibody. We can characterize these two possibilities as follows:

(a) the optimal amount of "external" antibody is identical for the hypothetical bell-shaped curve and for the summated relation between plaque number and "external" antibody. Furthermore, the maximum plaque number of the summated curve is the sum of the highest plaque number in the sigmoid curve and in the bell-shaped curve.

(b) the optimal amount of "external antibody" is less for the summated curve than for the bell-shaped curve. Furthermore, the maximum plaque number of the summated curve (summated curve, Fig. 3b) is smaller than the sum of the highest plaque number in the sigmoid and in the bell-shaped curve.

To distinguish the above alternatives, we have compared the maximum number of plaques by the overlay and by the incorporation technique. We have found that the plaque number obtained by these two techniques is identical if the plaques are obtained 8 days after an injection (top of Fig. 2). This can only occur if *optimal* "external" antibody does not inhibit plaques of high hemolytic capacity. This is compatible with the possibility discussed under (a) but not with that discussed under (b). We may therefore conclude that the relative low value for optimal antibody, found with plaque-forming cells a week after injection, is *not* an artefact of summation.

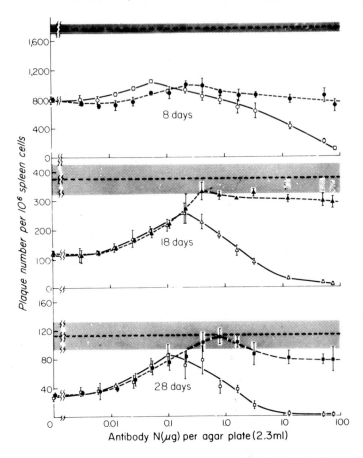

Figure 2. Changes with time in response to a single injection. The effect on plaque formation of "external" (anti-allotype) antibody *during* and *after* the release of "internal" antibody by plaque-forming cells [23].

Rabbits (homozygous at the A_b locus) received one i.v. injection of 6×10^9 sheep red blood corpuscles and were sacrificed 8, 18 or 28 days later. Purified antibody against the allotypic specificity of the light chain was either incorporated into the agar, together with spleen cells and sheep red cells (open symbols, full line) or was allowed to enter the agar by diffusion, two hours after sheep erythrocytes and spleen cells had been mixed with agar (closed symbols, broken line). Plaque counts are given for 10^6 sheep cells. Vertical bars indicate two standard deviations (95% confidence limit). Shaded areas indicate 95% confidence limit of the sum of the plaques observed (by the incorporation technique) in the absence of "external" antibody and in the presence of optimal "external" antibody. This sum is in excess of the plaque number found by the overlay technique when plaque-forming cells were examined 8 days after an injection. Thus, the enhanceable plaques are found in the incorporation technique as the difference between the plaque number in the absence of "external" antibody and the plaque number in the presence of optimal antibody. The above sum is identical with the number of plaques found by the overlay technique when plaque-forming cells were examined 28 days after an injection. Thus, the enhanceable plaques are found in the incorporation technique as the total number of plaques found in

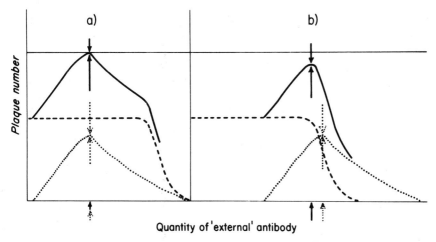

Figure 3. Schematic representation of the effect of "external" antibody on plaque formation [23].

The sigmoid curve, in broken lines, shows the effect of "external" antibody on plaques of high hemolytic capacity. The bell-shaped curve (dotted line) shows the effect of "external" antibody on the formation of plaques of low hemolytic capacity. (a) and (b) differ in the relative position of the two curves. The full lines show the summation of the curves. Arrows show optimal "external" antibody for the summated curve (→) and for the bell-shaped curve (--→). The optimal quantity of "external" antibody for the two curves is identical in (a) and different in (b). Horizontal line shows the sum of the highest plaque number of the sigmoid curve and of the bell-shaped curve. In (a) this sum is identical with the highest plaque number of the summated curve; in (b) the sum is greater than the highest plaque number of the summated curve.

Figure 2—continued

the presence of optimal antibody. For plaques obtained 18 days after a single injection, the situation is intermediate between that found in spleen cells obtained 8 days and 28 days after injection.

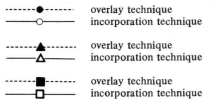

overlay technique	A^4/A^4 rabbit; 8 days after a single injection;
incorporation technique	"external" antibody against A4
overlay technique	A^5/A^5 rabbit; 18 days after a single
incorporation technique	injection; "external" antibody against A5
overlay technique	A^5/A^5 rabbit; 28 days after a single
incorporation technique	injection; "external" antibody against A5

The question arises whether this optimal quantity of antibody is affected by immunoglobulins, other than the plaque-forming antibodies. To examine this question, we tested the effect of "external" antibody on different numbers of plaque-forming cells, obtained from the same animal. We found that the number of plaques, observed with quantities of "external" antibody which were less than the optimal quantity, depended on the total number of cells. The dependence was less pronounced when the "external" antibody was in excess of optimal quantity (Figs. 4A and B). The optimal quantity of antibody was not appreciably affected by the total cell number, and hence by the total immuno-globulin in the test-system. It would therefore appear that the optimal quantity of antibody may serve as a relative measure of the amount of "internal" antibody released by individual plaque-forming cells.

Having so far examined properties of plaque-forming cells from animals which were homozygous at the A_b locus, we turn next to animals which were heterozygous at this locus.

The allotypic heterogeneity of plaque-forming cells.
(Donors heterozygous on A_b locus.)

In heterozygous A^4/A^5 rabbits, we could determine the number of direct plaques due to antibody of allotypic specificity A4, the number of direct plaques due to antibody of allotypic specificity A5, the number of plaque-forming cells which produced antibody of low hemolytic capacity and allotypic specificity A4, and finally, the number which produced antibody of low hemolytic capacity and of allotypic specificity A5.

The sum of the plaques inhibited by antibody to A4 and by antibody to A5 exceed by about 20% the number of plaques found in the absence of "external" antibody. It appeared that certain plaque-forming cells were affected by both of the two different antibodies. In fact, we found that antibody affected cells in two ways, one depending on its combining capacity with antigen, the other depending on other properties of the antibody molecule. It could be shown that plaque formation was not only inhibited by antibody, but also by normal immunoglobulin. This second type of interference became evident when we examined the effect on the plaque number of normal immunoglobulins which had the same allotypic specificity as the light chains of the "external" antibodies. Such immunoglobulins had no effect on the total number of enhanceable plaques, but reduced plaque formation when present in high concentration (Figs. 5A, B and C).

We have so far examined the interaction of the rabbit's plaque-forming cells with "external" antibody against the specificities present on most classes of immunoglobulins. A different situation may be seen in the mouse, with an allotypic specificity found on a relatively small portion of the total immuno-globulins and hence in the products of a relatively small proportion of

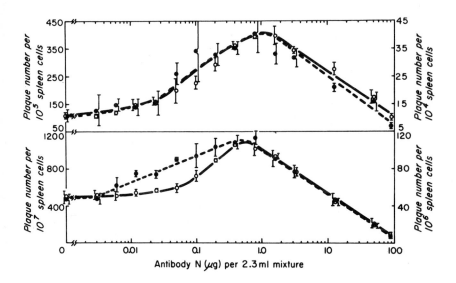

Figure 4A. The effect of the number of spleen cells on the interaction between plaques and "external" antibody.

Vertical bar shows two standard deviations

Top panel:
Spleen cells from A^4/A^4 rabbit, three days after 10 i.v. injections of 6 x 10^9 sheep erythrocytes on day 0, 2, 4, 28, 30, 32, 56, 58, 60 and 90.

————○————   plaque number per 10^5 spleen cells
------●-------   plaque number per 10^4 spleen cells

Bottom panel:
Spleen cells from A^4/A^4 rabbit, obtained 40 days after 10 i.v. injections of 6 x 10^9 sheep erythrocytes on day 0, 2, 4, 28, 30, 32, 56, 58, 60 and 90.

————○————   plaque number per 10^7 spleen cells
••••••••●••••••••   plaque number per 10^6 spleen cells

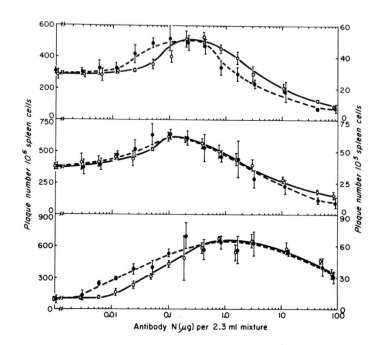

Figure 4B. The effect of the number of spleen cells on the interaction between plaques and "external" antibody.

Top and centre panels:
A^5/A^5 homozygous rabbits were tested six days after two weekly i.v. injections of 6×10^9 sheep erythrocytes. Vertical bar shows two standard deviations.

———○——— plaque number per 10^6 spleen cells
·······●······· plaque number per 10^5 spleen cells

Bottom panel:
A^4/A^4 homozygous rabbit was tested 19 days after 10 i.v. injections of 6×10^9 sheep erythrocytes on day 0, 2, 4, 28, 30, 32, 56, 58, 60 and 90. Vertical bar shows two standard deviations.

———○——— plaque number per 10^6 spleen cells
·······●······· plaque number per 10^5 spleen cells

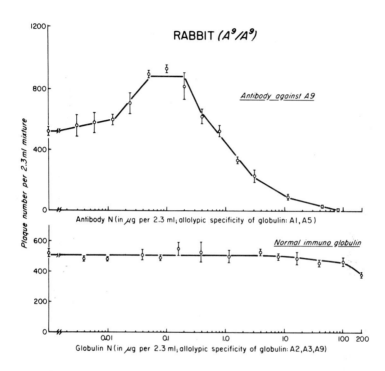

Figure 5A. The effect of antibody and of immunoglobulin on plaque number.
Spleen cells were obtained from an A^2/A^3, A^9/A^9 rabbit 6 days after 2 weekly i.v. injections of 6 × 10⁹ sheep erythrocytes. The number of plaques was determined in the presence of increasing amounts of specifically-purified antibody to A9 (top panel) and immunoglobulin separated on Porath columns (bottom panel). Vertical bar shows two standard deviations.

Panel	Immunoglobulin added to system		
	Antibody directed against	Allotypic specificity	
		Heavy chain	Light chain
Top	A9	A1	A5
Bottom	no known activity	A2, A3	A9

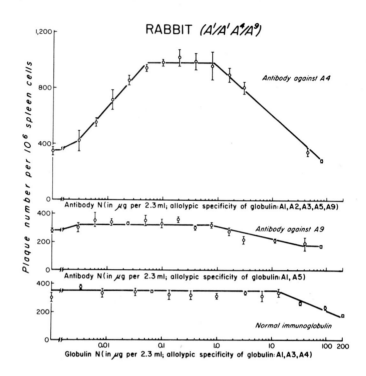

Figure 5B. The effect of antibody and of immunoglobulin on plaque number.

Spleen cells were obtained from an A^1/A^1, A^4/A^9 rabbit 6 days after 2 weekly i.v. injections of 6×10^9 sheep erythrocytes. The number of plaques was determined in the presence of increasing amounts of specifically-purified antibody to A4 (top panel), specifically purified antibody to A9 (centre panel) and immunoglobulin separated on Porath columns (bottom panel). Vertical bar shows two standard deviations.

Panel	Immunoglobulin added to system		
	Antibody directed against	Allotypic specificity	
		Heavy chain	Light chain
Top	A4	A1, A2, A3	A5, A9
Centre	A9	A1	A5
Bottom	no known activity	A1, A3	A4

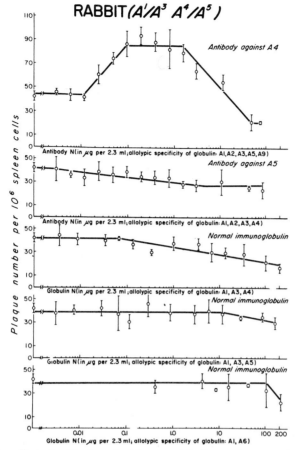

Figure 5C. The effect of antibody and of immunoglobulin on plaque number.

Spleen cells were obtained from an A^1/A^3, A^4/A^5 rabbit 6 days after 2 weekly i.v. injections of 6×10^9 sheep erythrocytes. The number of plaques was determined in the presence of increasing amounts of specifically-purified antibody to A4 (top panel), specifically-purified antibody to A5 (second panel from top) and immunoglobulins separated on Porath columns (third, fourth and fifth panels from top). Vertical bar shows two standard deviations.

Panel	Immunoglobulin added to system		
	Antibody directed against	Allotypic specificity	
		Heavy chain	Light chain
Top	A4	A1, A2, A3	A5, A9
Second from top	A5	A1, A2, A3	A4
Third from top	no known activity	A1, A3	A4
Fourth from top	no known activity	A1, A3	A5
Fifth from top	no known activity	A1	A6

antibody-forming cells. We employed as "external" antibody a murine antiserum directed against MuA2 and compared its effect with that of an antiserum of rabbit origin which was directed against mouse immunoglobulins. Since we employed whole sera it was necessary to examine the effect of normal sera and to correct for this effect. Rabbit antisera of broad specificity led to enhancement of plaques and to inhibition of plaques (Fig. 6A). The murine antibody, on the other hand, promoted enhancement of plaque-numbers but did not result in specific inhibition of plaque formation (Fig. 6B). It was thus clear that only a proportion of immunoglobulins, and only those which produced enhanceable plaques, could be affected by the murine antibody against MuA2. This confirms the previously reported presence of MuA2 on circulating γG and its absence on circulating γM molecules [5] and will become relevant in the discussion of the "Pre-Productive Cell".

We have so far considered factors which determine the effect of antibodies on plaque-formation. We shall now turn to interaction between alleles.

Gene interaction

Dray and Nisonoff [22] have shown that 82% of the total immunoglobulins of an A^5/A^5 rabbit carry the A5 allotypic specificity and that 91% of the total immunoglobulins of an A^4/A^4 rabbit carry the A4 specificity.

Thus, in animals homozygous on the A_b locus, the gene product of A_b is found on a majority of immunoglobulins. We may consider this state of affairs as a reflection of a competition for antigen capture by receptors of A_b origin. This could be due to numerical preponderance of such receptors. The preponderance of the product of the A_b locus is somewhat greater in A^4/A^4 animals. One might therefore expect in heterozygous A^4/A^5 animals a slight preponderance of the product of the A^4 gene over that of the A^5 gene. Surprisingly, this preponderance was found to be almost threefold [22]. This problem has been examined by us in terms of the number of cells forming A4 and A5 antibody respectively. We determined direct plaques and enhanceable plaques and, on the average, there were three times as many A^4 as there were A^5 plaques [1, 23]. This cellular ratio is in excellent agreement with the molecular ratio in the circulation [22] and indicates that we are not dealing with a difference in output of A4 and A5 immunoglobulin by heterozygous and by homozygous cells, but with a difference in the number of cells which produce A4 and A5 respectively. The extent of the competitive advantage of the A^4 over the A^5 gene was thus much larger than one would have expected from the relative immunoglobulin concentrations of homozygous animals. This focused our attention on the general problem of the mutual effects of different alleles (A^4, A^5, A^6, A^9) of the A_b locus, and we will now turn to this extension of our investigation.

The foregoing analysis of the "incorporation" technique has shown that we can determine with the highest precision relative enhanceable plaque numbers in

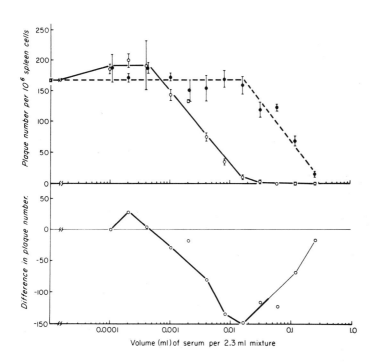

Figure 6A. Enhanceable and inhibitable (direct) plaque-forming cells in the mouse-spleen—effect of RABBIT antisera against mouse immunoglobulins.

Spleen cells were obtained from a mouse of strain C57BL/6J ($\male$, 74 days old). The mouse was injected i.v. with 4×10^8 sheep erythrocytes and was sacrificed four days later. The number of plaques was tested by the incorporation assay with increasing quantities of the anti-mouse γ globulin serum of rabbit origin and with normal rabbit serum.

Top panel:

———o———   plaque number as a function of increasing quantities of anti-mouse γ globulin (antiserum of rabbit origin)

------●------   plaque number as a function of increasing quantities of normal rabbit serum

Bottom panel:

———o———   Difference in plaque number in the presence of antiserum and of normal serum

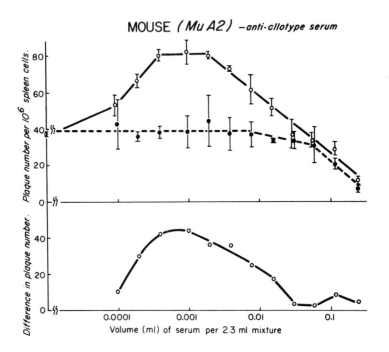

Figure 6B. Enhanceable plaque-forming cells in the mouse spleen—effect of anti-MuA2 serum (from BALB/cJ mice).

Spleen cells were obtained from a mouse of strain C57BL/6J (♂, 68 days old). The mouse was injected i.v. with 4 × 10⁸ sheep erythrocytes on day 0, 3, 7 and 10 and sacrificed on day 14. The number of plaques was tested by the incorporation of quantities of anti-MuA2 serum (from BALB/cJ mice) and of normal BALB/cJ mouse serum.

Top panel:

———○———   Plaque number as a function of increasing quantities of anti-MuA2 serum (from BALB/cJ mice)

------●------   Plaque number as a function of increasing quantities of normal BALB/cJ mouse serum

Bottom panel:

———○———   Difference in plaque number in the presence of antiserum and of normal serum rabbits injected with two doses of sheep red cells and assayed within 6 days after injection. We therefore chose these conditions. We developed plaques with specifically purified anti-allotype antibodies from antisera, which were extensively preabsorbed to remove cross-reactive antibodies.

We determined the total number of enhanceable plaques in animals of genotype A^4/A^5, A^4/A^6, A^4/A^9, A^5/A^6 and A^6/A^9. It will be seen that there is very marked interaction between the genes and that there is a definite dominance with products of A^4 over those of other alleles (Fig. 7). Very pronounced dominance is also observed of A^6 over A^9. Occasionally the gene products are equivalent and this is best illustrated in the case of A^5/A^6.

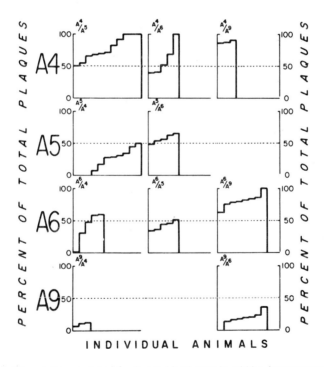

Figure 7. The relative numbers of enhanceable plaques in rabbits, heterozygous at the A_b locus.

Spleen cells from rabbits of allotypic genotype A^4/A^5, A^4/A^6, A^4/A^9, A^5/A^6 and A^6/A^9 were tested. Rabbits received two weekly i.v. injections of 6×10^9 sheep erythrocytes. Cells were obtained six days after the last injection. The number of enhanceable plaques was determined by the incorporation technique and with appropriate specifically-purified antibodies. Vertical bars indicate the percentage of enhanceable plaques of a given allotypic specificity (e.g. for A^4/A^5 the percentage for enhanceable A5 plaques was obtained as enhanceable A5 plaques $\times$ 100/enhanceable A5 + enhanceable A4 plaques).

Allelic exclusion

The individual antibody-forming cells of a heterozygous animal produce immunoglobulins of only one allotypic specificity. In other words, in each individual cell one of the allotypic genes is silent. Is this also the case in the cells of homozygous animals? This can be assessed for plaques formed by "internal" antibody of *low* hemolytic capacity by comparing the output of A4 specificity by plaque-forming cells of A^4/A^4 and A^4/A^5 rabbits. The quantity of "external" antibody which is required for maximal enhancement is clearly related to the output of "internal" antibody. If optimal antibody varies over the same range for plaques from homozygous and heterozygous rabbits, the output of "internal" antibody also lies within the *same range*. Six days after two injections, the optimal quantity was 0.09072 ± 0.032 µg antibody-nitrogen for homozygous plaque-forming cells and 0.0998 ± 0.034 for heterozygous plaque-forming cells (Fig. 8). This is compatible with a 1:1 ratio of cell output. The chance of this ratio being 2:1 is 20%. The quantity of "external" antibody for the upper limit of plaque inhibition was 0.492 ± 0.14 µg N antibody for homozygous and 0.788 ± 0.15 for heterozygous cells. There is a chance of less than 1% that this ratio could be 2:1. We attempted to assess the relative output of homozygous and heterozygous cells by additional criteria. We can examine this question in terms of the relation between plaque numbers and quantity of "external" antibody (incorporation technique) in the zone in which the "external" antibody is in excess, i.e. for amounts which *exceed* that of the optimal "external" antibody. In this range the logarithms of "external" antibody and plaque numbers are linearly related. The slope and the position of this curve reflects the relative proportion of plaque-forming cells which produce different amounts of "internal" antibody. The position of the curve can be defined in terms of the quantity of "external" antibody which reduces to 50% the total plaques visualized in the presence of optimal antibody. In both these respects the plaque-forming cells of homozygous and heterozygous animals were comparable (Table 1). We may conclude that the cell output of cells from heterozygous and homozygous animals is also comparable and, therefore, that *only one gene is active* in antibody-forming cells of homozygous as well as in cells from heterozygous animals.

The silence in A^4/A^5 heterozygotes of one of the two alleles of the light chain specificities is but one instance of what appears to be a general rule for the distribution of these two allotypes and, indeed, for the distribution of all classes of immunoglobulins [14, 15, 24-26]. We are thus faced with the problem of two genes active in the animal, as a whole, but of which only one is expressed by most or all individual antibody-forming cells. In general this has so far been observed with sex-linked gene-products [27-31], but never with products of somatic genes (but see [31] and [32]). It would therefore appear that we should look for a mechanism which does not involve sex-linkage and yet leads to dosage

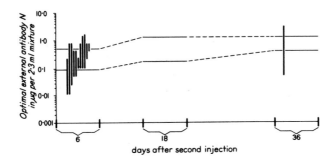

Figure 8. The consumption of "external" antibody by spleen cells from rabbits homozygous at the A_b locus and from animals heterozygous at that locus.

Each vertical bar indicates results from incorporation assays with specifically-purified antibody against A4 and with spleen cells from A^4/A^5 rabbits. All rabbits received two injections with sheep erythrocytes and were tested thereafter at the times shown on the horizontal axis. The lower limit of the vertical bars shows optimal quantity of antibody, the upper limit indicates the quantity of "external" antibody at which plaque inhibition begins to be significant. The lines running from left to right indicate the corresponding quantities determined with cells from homozygous rabbits.

Table 1. Amount of "external" antibody required for inhibition of 50% of plaques.

Designation	Allotype	b	D^E_{50}
329	A^4/A^4	3·12	1·2
344		3·58	5·0
350		2·91	2·5
320	A^4/A^5	1·78	2·6
343		3·25	3·7
314		3·16	4·9

"External" antibody was directed against allotypic specificity A4. Animals received two injections with 6×10^9 red cells and were tested 13 days after the initiating injection. b is the slope of the logarithm of the plaque number as a function of the logarithm of the quantity of "external" antibody. The slope is determined for quantities of "external" antibody in excess of the quantity required for maximal enhancement. D^E_{50} is the amount of "external" antibody (in μg N) required to reduce the maximum number of plaques (in the presence of optimal antibody) by 50%.

compensation. We may perhaps find such a mechanism if there were hetero-geneous, antibody-like but non-induced *receptors* [33-35] on cells. The cells would not release antibody until contact between receptor and antigen initiated exclusive production of antibody which resembles the occupied receptor. This concept of heterogeneous receptors on the pre-committed cell would allow for the formation of more than one type of immunoglobulin if more than one cell receptor were occupied at the same time. Such an event would be rare *in vivo* [36-38], but might occur more frequently *in vitro* [39, 68]. We shall return to the receptor-hypothesis after the presentation of experimental evidence which may encourage the assumption that cell receptors exist and which allows us to define certain broad limits of the properties of these receptors.

CELLS IN THE PRE-PRODUCTIVE STATE

Change in phenotypic expression

Neonatal administration of antibody directed against a particular allotypic specificity prevents the formation of antibody of that allotypic specificity. This occurs in newborn animals which have very few cells able to proceed to antibody formation [10, 40], but have cells which can react with antigen, though this results in tolerance. The animal, at this stage, had no demonstrable circulating autologous immunoglobulins. What then is the target of the passively adminis-tered anti-allotype serum and the mechanism which triggers alteration of phenotype? Are there other known biological processes of this type?

Expression of cell membrane-antigens can be altered by contact with antibody (serotype transformation [41], modulation [42]). Suppression is the only instance of soluble, circulating antigens being thus affected [2, 43-46]. Induction of suppression might resemble modulation [42] and depend on a primary interaction between anti-allotype antibody and a cell of the immune apparatus. One could visualize non-induced antibody molecules, carrying allo-typic specificity, located on the surface of uncommitted cells and capable of combining with antigen or with anti-allotype antibody [1, 2, 23, 33, 35, 47, 48]. Commitment and/or antibody production would be triggered by a signal which emanates after combination between antigen and receptor (non-induced cellbound antibody). On the other hand, suppression would result after com-bination between receptor and anti-allotype antibody. On the basis of this working hypothesis three mechanisms deserve consideration:

1. Complement-mediated death of cells with which anti-allotype antibody has combined [49].
2. Blocking of receptor sites so that antigen cannot combine with them ("blind-folding" [50, 51]) or
3. An "inadequate signal" which follows combination between *receptor* and anti-allotype antibody (rather than antigen) and which would result in abortive and non-productive differentiation [2, 23, 46, 47].

Suppression in the absence of the complete hemolytic complement system

We shall describe experiments designed to test the first of these three pos-
sibilities. To this end, we have used various hybrids which either possess or lack
MuBl [52, 53], the $C'5$ component of complement [54, 55]; animals lacking
MuBl lack the complete hemolytic complement system. All hybrids were

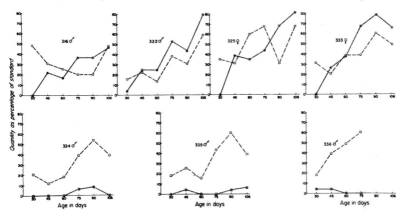

Figure 9. Neonatal injections with anti-MuA2 serum of MuB1-positive hybrids between
MuA2-positive paternal and MuA1-positive maternal animals. Hybrids: NBL/N♂X CBA/J ♀.

Description	Symbol	Allotypic Specificity in serum	
316 ♂ 322 ♂ 325 ♀ 333 ♀	O------------O ●————————●	MuA1 MuA2	Animals not injected at birth
334 ♂ 335 ♂ 336 ♂	□-----------□ ■————————■	MuA1 MuA2	Animals injected at birth with anti-MuA2 serum

offspring of matings between mice homozygous for allotypic specificity MuA2
[56-58] and mice homozygous for MuA1 [56, 59]. Hybrids were neonatally
injected with antibody directed against the allotypic specificity of their male
parent. We shall also describe experiments in which the effect of specific
antibody on a circulating antigen, other than an immunoglobulin, was tested.

In offspring between MuA2-positive fathers and MuA1-positive mothers,
decline of the maternal allotypic specificity extended beyond the 30th day of
life and obscured the early detection of autologously-synthesized immunoglobulin of the same specificity. A subsequent increase in the concentration of
this immunoglobulin may be observed as early as the 45th day of life or as late
as the 90th day of life (broken lines, Fig. 9). On the other hand, the
immunoglobulin carrying the paternal allotypic specificity could be seen to

increase from the 30th day of life and was usually still on the increase when the animal had reached the 100th day of its life (full lines, Fig. 9). Passive administration of anti-MuA2 serum at birth brought about a considerable reduction in the amount of circulating immunoglobulin of MuA2 specificity and this reduction was maintained throughout the period of observation, i.e. up to the 106th day of life, (bottom of Fig. 9). There was no compensatory increase in the concentration of MuA1 (cf. [47, 49]).

The animals used in the above experiments were MuB1-positive. If MuB1-negative hybrids (MuA2-positive fathers and MuA1-positive mothers) were injected at birth with antibody directed against MuA2, suppression of the synthesis of MuA2 was found and persisted up to the 90th day. As in the animals which possessed complement in their circulation, there was no compensatory increase in circulating MuA1 (Fig. 10). This suppression was not only observed with unheated anti-MuA2 sera, which contained MuB1, but also with heated anti-MuA2 sera in which MuB1 was destroyed (Fig. 11).

Clearly, suppression was unaffected by the presence or absence of the complete hemolytic complement system [49].

To test the effect of neonatally-administered antibody, directed against a circulating antigen which was not an immunoglobulin, we injected MuB1-positive offspring of MuB1-negative mothers with antibody against MuB1.

The lack of detectable consequences when MuB1-positive offspring of MuB1-negative mothers were injected with antibody to MuB1 contrasted sharply with the results reported above. Animals were injected with antibody, beginning at twelve hours after birth and continuing up to the 20th day after birth. Concentrations of MuB1 were normal, as early as 10 days after the last injection. This can be seen in Fig. 12 which also shows the marked sex-associated differences in MuB1 concentration, which is in accordance with previous observations [52, 59, 60]. The level of circulating MuB1 in such animals was no more affected by these injections than was that of neonatally-injected MuB1-positive offspring of MuB1-positive parents (Fig. 13).

Suppression reveals a feature in the formation of antibody which is not found in the formation of other proteins released into the blood stream. There was a striking contrast between the long-lasting delay in the appearance of circulating immunoglobulins, carrying an allotypic specificity against which neonatally-injected antibody was directed, and the absence of persisting reduction in MuB1 concentration after exposure to antibody directed against this antigen.

Let us now return to the mechanism whereby suppression may be induced. The assumption that productive-commitment was mediated by receptors (surface-bound allotypic specificity of uncommitted cells), has been invoked in the discussion of allelic exclusion. The involvement of such receptors in suppression may gain support from the dramatic blast-response *in vitro* of lymphoid cells to allotypic antibodies [4, 61-63].

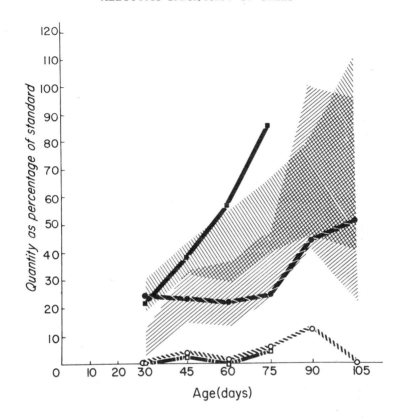

Figure 10. Neonatal injections with anti-MuA2 serum of MuB1-negative hybrids between MuA2-positive paternal and MuA1-positive maternal animals [49]. Hybrids: NBL/N ♂ X DBA/2J ♀.

Designation	Symbol	Allotypic specificity in serum	
346 ♂	○〰〰○ ○▬▬○	MuA2 MuA1	Animals injected at birth with anti-MuA2 serum
347 ♀	□▬▬□ □▬▬□	MuA2 MuA1	
	(hatched box)	MuA2	95% confidence limit of allotype-concentration in nine mice which were not injected at birth
	(hatched box)	MuA1	

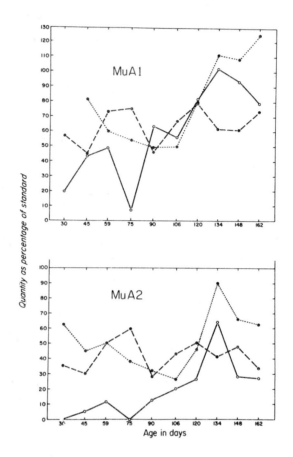

Figure 11. Neonatal injections with anti-MuA2 serum of MuB1-negative hybrids between MuA2-positive paternal and MuA1-positive maternal animals [49].
Hybrids: NBL/N ♂ X DBA/2J ♀.

Designation	Symbol	
		Animal injected at birth with heated (56°C, 1 h) anti-MuA2 serum
374 ♀	○————○	
375 ♀	●•••••••••••	Animals not injected at birth
373 ♂	●------------●	

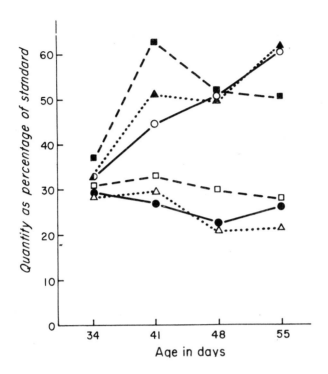

Figure 12. Neonatal injections with MuB1-antiserum of MuB1-positive hybrids between MuA2-positive paternal and MuA1-positive maternal animals [49]. Hybrids: C57BL/6J ♂ X A/J ♀.

Designation	Symbol	Allotypic specificity in serum	
237 ♂	○————○		Animals injected from birth with 0·2 ml MuB1-antiserum daily up to the 20th day of age
240 ♀	●————●	MuB1	
238 ♂	■----------■		Animals not injected at birth
239 ♂	▲··········▲		
241 ♀	□----------□		
242 ♀	△··········△		

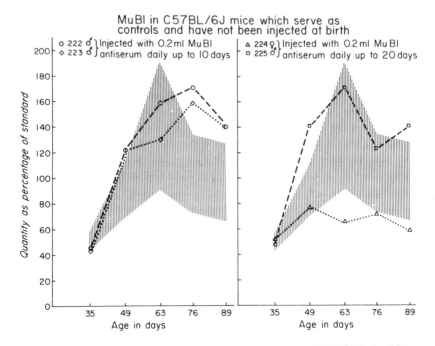

Figure 13. Neonatal injections with MuB1-serum of homozygous (C57BL/6J) mice [49].

Designation	Symbol	Allotypic specificity in serum	
222 ♂	○------------○	}	Animals injected from birth with 0·2 ml MuB1-antiserum, daily, up to the 10th day of age
223 ♂	◇··············◇	} MuB1	
224 ♀	△··············△		Animals injected daily from birth with 0·2 ml MuB1-antiserum up to the 20th day of age
225 ♂	□------------□	}	
	▦		95% confidence limit for relative concentration of MuB1 in eleven mice which were not injected at birth

These experiments certainly show that allotypic specificity resides at or near the surface of some lymphoid cells. They also indicate that the interaction of antibody with these molecules can stimulate differentiation. Is it possible that blast transformation is caused by circulating immunoglobulins which have become attached to cells? Gell and Sell have considered this possibility and have excluded it by showing blast transformation with cells from newborn animals, which lack circulating autologous antibody molecules. Thus, it seems reasonably certain that cells synthesize membrane components with allotypic specificity. Still, there is no evidence that cells which undergo blast-transformation are involved in the antibody-forming process. However, it is difficult to imagine any other function for such cells and it therefore seems reasonable to assume that these cells are pre-productive and that membrane-bound non-induced molecules with allotypic specificity play a part as antigen-receptors. We must next ask ourselves whether it is likely that the synthesis of membrane-components could be inhibited by combination with antibody. In fact, there are two intriguing instances of this type of process and one of these has been observed in the lymphoid system, among thymus cells. We shall return to this cell population when presenting our studies of "Progenitor Cells" and shall confine ourselves here to their antibody-mediated transformation.

We have already mentioned that both the serotype-antigens of *Paramecium* (serotype transformation [41, 64]) and the TL antigens of the thymus (modulation [42]) are known to undergo changes after contact with specific antibody. In these phenomena, as in suppression, the lost antigen is the product of a known gene and in neither case can the loss of antigen be attributed to genetic mutation. Modulation, but not serotype-transformation, resembles suppression in that the loss of the antigen occurs much more quickly than the ultimate re-acquisition of the antigen. We have shown above that suppression does not depend on the complete hemolytic complement system; in this respect, too, suppression resembles modulation [42, 49].

Since cell death, mediated by the complete hemolytic complement system, is not responsible for suppression, it remains to be seen whether "blind-folding" or abortive transformation may play a part in this antibody-induced change of phenotypic expression. At this stage we do not possess the information which would allow us to distinguish between these alternatives or even to assure us of their applicability.

Compensation

We have so far considered the effect of suppression on the directly affected immunoglobulin; we shall now examine the effect on other, non-suppressed, immunoglobulins. In rabbits, the product of the allele of the suppressed immunoglobulin increases, though it does not always reach the serum concentration of homozygous animals (Fig. 14). If the products of both alleles are suppressed, another type of immunoglobulin appears in increased concentration [65]. It is clear that "blind-folding" of pre-productive cells with heterogeneous receptors (multipotential cell), or abortive differentiation of cells with homogeneous receptors, could account for this observation. In the first case, blind-folding would increase the chance of a receptor, other than the blocked one, being occupied by an antigen. In the second case, abortive differentiation would exhaust the supply of one type of pre-productive cell, to be replaced by other types of pre-productive cells.

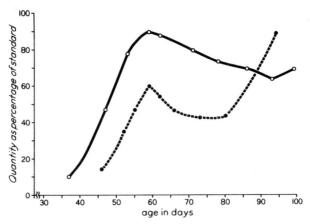

Figure 14. Compensation of allotype concentration in suppressed rabbits.

The same alternatives would be adequate to account for the finding that the suppression of MuA2 does not affect the concentration of MuA1. This allotypic specificity is found on a relatively small proportion of molecules, hence, blind-folding of a multipotential cell would not have a profound effect on the probability of other receptors being occupied by an antigen, nor would the exhaustion of the stem cells of a unipotential cell create a substantial provocation for replacement by other types.

We have thus made the alternatives, stated in the previous page, more precise without being able to decide between them.

PROGENITOR CELLS

We have so far examined the interaction of the genes controlling allotypic specificity in productive cells, and the evidence for allotypic specificity in preproductive cells. We shall now present evidence for cells which are related to these two stages in cell progression and which represent an earlier stage of the cell progression.

Cell transfer experiments

We shall now turn to the identification of the cell populations which are progenitors of cells with allotypic specificity and which are responsible for the ultimate appearance of molecules carrying allotypic specificity in the circulation. This question has been examined in the following way; newborn animals, of a given genotype (say A^4/A^4), were injected with antigen-treated cells from donors whose genotype differed from that of the recipient (say A^5/A^5). When antibody to the antigen could be found in the recipient animals, it was invariably of recipient-type, but we also detected immunoglobulins which were the product of donor cells (Fig. 15). However, the kinetics of the appearance of this donor immunoglobulin differed vastly with the type of cell populations that had been administered to the newborn animals.

The donor allotypic specificity could be observed in most recipients for a period of 4-10 weeks, with a continuous decline in concentration until it escaped detection. The half-life of disappearance, measured by agglutination inhibition, was about 7 days (not corrected for increasing body weight, Fig. 15 I), a half-life quite similar to that found when immunoglobulins were passively transferred [66, 67]. Transfer of different cell populations led to remarkable and significant differences in the frequency with which allogeneic immunoglobulin could be detected and in the quantity of donor allotypic specificity. In 14-day-old rabbits, donor allotype was found in 12/25 animals which had received thymus cells and in 26/26 and 34/35 animals which had been given lymph node cells and mononuclear peritoneal exudate cells, respectively. There was very little donor immunoglobulin if thymus cells had been administered and much more if mononuclear peritoneal exudate cells or lymph node cells had been given (Fig. 16). It thus appeared as if mononuclear peritoneal exudate cells and lymph node cells could produce molecules with allotypic specificity quite soon after injection into the animal, but that this synthetic capacity was being lost after less than two weeks residence of the donor cells in the recipient.

Chimerism

The continuous decline of allotypic specificity of donor type, so far described, was observed in most, but not in all, recipients. In some animals there was a rapid increase of donor allotypic specificity which continued up to the 45th to 60th day of life and finally resulted in a stabilized concentration of the "foreign" allotype which was quite similar to that found in normal heterozygous animals (Fig. 17). The stabilized level was maintained throughout the period of observation. This active synthesis of donor immunoglobulins was most frequently observed in animals which had received thymus cells (Fig. 16), occasionally in animals which had received lymph node cells (Fig. 16), but never in animals which had received mononuclear peritoneal exudate cells. In the case of animals which had received thymus cells, the stabilized concentration was

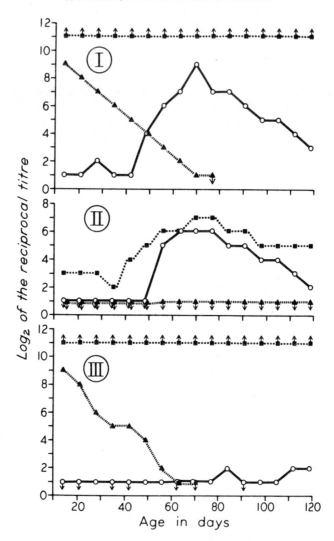

Figure 15. Examination of the cellular origin of the antibody to HA detectable in the serum of a rabbit (No. 2115B) injected with HA, taken up by mononuclear peritoneal exudate cells. I. Titers of antibody to human serum albumin and allotypic specificities in the serum. II. Titers of antibody to human serum albumin and allotypic specificities in the eluate obtained by absorption of serum on cellulose conjugated with HA and elution at pH 3·0. III. Titers of antibody to HA and allotypic specificities in the supernatant after absorption with cellulose conjugated with HA [67].

········■········	Reciprocal titer of the recipient-type allotypic specificity.
········▲········	Reciprocal titer of donor-type allotypic specificity.
———○———	Reciprocal titer of antibody to HA

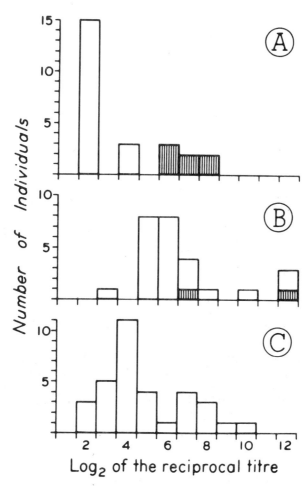

Figure 16. Presence of donor-type allotypic specificity in the sera of 14-day-old rabbits [67]. A. Rabbits injected with thymus cells. B. Rabbits injected with lymph node cells. C. Rabbits injected with mononuclear peritoneal exudate cells. Hatched areas represent individuals in which the donor-type allotypic specificity was present throughout life (chimeras).

close to that of untreated heterozygotes (A^4/A^5) and was 10–20% of this value in animals which had been injected with lymph node cells. The increase in foreign immunoglobulin occurred later in animals which had received lymph node cells and was preceded by a phase in which the molecules of donor allotypic specificity decreased (Fig. 17).

In order to examine the location of donor cells in animals which, though genotypically A^4/A^4, have acquired the capacity to produce immunoglobulins of allotype A5, we transplanted cells from such animals to newborn rabbits of allotype A^4/A^4. The acquired allotypic specificity (A5) could be detected in the recipients when lymph node cells or spleen cells were transferred but not when thymus cells or bone marrow cells were transferred (Table 2).

Table 2. Secondary transfer*

Donor cells	Presence of A5 in the recipient† Cells incubated with		Presence of antibody to HA ‡
	HA	–	
Thymus cells	0/4	0/5	3/4
Lymph node cells	7/10	3/3	9/9
Spleen cells	3/3	–	2/2
Bone marrow cells	0/3	0/4	1/2

* Newborn rabbits of allotype A^4/A^4 were injected with cells from adult donors. The donors were genotypically A^4/A^4 but had acquired the capacity to produce immunoglobulins of allotype A5 as a consequence of neonatal transfer.

† On the 14th day of life.

‡ In newborn animals which received donor cells that which had been incubated with HA.[131]I *in vitro*. Animals were considered as responders if antibody had been formed during the first 35 days of life.

We have thus found that peritoneal exudates and lymph nodes contain cells which can, in a relatively short period of time, produce allotypically-marked molecules but have a relatively short productive life in the body. We have seen that certain thymus cells contain the information which can result in the appearance of allotypic specificities and that the lymph node contains a similar population of cells but clearly in smaller numbers [66, 67].

At present our distinction between progenitor and pre-productive cells is based on the location in the thymus of the progenitor cell. It remains to be seen whether the progenitor cell is sensitive to suppressing anti-allotype antibody. The answer to this question has to await the transfer of thymus cells from suppressed animals.

In summary, we have seen that populations of productive cells can be subdivided in terms of the hemolytic capacity and allotypic specificity of their antibody, that the average cell output of homozygous and heterozygous cells is

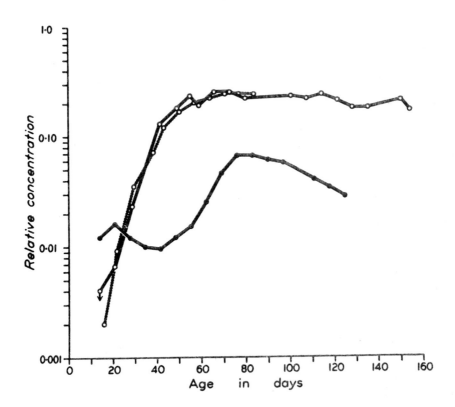

Figure 17. Concentration of donor allotypic protein (immunoglobulin) in the serum of rabbits injected at birth with nucleated cells. Comparison between concentration of allotypic immunoglobulin in chimeric animals and in normal heterozygotes. Allotype of recipient animals was A5 and allotype of donor animals was A4. Allotype concentration was measured by a single diffusion method [67].

——○——	Concentration of allotypic protein of donor type in a rabbit injected at birth with thymus cells.
——●——	Concentration of allotypic protein of donor type in a rabbit injected at birth with lymph node cells.
------○------	Concentration of allotypic immunoglobulin in normal heterozygous animal.

similar, and that there is some interaction between alleles, resulting in a regular numerical dominance of cells making immunoglobulin of certain allotypes over cells making immunoglobulins of another allotypic specificity. Next, we have shown that pre-productive cells are affected by anti-allotype antibody, that this does not depend on the presence of the complete hemolytic complement system, and that this may lead to a compensatory increase of other immuno-globulins when the suppressed allotypic specificity is ubiquitous (A_b locus of the rabbit) but not when it is confined to a narrow section of immunoglobulin (MuA). Finally, we have demonstrated that allotypic specificity can be trans-ferred with thymus cells, which may therefore be regarded to contain progenitors of the pre-productive cells. Such progenitor cells are also found in the lymph nodes, though in smaller numbers.

ACKNOWLEDGEMENT

We wish to thank Mrs. S. W. Koh and Miss P. Javier for their competent and conscientious technical assistance and Dr. C.-Y. Wu for his statistical advice.

This investigation was supported by grants from The Banting Research Foundation, Medical Research Council (MT 832), National Cancer Institute of Canada, Ontario Cancer Treatment and Research Foundation (145) and the Ontario Heart Foundation (1-23).

REFERENCES

1. Chou, C.-T., Cinader, B. and Dubiski, S., *Cold Spring Harb. Symp. quant. Biol.* **32** (1967) 317.
2. Dubiski, S., *Cold Spring Harb. Symp. quant. Biol.* **32** (1967) 311.
3. Gell, P. G. H., *in* "Regulation of the Antibody Response ", (edited by B. Cinader), Charles C. Thomas, Springfield, Ill. 1968. (In press.)
4. Gell, P. G. H., *Cold Spring Harb. Symp. quant. Biol.* **32** (1967) 441.
5. Herzenberg, L. A. and Warner, N. L., *in* "Regulation of the Antibody Response", (edited by B. Cinader), Charles C. Thomas, Springfield, Ill. 1968. (In press.)
6. Mitchison, N. A., *in* "Regulation of the Antibody Response", (edited by B. Cinader), Charles C. Thomas, Springfield, Ill. 1968. (In press.)
7. Osoba, D., *in* "Regulation of the Antibody Response", (edited by B. Cinader), Charles C. Thomas, Springfield, Ill. 1968. (In press.)
8. Potter, M., *in* "Regulation of the Antibody Response", (edited by B. Cinader), Charles C. Thomas, Springfield, Ill. 1968. (In press.)
9. Smithies, O., *Cold Spring Harb. Symp. quant. Biol.* **32** (1967) 161.
10. Šterzl, J. and Silverstein, A. M., *Adv. Immun.* **6** (1967) 337.
11. Till, J. E., McCulloch, E. A., Phillips. R. A. and Siminovitch, L., *Cold Spring Harb. Symp. quant. Biol.* **32** (1967) 461.

12. Wilson, D. B. and Billingham, R. E., *Adv. Immun.* **7** (1967) 189.
13. Bernier, G. M. and Cebra, J. J., *J. Immun.* **95** (1965) 246.
14. Chiappino, G. and Pernis, B., *Pathologia. Microbiol.* **27** (1964) 8.
15. Pernis, B. and Chiappino, G., *Immunology* **7** (1964) 500.
16. Dresser, D. W. and Wortis, H. H., *Nature, Lond.* **208** (1965) 859.
17. Ingraham, J. S., Biegel, A. A. and Todd, C. W., *Fedn Proc. Fedn Am. Socs exp. Biol.* **24** (1965) 180.
18. Šterzl, J. and Říha, I., *Nature, Lond.* **208** (1965) 858.
19. Weiler, E., *Proc. natn. Acad. Sci. U.S.A.* **54** (1965) 1765.
20. Weiler, E., Melletz, E. W. and Breuninger-Peck, E., *Proc. natn. Acad. Sci. U.S.A.* **54** (1965) 1310.
21. Říha, I., *Folia microbiol, Praha* **9** (1964) 304.
22. Dray, S. and Nisonoff, A., *Proc. Soc. exp. Biol. Med.* **113** (1963) 20.
23. Chou, C.-T., Cinader, B. and Dubiski, S., *Int. Archs Allergy appl. Immun.* **32** (1967) 583.
24. Bernier, G. M. and Cebra, J. J., *Science, N.Y.* **144** (1964) 1590.
25. Pernis, B., Chiappino, G., Kelus, A. S. and Gell, P. G. H., *J. exp. Med.* **122** (1965) 853.
26. Mellors, R. C. and Korngold, L., *J. exp. Med.* **118** (1963) 387.
27. Lyon, M. F., *Am. J. hum. Genet.* **14** (1962) 135.
28. Davidson, R. G., Nitowski, H. M. and Childs, B., *Proc. natn. Acad. Sci. U.S.A.* **50** (1963) 481.
29. Beutler, E., *Cold Spring Harb. Symp. quant. Biol.* **29** (1964) 261.
30. Demars, R. and Nance, W. E., *in* "Retention of Functional Differentiation in Cultured Cells", Wistar Institute Symposium Monograph. No. 1, (edited by V. Defendi), Wistar Institute Press, Philadelphia, 1964, p. 35.
31. Grüneberg, H., *Ann. hum. Genet.* **30** (1967) 239.
32. Fudenberg, H. H. and Hirschhorn, K., *Science, N.Y.* **145** (1964) 611.
33. Braun, W. and Cohen, E. P., *in* "Regulation of the Antibody Response", (edited by B. Cinader), Charles C. Thomas, Springfield, Ill. 1968. (In press.)
34. Cinader, B., *in* "Regulation of the Antibody Response", (edited by B. Cinader), Charles C. Thomas, Springfield, Ill. 1968. (In press.)
35. Yoshimura, M. and Cinader, B., *J. Immun.* **97** (1966) 959.
36. Attardi, G., Cohn, M., Horibata, K. and Lennox, E. S., *J. Immun.* **92** (1964) 346.
37. Attardi, G., Cohn, M., Horibata, K. and Lennox, E. S., *J. Immun.* **93** (1964) 94.
38. Mäkelä, O., *Cold Spring Harb. Symp. quant. Biol.* **32** (1967) 423.
39. Fahey, J. L. and Finegold, I., *Cold Spring Harb. Symp. quant. Biol.* **32** (1967) 283.
40. Šterzl, J., *Cold Spring Harb. Symp. quant. Biol.* **32** (1967) 493.
41. Beale, G. H., *Int. Rev. Cytol.* **6** (1957) 1.
42. Old, L. J., Stockert, E., Boyse, E. A. and Kim, J. H., *J. exp. Med.* **127** (1968) 523.
43. Dray, S., *Nature, Lond.* **195** (1962) 677.
44. Mage, R. and Dray, S., *J. Immun.* **95** (1965) 525.
45. Mage, R., Young, G. O. and Dray, S., *J. Immun.* **98** (1967) 502.
46. Dubiski, S., *in* "Regulation of the Antibody Response", (edited by B. Cinader), Charles C. Thomas, Springfield, Ill. 1968. (In press.)

47. Herzenberg, L. A., Goodlin, R. C. and Rivera, E. C., *J. exp. Med.* **126** (1967) 701.
48. Eisen, H. N., Little, J. R., Osterland, C. K. and Simms, E. S., *Cold Spring Harb. Symp. quant. Biol.* **32** (1967) 75.
49. Cinader, B. and Dubiski, S., *J. Immun.* **101** (1968) 1236.
50. Levey, R. H. and Medawar, P. B., *Ann. N.Y. Acad. Sci.* **129** (1966) 164.
51. Levey, R. H. and Medawar, P. B., *Proc. natn. Acad. Sci. U.S.A.* **56** (1966) 1130.
52. Cinader, B., Dubiski, S. and Wardlaw, A. C., *J. exp. Med.* **120** (1964) 897.
53. Cinader, B., Dubiski, S., and Wardlaw, A. C., *in* "Studies in Rheumatoid Diseases", Proceedings of the Third Canadian Conference on Research in the Rheumatic Diseases, University of Toronto Press, Toronto, 1966, p. 202.
54. Nilsson, U. R. and Müller-Eberhard, H. J., *J. exp. Med.* **125** (1967) 1.
55. Müller-Eberhard, H. J., *Adv. Immun.* **8** (1968) 2.
56. Dubiski, S. and Cinader, B., *Nature, Lond.* **197** (1963) 705.
57. Dubiski, S. and Cinader, B., *Can. J. Biochem. Physiol.* **41** (1963) 1311.
58. Kelus, A. and Moor-Jankowski, J. K., *Nature, Lond.* **191** (1961) 1405.
59. Dubiski, S. and Cinader, B., *Proc. Soc. exp. Biol. Med.* **122** (1966) 775.
60. Urbach, G. and Cinader, B., *Proc. Soc. exp. Biol. Med.* **122** (1966) 779.
61. Sell, S. and Gell, P. G. H., *J. exp. Med.* **122** (1965) 423.
62. Gell, P. G. H. and Sell, S., *J. exp. Med.* **122** (1965) 813.
63. Sell, S. and Gell, P. G. H., *J. exp. Med.* **122** (1965) 923.
64. Finger, I., *in* "The Control of Nuclear Activity", (edited by L. Goldstein), Prentice-Hall Inc., Englewood Cliffs, N.J., 1967, p. 378.
65. Dubiski, S., *Nature, Lond.* **214** (1967) 1365.
66. Chou, C.-T., Dubiski, S. and Cinader, B., *Nature, Lond.* **211** (1966) 34.
67. Chou, C.-T., Dubiski, S. and Cinader, B., *J. exp. Med.* **126** (1967) 305.
68. Kamei, H. and Moore, G. E., *Nature, Lond.* **215** (1967) 860.

FEBS Symposium, Volume 15, 1969, pp. 169-175

The N-terminal Amino Acid Sequence in a
κ-type Mouse Light Chain

F. MELCHERS

The Salk Institute for Biological Studies, La Jolla, California, U.S.A.
and Max-Planck-Institut für Molekulare Genetik, Berlin, Germany*

Amino acid sequence analysis of human and mouse light chains have revealed two main structural characteristics:

1. Among light chains of a given type (e.g. κ) the N-terminal half of the polypeptide chain is variable, while the C-terminal half is invariable [1].
2. Among light chains of a given type, there seem to be subtypes [2, 3]. For κ-type mouse light chains, two subtypes $κ_I$ and $κ_{II}$ have been proposed [3]. But three subtypes $κ_I$, $κ_{II}$ and $κ_{III}$ have been suggested for human κ light chains.

We suggest that the light chain of MOPC46 is also an example of a third mouse subtype. We report the N-terminal sequence to residue 39 of the κ-type light chain produced by the plasma cell tumor MOPC46 in Balb/c-mice (M. Potter, NIH, Bethesda, Md., U.S.A.). Carbohydrate has been found in this light chain [4] attached covalently to residue 28. Moreover, the sequence of this N-terminal region suggests this light chain is not of subtype $κ_I$ or $κ_{II}$.

RESULTS

Light chain protein, precipitated from urine of MOPC46-plasma cell-tumor bearing Balb/c-mice by adding $(NH_4)_2SO_4$ to 70% saturation, showed electrophoretic heterogeneity in starch gels. One set of three bands and another of five bands could be detected (Fig. 1).

By gel filtration on Sephadex G-100 and ultracentrifugation, the first set of bands was shown to be light chain monomers, while the second proved to be dimers, all of them being serologically indistinguishable from each other. Purification of the light chain protein by column chromatography on DEAE-cellulose resulted in a separation of the various monomeric and dimeric forms (Fig. 1). Analysis of the purified bands showed them to have the same amino acid composition and revealed, surprisingly, carbohydrate. The monomer forms

* Present address

169

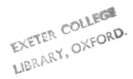

I, II, and III (Fig. 1), all contained the following residues per mole of light chain: 4 mannoses, 4 galactoses, 2 fucoses, and 6 glucosamines. The bands differ in their content of N-glycolyl-neuraminic acid, band III having 2, band II 1, and band I no sialic acid residues per mole of light chain. Furthermore, it was shown that the five dimeric forms of the light chain were composed of each of the possible combinations of the three monomeric forms.

These results made it very probable that the heterogeneity of MOPC46 light chain in electrophoresis and chromatography was due solely to a different content of sialic acid.

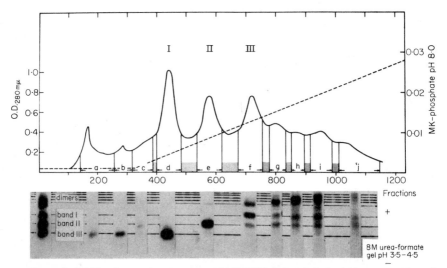

Figure 1. Purification and separation of MOPC46 light chain by chromatography of 3600 OD$_{280m\mu}$-Units MOPC46 protein on a 4·5 × 109 cm DEAE-cellulose column using a linear gradient of 0·001 M to 0·04 M K-phosphate-buffer, pH 8·0. Electrophoresis was performed in 8 M Urea-formate starch gels [5].

Further structural studies were carried out to determine whether all carbohydrate, including the sialic acids, is attached at a single residue of the polypeptide chain and, if so, to identify this residue and its position.

Digestion of a mixture of all the monomeric and dimeric forms of the light chain with trypsin yielded 3 glycopeptides T_I, T_{II}, and T_{III} (Fig. 2). Digestion with chymotrypsin gave 3 glycopeptides C_I, C_{II}, and C_{III}. Isolated monomeric forms of the light chain band I, II or III gave only one tryptic glycopeptide, T_I, T_{II} or T_{III}, or one chymotryptic peptide, C_I, C_{II} or C_{III}. The three glycopeptides all have the same amino acid composition, contain 4 mannose, 4 galactose, 2 fucose, and 6 glucosamine residues per mole, and differ in their content of N-glycolyl-neuraminic acid. T_{III} had 2, T_{II} had 1, and T_I had no sialic acid residues. These results show that all carbohydrate found in MOPC46 light chain is attached to the glycopeptides T_I, T_{II}, and T_{III}. They make it seem likely that all carbohydrate is attached at a single residue position of the polypeptide chain and that the sialic acid causing the electrophoretic and chromatographic heterogeneity of the light chain is bound to this carbohydrate group.

The amino acid composition of the glycopeptides is such as to indicate that they do not come from the invariable half of a κ-type mouse light chain [7]. From the analyses and homologies with other light chains we furthermore

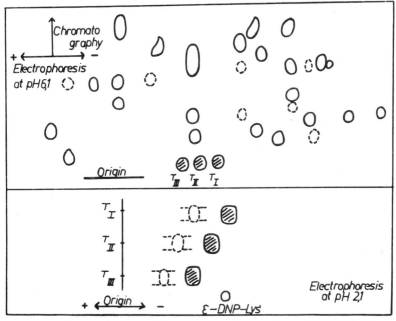

Figure 2. Separation of the tryptic peptides of aminoethylated MOPC46 light chain (mixture of all monomeric and dimeric forms) by ascending chromatography [6] and electrophoresis at pH 6·1 (pyridine/acetic acid/H$_2$O, 10:1:69, v/v/v). The glycopeptides are marked T_I, T_{II}, T_{III}.

suspected them to be localized between positions 22 and 39 of the variable portion of κ-type mouse light chains (numbering of mouse 41 [7]). The actual N-terminal amino acid sequence of MOPC46 light chain (Fig. 3) was established as follows:

1. The mixture of all monomeric and dimeric forms of the light chain was subjected to Edman-degradation for 13 steps. The yields of the first four PTH-amino acids (Asp 93%, Ile 88%, Val 87%, Leu 80%) indicated that the mixture, although electrophoretically and chromatographically heterogeneous, had the same N-terminal end.

2. A peptide (N_t) was obtained from tryptic digests of the light chain protein. Analysis of its N-terminus and of its 4 chymotryptic peptides

(CN$_t$ 1-4) proved it to be the N-terminal peptide of MOPC46 light chain from positions 1-24.

3. Peptide CN$_t$4, Ser-AECys-Arg, is the overlapping peptide between the N-terminus N$_t$ and the three chymotryptic glycopeptides C$_I$, C$_{II}$, C$_{III}$, for C$_I$, C$_{II}$ and C$_{III}$ upon digestion with trypsin yielded the peptide (TC$_{1 (I-III)}$) Ser-AECys-Arg.

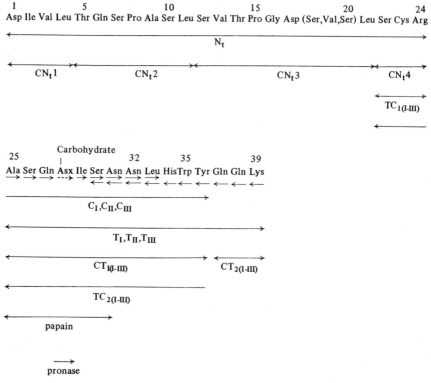

Figure 3. The elucidation of the N-terminal amino acid sequence of MOPC46 light chain. Between arrows are peptides obtained by the various enzymic digestions: → represent Edman-degradation steps, ← Carboxypeptidase B digestion.

4. Digestions with exopeptidases, pronase and papain, and Edman-degradations of the three tryptic glycopeptides T$_I$, T$_{II}$, and T$_{III}$, established the amino acid sequence around the attachment point of carbohydrate at position 28. The results are summarized in Fig. 3.

In these sequence determinations several unusual reactions were observed with these glycopeptides:

1. Trypsin does not cleave the peptide bond followed by the carboxyl group of AECys at position 23.

2. Chymotrypsin does not hydrolyse the peptide bond followed by the carboxyl group of Leu at position 33.

3. Aminopeptidase does not cleave the tryptic glycopeptides T_I, T_{II}, and T_{III}.

4. Edman-degradations of glycopeptide T_I proceeded without difficulty as far as Leu at position 33, but only to Gln at position 27 for glycopeptides T_{II} or T_{III}. When the sialic acid was removed from T_{II} and T_{III} by neuraminidase, Edman-degradation proceeded down to Leu at position 33. No explanation can be given as to why the glycopeptides containing sialic acid are resistant to Edman-degradation at the point of carbohydrate attachment.

5. Carboxypeptidase A cleaves glycopeptides T_I, T_{II}, and T_{III} to single amino acids within two hours, although this is unexpected because of the C-terminal basic amino acid.

6. Carboxypeptidase B cleaves off the carboxyterminal Lys, as expected, but then degrades T_I, T_{II}, and T_{III} further from the carboxyterminal end as far as Ser at position 30. By this additional activity of the enzyme on the tryptic glycopeptides, His could be placed between Leu and Trp-Tyr at position 34.

By repeated pronase digestion of T_I, T_{II}, and T_{III}, Asp or Asn was found as the amino acid to which carbohydrate is attached. By analysis of the fragments obtained from papain digestion of T_I, T_{II}, and T_{III}, this attachment point could be localized at position 28.

CONCLUSIONS

Our studies with the light chain produced by the plasma cell tumor MOPC46 have shown that this protein contains carbohydrate. Its heterogeneity observed in electrophoresis and chromatography can be explained by a difference in the number of N-glycolyl-neuraminic acid residues attached to the carbohydrate group. Three glycopeptides are obtained, each from tryptic or chymotryptic digestion of the light chain. All of the three glycopeptides have the same amino acid sequence, the same hexose- and hexosamine-content and differ only in their content of sialic acid. The carbohydrate group is attached covalently, probably as an N-glycoside and via N-acetyl-glucosamine, to Asn or Asp at position 28 of the N-terminal portion of the light chain. It should be noted that a high degree of variability has been observed in this part of the variable region of κ-type light chains [8].

The amino acid sequence published here corrects one published earlier [9]. It agrees well with data published by Coleman and co-workers [10] and supports a hypothesis by Neuberger and Marshall [11] suggesting that Asn-X-$\frac{Ser}{Thr}$ is the amino acid sequence recognized by the enzyme which attaches the "first" N-acetyl-glucosamine residue in the carbohydrate group. X may be any amino acid.

Comparison with two other κ-type light chains in Balb/c-mice (Fig. 4) reveals that MOPC46 light chain has an N-terminal sequence similar to mouse 70, a characteristic feature of the proposed κ_I-subtype, while it has the same deletion of 4 amino acids next to position 28 as mouse 41, a characteristic feature of the κ_{II}-subtype. The amino acid sequence of MOPC46 light chain, on the other hand, shows that it cannot be the product of a gene originated by a crossover between the proposed κ_I- and κ_{II}-subtype genes. We suggest rather that it may represent a third subtype κ_{III} in mouse, as has been proposed for human κ-type light chains [2].

		1	5	10	15	20	25
κ_I	M 41	Asp Ile Gln Met Thr Gln Ser Pro Ser Ser Leu Ser Ala Ser Leu Gly Glu Arg Val Ser Leu Thr Cys Arg Ala					
κ_{II}	M 70	Asp Ile Val Leu Thr Gln Ser Pro Ala Ser Leu Ala Val Ser Leu Gly Gln Arg Ala Thr Ile Ser Cys Arg Ala					
	M 46	Asp Ile Val Leu Thr Gln Ser Pro Ala Ser Leu Ser Val Thr Pro Gly Asp(Ser,Val,Ser)Leu Ser Cys Arg Ala					

	30	35
M 41	Ser Gln - - - - - - - - - - - - Asx Ile Gly Ser Leu Ser Asx Trp Leu Glx Glx Gly	
	28a b c d e 30	
M 70	Ser Glu Ser Val Asx Asx Ser Gly Ile Ser Phe Met Asn(Trp,Phe,Glx)Glx Lys	
	Carbohydrate	
M 46	Ser Gln - - - - - - - - - - - Asx Ile Ser Asn Asn Leu His Trp Tyr Gln Gln Lys	

M 41 and M 70 from Gray, Dreyer and Hood [7].

	1	5	10	15	20
I	Asp Ile Gln Met Thr Gln Ser Pro Ser Ser Leu Ser Ala Ser Val Gly Asp Arg Val Thr Ile Thr Cys Gln				
II	Asp Ile Val Leu Thr Gln Ser Pro Leu Ser Leu Pro Val Thr Pro Gly Glu Pro Ala Ser Ile Ser Cys Arg				
III	Glu Ile Val Leu Thr Gln Ser Pro Gly Thr Leu Ser Leu Ser Pro Gly Glu Arg Ala Thr Leu Ser Cys Arg				

I, II, III from Milstein [2].

Figure 4. Comparison of the N-terminal amino acid sequence of MOPC46 light chain to other known sequences of mouse and human κ-type light chains.

ACKNOWLEDGEMENT

This work was supported by U.S. Public Health Service Grant No. AI-06544 to Dr. E. S. Lennox.

REFERENCES

1. Hilschmann, N. and Craig, L. C., *Proc. natn. Acad. Sci. U.S.A.* **53** (1965) 1403.
2. Milstein, C., *Nature, Lond.* **216** (1967) 331.
3. Hood, L., Gray, W. R., Sanders, B. G. and Dreyer, W. J., *Cold Spring Harb. Symp. quant. Biol.* **32** (1967) 133.
4. Melchers, F., Lennox, E. S. and Facon, M., *Biochem. biophys. Res. Commun.* **24** (1966) 244.

5. Edelman, G. M. and Poulik, M. D., *J. exp. Med.* **113** (1961) 861.
6. Weigert, M. G. and Garen, A., *J. molec. Biol.* **12** (1965) 448.
7. Gray, W. R., Dreyer, W. J. and Hood, L., *Science, N.Y.* **155** (1967) 465.
8. Putnam, F. W., Titani, K., Wikler, M. and Shinoda, T., *Cold Spring Harb. Symp. quant. Biol.* **32** (1967) 9.
9. Melchers, F. and Knopf, P. M., *Cold Spring Harb. Symp. quant. Biol.* **32** (1967) 255.
10. Coleman, T. J., Marshall, R. D. and Potter, M., *Biochim. biophys. Acta* **147** (1967) 396.
11. Neuberger, A. and Marshall, R. D., *in* "Symposium on Foods, Carbohydrates and their Roles", The Avi Publishing Co. Inc., Westport, Connecticut, 1968.

FEBS Symposium, Volume 15, 1969, pp. 177-182

Sequence Studies on a γ4 Immunoglobulin Chain

J. R. L. PINK and C. MILSTEIN

M.R.C. Laboratory of Molecular Biology, Cambridge, England

The sequence around the half cystine of the Fd fragment of heavy chains involved in binding the light chains has been shown to be identical in several γ1 heavy chains but to differ in a γ4 chain (Vin)* and a μ chain [1]. In fact, the difference between the γ4 and the γ1 sequences seemed so great that we decided to carry out more extensive amino acid sequence studies on the γ4 chain of protein Vin. More recent studies, discussed in another paper in this symposium [3], have shown that the interchain bridges of different human γ chains are especially characteristic of each class of chain. In this paper we report some results of the sequence studies on γ4 chain Vin, and compare it with other heavy chains. This comparison indicates that, so far, the greatest differences between γ1 and γ4 chains (apart from the interchain bridges) occur at the N-terminal section of the Fd fragment. The portions of the Fc fragment investigated are extremely similar to known segments of the γ1 chains.

Vin heavy chain contains approximately 26 lysine and 13 arginine residues, 11 cysteines and 5 methionines, in a total of 450 residues. From a tryptic digest of the totally carboxymethylated heavy chain, peptides accounting for 20 of the lysines and 10 of the arginines have been isolated. These include peptides accounting for 11 unique cysteine sequences [4, 5]. Most of these peptides have been assigned to cyanogen bromide fragments obtained from the intact molecule. The cyanogen bromide products were separated on Sephadex G-100 in 6 M urea, 0.2 M formic acid, giving the profile shown in Fig. 1. Figure 2 shows the positions of cyanogen bromide cleavages and the probable positions of disulphide bridges in Vin [5].

Fraction CB5 (Fig. 1) contained an 18-residue peptide, CB5a, derived from the C-terminal end of the heavy chain; it was identical in composition to C-terminal fragments previously obtained from other γ4 chains by Prahl [6]. CB5 also contained a 16-residue peptide, CB5b, whose composition and N-terminus suggest that it is derived from the N-terminal end of Vin λ light

---

*Contrary to previous results (see [1]), protein Vin has now been shown to be an IgG4 protein, both by chemical [2], and antigenic (kindly performed by E. C. Franklin and by H. G. Kunkel) typing.

chains. CB5b is aligned to give maximum homology with the N-terminus of another λ light chain (protein X) [7] in Table 1.

Fractions CB4 and CB3 were identified (by characterization of their Ccm peptides) as being derived from the Fc region of the molecule. CB4 is, roughly, the C-terminal half of the Fc fragment, and CB3 its N-terminal portion (see Fig. 2). Each fragment contains a single disulphide bridge. The peak CB2 contains the

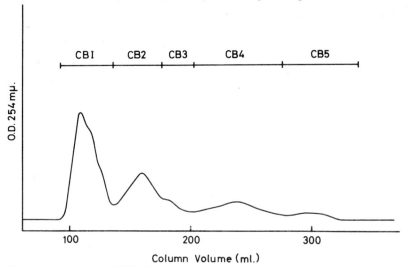

Figure 1. Separation of CNBr fragments of protein Vin (on Sephadex G-100 in 6 M urea, 0·2 M formic acid).

four Ccm residues of the Fc fragment, and probably includes an unsplit methionine residue.

Peak CB1 corresponds roughly to an Fab fragment. On reduction and carboxymethylation of CB1, three fragments were obtained and were separated on Sephadex G-100 in 5% formic acid. One large aggregating fragment, CB1a,

Table 1. The N-terminal portion, CB5b, of Vin λ chain compared with another λ chain (protein X) [7].

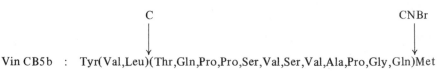

Positions of chymotryptic and cyanogen bromide cleavage in protein Vin are indicated by letters C and CNBr. Residues within the brackets are arranged to give maximum homology with protein X.

corresponds to the cyanogen bromide Fd-like fragment of the heavy chain; it was obtained almost free of light chains by a second run on Sephadex G-100 in 0·5% formic acid. A second peak, CB1b, was a large fragment from the light chain, and a third small fragment, CB1c, was derived from the N-terminus of the heavy chain. Both CB1c and the heavy chain have N-terminal Glx. We have been able to find only five fragments in good yield from the heavy chain, although it contains five methionines. A theoretical sixth fragment should be produced, but was not found, perhaps because cyanogen bromide cleavage at one methionine is very inefficient.

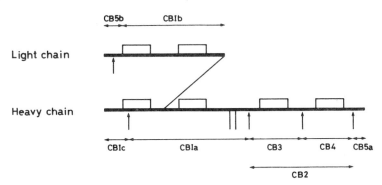

Figure 2. Positions of CNBr splits (↑) in protein Vin half-molecule. Vin heavy chain probably contains five methionines, but positions of only four cleavage points have been established. The positions of the half-cystine residues in fragment CB1a are assigned on the basis of comparison with light chains, or with rabbit IgG [19].

Fragment CB1c was 34 residues long and was similar to fragments obtained from a γ1 protein (Daw) by Piggot and Press [8], and from rabbit IgG by Wilkinson [9]. Its N-terminus is not blocked, whereas most immunoglobulin heavy chains studied so far have had Pca as the N-terminus. The sequences of fragments from Vin and Daw are compared in Table 2. There are a large number of differences between the two fragments, especially when considered at the nucleotide level; 9 (underlined in Table 2) of the 19 amino acid substitutions correspond to double base changes. (The change from Pca to Glu at the N-terminal position is counted as a single base substitution.)

Does this degree of difference between γ1 and γ4 proteins also exist between their respective Fc fragments? Some of the tryptic peptides obtained from the intact heavy chain of Vin were shown to be present in the "Fc-like" cyanogen bromide fragment CB2. They could be aligned by comparison with rabbit Fc fragment [10] (see Table 3). The alignment is partly confirmed by the isolation of peptic overlap peptides derived from cleavages shown in Table 3. The Fc fragments of rabbit, γ1, and γ4 are clearly very similar.

This sequence contains the Gm a⁻-like peptide of γ4 proteins described by

Frangione *et al.* [11]. We believe the γ4 sequence in this region differs from the corresponding γ1 Gm a⁻ sequence by a single amino acid substitution (Arg → Gln at position 92), since we have isolated the Gm-specific peptide from a γ1 Gm a⁻ protein (the heavy chain disease protein Cra) and shown it to have the sequence Glu-Glu-Met-Thr-Lys (Table 3). In addition, Waxdal *et al.* [12] have reported a similar sequence from another γ1 Gm a⁻ protein (Eu).

Our γ1 Gm a⁻ sequence and that of Waxdal *et al.* differ from the Gm a⁻ sequence Met-Glu-Glu-Thr-Lys (not included in Table 3) proposed by Thorpe

Table 2. N-terminal sequence of a γ4 and a γ1 Ig chain.

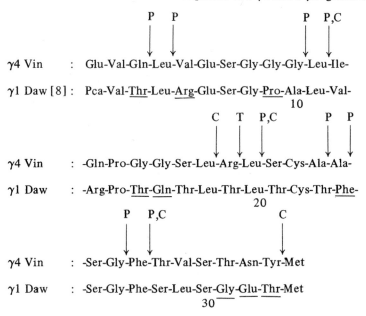

Positions of chymotryptic, peptic, and tryptic cleavage in protein Vin are indicated by letters C, P and T, respectively. Pca is pyrrolidone carboxylic acid.

and Deutsch [13]. These authors also reported a Gm a+ sequence (Table 3); this differs by four base changes from their Gm a⁻ sequence, but by only two base changes from our γ1 Gm a⁻ sequence and that of Waxdal *et al.* (Table 3).

The number of differences between γ1 Gm a⁻ chains and γ4 chains in the Fc region (cyanogen bromide fragments CB2 and CB5a) is small—so far only 5 amino acid substitutions out of 64 positions, none of which are double base changes. (The data on γ1 chains are derived from refs. 12-15.) This is in sharp contrast to the comparison of the 34 residue N-terminal fragments of Daw (γ1) and Vin (γ4) (Table 2). These are almost as different as are κ and λ chains in their N-terminal portions. In fact, the Daw (γ1) fragment is more like the rabbit (Aal allotype) fragment [9] than the Vin (γ4) fragment.

Lennox and Cohn [16] have proposed that different classes of heavy chain may share the same germ-line variable gene, but the results discussed above make

Table 3. Sequences of portions of the Fc fragment.

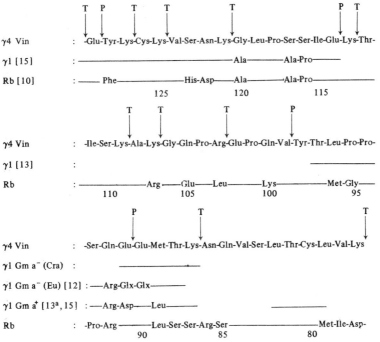

Positions of peptic and tryptic cleavage in protein Vin are indicated by letters P and T, respectively. The alignment of peptides in this chain is based partly on a comparison with the rabbit Fc sequence (Rb). Residues are numbered from the C-terminal end of the chain.

ª The γ1Gm a⁻ sequence reported by these authors [13] is not included, for reasons discussed in the text.

it unlikely that Vin and Daw N-terminal sections are in fact derived from the same germ-line gene. It is, however, not excluded that a pool of genes coding for the variable sections may be shared by the different types of heavy chains. Such pools of variable region genes seem to be involved in the variability of κ chains [17, 18], but the λ chains do not share the same pool. It is hoped that further studies on γ4 chains will help to solve this problem.

REFERENCES

1. Pink, J. R. L. and Milstein, C., *Nature, Lond.* **214** (1967) 92.
2. Frangione, B., Milstein, C. and Franklin, E. C., *Fedn Proc. Fedn Am. Socs exp. Biol.* **27** (1968) 559.
3. Milstein, C., this volume, p. 43.
4. Pink, J. R. L. and Milstein, C., *Nature, Lond.* **216** (1967) 941.
5. Milstein, C., Frangione, B. and Pink, J. R. L., *Cold Spring Harb. Symp. quant. Biol.* **32** (1967) 31.
6. Prahl, J. W., *Biochem. J.* **105** (1967) 1019.
7. Cohen, S. and Milstein, C., *Adv. Immun.* **7** (1967) 1.
8. Piggot, P. J. and Press, E. M., *Biochem. J.* **104** (1967) 616.
9. Wilkinson, J. M., this volume, p. 183.
10. Hill, R. L., Delaney, R., Fellows, R. E. and Lebovitz, H. E., *Proc. natn. Acad. Sci. U.S.A.* **56** (1966) 1762.
11. Frangione, B., Franklin, E. C., Fudenberg, H. H. and Koshland, M. E., *J. exp. Med.* **124** (1966) 715.
12. Waxdal, M. J., Konigsberg, W. H. and Edelman, G. M., *Biochemistry, N.Y.* **7** (1968) 1967.
13. Thorpe, N. O. and Deutsch, H. F., *Immunochemistry* **3** (1966) 329.
14. Press, E. M., Piggot, P. J. and Porter, R. R., *Biochem. J.* **99** (1966) 356.
15. Frangione, B., Milstein, C. and Franklin, E. C., *Biochem. J.* **106** (1968) 15.
16. Lennox, E. S. and Cohn, M., *A. Rev. Biochem.* **36** (1967) 365.
17. Hood, L., Gray, W. R., Sanders, B. G. and Dreyer, W. J., *Cold Spring Harb. Symp. quant. Biol.* **32** (1967) 133.
18. Milstein, C., *Nature, Lond.* **216** (1967) 5113.
19. Cebra, J. J., Steiner, L. A. and Porter, R. R., *Biochem. J.* **107** (1968) 79.

and Vin (γ4) (Table 2). These are almost as different as are κ and λ chains in their N-terminal portions. In fact, the Daw (γ1) fragment is more like the rabbit (Aal allotype) fragment [9] than the Vin (γ4) fragment.

Lennox and Cohn [16] have proposed that different classes of heavy chain may share the same germ-line variable gene, but the results discussed above make

Table 3. Sequences of portions of the Fc fragment.

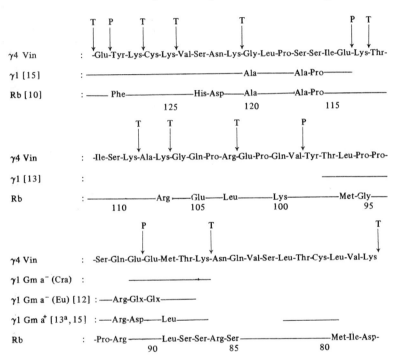

Positions of peptic and tryptic cleavage in protein Vin are indicated by letters P and T, respectively. The alignment of peptides in this chain is based partly on a comparison with the rabbit Fc sequence (Rb). Residues are numbered from the C-terminal end of the chain.

[a] The γ1Gm a⁻ sequence reported by these authors [13] is not included, for reasons discussed in the text.

it unlikely that Vin and Daw N-terminal sections are in fact derived from the same germ-line gene. It is, however, not excluded that a pool of genes coding for the variable sections may be shared by the different types of heavy chains. Such pools of variable region genes seem to be involved in the variability of κ chains [17, 18], but the λ chains do not share the same pool. It is hoped that further studies on γ4 chains will help to solve this problem.

REFERENCES

1. Pink, J. R. L. and Milstein, C., *Nature, Lond.* **214** (1967) 92.
2. Frangione, B., Milstein, C. and Franklin, E. C., *Fedn Proc. Fedn Am. Socs exp. Biol.* **27** (1968) 559.
3. Milstein, C., this volume, p. 43.
4. Pink, J. R. L. and Milstein, C., *Nature, Lond.* **216** (1967) 941.
5. Milstein, C., Frangione, B. and Pink, J. R. L., *Cold Spring Harb. Symp. quant. Biol.* **32** (1967) 31.
6. Prahl, J. W., *Biochem. J.* **105** (1967) 1019.
7. Cohen, S. and Milstein, C., *Adv. Immun.* **7** (1967) 1.
8. Piggot, P. J. and Press, E. M., *Biochem. J.* **104** (1967) 616.
9. Wilkinson, J. M., this volume, p. 183.
10. Hill, R. L., Delaney, R., Fellows, R. E. and Lebovitz, H. E., *Proc. natn. Acad. Sci. U.S.A.* **56** (1966) 1762.
11. Frangione, B., Franklin, E. C., Fudenberg, H. H. and Koshland, M. E., *J. exp. Med.* **124** (1966) 715.
12. Waxdal, M. J., Konigsberg, W. H. and Edelman, G. M., *Biochemistry, N.Y.* **7** (1968) 1967.
13. Thorpe, N. O. and Deutsch, H. F., *Immunochemistry* **3** (1966) 329.
14. Press, E. M., Piggot, P. J. and Porter, R. R., *Biochem. J.* **99** (1966) 356.
15. Frangione, B., Milstein, C. and Franklin, E. C., *Biochem. J.* **106** (1968) 15.
16. Lennox, E. S. and Cohn, M., *A. Rev. Biochem.* **36** (1967) 365.
17. Hood, L., Gray, W. R., Sanders, B. G. and Dreyer, W. J., *Cold Spring Harb. Symp. quant. Biol.* **32** (1967) 133.
18. Milstein, C., *Nature, Lond.* **216** (1967) 5113.
19. Cebra, J. J., Steiner, L. A. and Porter, R. R., *Biochem. J.* **107** (1968) 79.

FEBS Symposium, Volume 15, 1969, pp. 183-186

N-terminal Amino Acid Sequences in the Heavy Chain of Immunoglobulin G from Rabbits of Different Allotype

J. M. WILKINSON

Department of Biochemistry, University of Oxford, Oxford, England

The heavy chain of rabbit IgG contains no free α-amino group. It has been shown previously [1] that the N-terminal amino acid is pyrrolidone carboxylic acid (PCA), while the sequence following it is a mixture of PCA-Ser-Val-Glu, PCA-Ser-Leu-Glu and PCA-Gln in the ratio of 5:2:2. Further, a tryptic peptide was isolated from the Fd fragment which is an extension of the major component and has the sequence PCA-Ser-Val-Glu-Glu-Ser-Gly-Gly-Arg.

In an attempt to extend these sequences further, Fd was cleaved at the methionine residues with CNBr and a fragment of molecular weight about 4000 was isolated after reduction of disulphide bonds [2]. The composition of this fragment was very similar to that of the N-terminal fragment isolated from a pathological human IgG by Piggot and Press [3], but the yield was only about 30% from either Fd or heavy chain. Initial sequence studies showed this fragment to be N-terminal and to contain the N-terminal tryptic peptide isolated from the Fd fragment.

Subsequent study by Prahl and Porter [4] of the products of CNBr cleavage of heavy chain of IgG from rabbits homozygous for one of the alleles at the *a* locus showed considerable differences in both the yields and amino acid compositions of the N-terminal fragments obtained. The yields obtained were 57%, 21% and 45% for the Aa1, Aa2 and Aa3 heavy chains respectively, these being calculated by Prahl and Porter [4] relative to the recovery of the Fc CNBr fragment C4a, which is present in high yield in all allotype preparations. These results differ from those of Koshland [5], who isolated these fragments from Aa1 and Aa3 heavy chains and found them to be present in molar yield; the reason for this discrepancy, however, is unclear. As the yield of the Aa2 fragment is low, insufficient material was available for sequence work and so attention was concentrated on the Aa1 and Aa3 fragments.

The compositions of the Aa1 and Aa3 fragments are given in Table 1, and these show several striking differences, notably in the lysine and arginine contents, and there are also a number of amino acids present in non-integral amounts.

Investigation of the N-terminal sequence of these fragments by digestion with pronase showed that the Aa3 fragment contained the sequence originally designated PCA-Gln while the Aa1 fragment did not. Accordingly, the N-terminal pronase peptides from the three allotype heavy chains were investigated by the technique used previously [1] and the proportions of the three peptides found are shown in Table 2. The peptide thought to be PCA-Gln has now been shown to be PCA-Glu-Gln after reinvestigation of the larger amounts available. This

Table 1. Composition of N-terminal CNBr fragment from Aa1 and Aa3 heavy chain (moles of amino acid per mole of peptide are given).

	Aa1	*Aa3*
Lys	0·0	1·0
Arg	1·0	0·2
Asp	0·7	1·6
Thr	5·1	2·9
Ser	5·1	4·9
Glu	3·0	3·9
Pro	2·4	1·4
Gly	4·6	4·8
Ala	0·9	1·7
Val	2·3	1·6
Ile	0·3	0·3
Leu	4·5	3·8
Tyr	1·0	1·4
Phe	1·0	1·6
CMCys	0·9	0·8
HOSer	1·1	0·9
Total	33·9	32·8

sequence, while present in the Aa3 heavy chain, is not unique to it, occurring also in the Aa2 heavy chain in a small percentage of molecules. The relative amounts of Aa1, Aa2 and Aa3 allotype molecules in the pooled serum used for the initial studies have been determined by Oudin (private communication) and are 56%, 10% and 34% respectively. Thus the Aa1 allotype is predominant in the pooled serum and this accounts for the original conclusion that the N-terminal sequence is not allotype-related [1].

Determination of the sequence of the Aa1 and Aa3 N-terminal CNBr fragments, which is shown in Fig. 1, has confirmed and extended the results of the N-terminal sequence studies. These sequences are from only that fraction of heavy chain molecules possessing a methionine at position 34; however, the finding of the N-terminal pronase peptides in approximately the same ratios in the fragments as in the whole chains, and the fact that the N-terminal tryptic peptide, PCA-Ser-Val-Glu-Glu-Ser-Gly-Gly-Arg, is present in high yield from Aa1 heavy chain but absent from the Aa3 heavy chain, would suggest that the sequences of the fragments are typical of the whole heavy chain population.

Table 2. Relative yields of N-terminal peptides from the heavy chain of rabbits of different allotype.

Peptide	Aa1	Aa2	Aa3
PCA-Ser-Val-Glu	80%	45%	—
PCA-Ser-Leu-Glu	20%	45%	65%
PCA-Glu-Gln	—	10%	35%

A considerable area of identical sequence has been found, particularly around the disulphide bond at position 22. These identical positions are shown in Fig. 1, where the two rabbit sequences are also compared with the sequence of the pathological human heavy chain, Daw [3]. The extent of homology between the two rabbit sequences is some 60% which is of the same order as that between either one and the human sequence.

Figure 1 shows the differences in sequence between the Aa1 and Aa3 heavy chains. In the first 34 residues there are 14 positions at which differences are

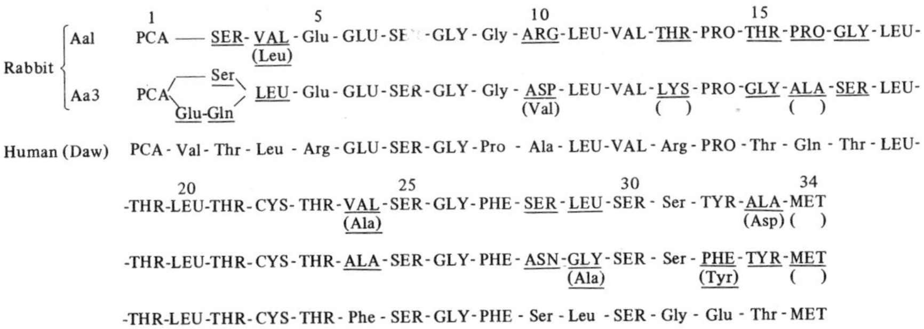

Figure 1. N-terminal sequences of heavy chains from rabbit and man. Amino acid residues shown in capitals indicate those common to all three sequences. Residues underlined are those which vary between the rabbit Aa1 and Aa3 sequences, while those in brackets are minor variants in each sequence. The bar at position 2 in the rabbit sequences indicates a presumed deletion. Sequence of human protein Daw is from Piggot and Press [3].

found and at 11 of these there are at least two variants in one chain or the other; the alternatives at positions 13 and 16 in the Aa3 sequence have not yet been identified but are almost certainly present. The ratios of the variant amino acids

7

within either sequence vary from 8:2 to 5:5, which would seem to rule out their being due to the 15-20% of allotypically unreactive heavy chains present.

It is clear that these differences are allotype-related, but it is not possible to decide whether they are responsible for the differences in antigenic specificity. It may be that these form the molecular basis of the antigenic subdivision of the allotypes found by Oudin [6] and others.

ACKNOWLEDGEMENT

I would like to thank Professor R. R. Porter, F.R.S., for his advice and encouragement during this work, and Dr. A. S. Kelus for his generous supply of allotypically-defined rabbit sera. This work was supported by the Medical Research Council.

REFERENCES

1. Wilkinson, J. M., Press, E. M. and Porter, R. R., *Biochem. J.* **100** (1966) 303.
2. Press, E. M., Givol, D., Piggot, P. J., Porter, R. R. and Wilkinson, J. M., *Proc. R. Soc.* Ser. B, **166** (1966) 150.
3. Piggot, P. J. and Press, E. M., *Biochem. J.* **104** (1967) 616.
4. Prahl, J. W. and Porter, R. R., *Biochem. J.* **107** (1968) 753.
5. Koshland, M. E., *Cold Spring Harb. Symp. quant. Biol.* **32** (1967) 119.
6. Oudin, J., *Proc. R. Soc.* Ser. B, **166** (1966) 207.

FEBS Symposium, Volume 15, 1969, pp. 187-191

Heavy Chain Heterogeneity of γG Immunoglobulins in the Pig

J.-J. METZGER and M. FOUGEREAU

Laboratoire d'Immunologie de l'I.N.R.A., Thiverval-Grignon, France

Sub-class heterogeneity has been described in human [1], mouse [2], guinea-pig [3], and sheep [4] γG immunoglobulins and has been assigned to the heavy polypeptide chains. Sub-class type heterogeneity has also been reported for the light chains of most animal species so far tested, and recently, Franěk and Zorina [5] have identified two types of light chains (λ and π) in pig γG immunoglobulins. So far, heavy chain heterogeneity in pig γG immunoglobulins has not been thoroughly investigated [6]. In the present communication, identification of two sub-classes of γG immunoglobulin in the pig is reported.

EXPERIMENTAL PROCEDURES

Crude immunoglobulin fraction was first prepared by salt precipitation of normal pooled sera, according to the procedure described by Kekwick [7]. γG immunoglobulin was then isolated by chromatography on DEAE-cellulose, equilibrated with a phosphate buffer 0·01 M, pH 7·8. Re-running of the γG immunoglobulin on DEAE-cellulose, using 5×10^{-4} M phosphate buffer as initial eluting agent allowed separation of the slow γG2 component. Antisera were prepared by injecting rabbits with the crude immunoglobulin fraction emulsified in complete Freund's adjuvant. With one antiserum (No. 250) out of a total of 15 injected rabbits, it was possible to identify two discrete components in the γG immunoglobulin fraction, which were shown to differ both in their antigenic properties and electrophoretic mobilities.

Isolation of tryptic peptides containing cysteinyl residues involved in the interchain disulfide bonds was achieved by means of two-dimensional high-voltage electrophoresis [8] after the immunoglobulin molecule had been reduced and carboxymethylated with [14C]iodoacetamide.

Other technical details have been reported elsewhere [9].

RESULTS AND DISCUSSION

Isolation of the γG immunoglobulin molecule and that of the slowest fraction is presented in Fig. 1. The fast component could not be successfully separated. Physicochemical properties of both components appear to be similar, by the following criteria; sedimentation constant, molecular weight, hexose content,

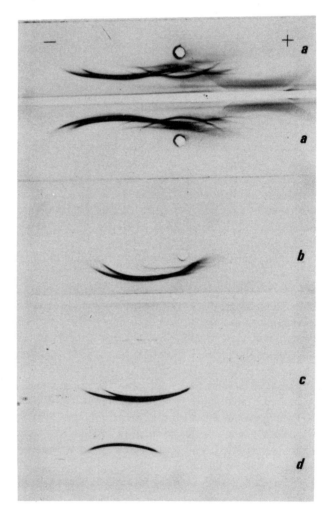

Figure 1. Separation by immunoelectrophoresis of the two sub-classes of pig γG immunoglobulin. (a) Pig normal pooled serum. (b) Crude immunoglobulin fraction prepared by salt precipitation. (c) Pig γG immunoglobulin isolated by chromatography on DEAE-cellulose equilibrated in phosphate buffer 0·01 M, pH 7·8. (d) Purified γG2 fraction. In the troughs: rabbit anti-whole pig serum. (Reproduced by permission of Recherches Véterinaires.)

electrophoretic behaviour on starch-gel in urea-formate buffer of the whole molecules, and also of the polypeptide chains. Both share identical antigenic determinants, as detected by all antisera but one. These results indicate that both components belong to the γG class. A specific determinant of the fast moving fraction was, however, detected when using rabbit antiserum No. 250. Differences in the primary structures were shown to occur on the heavy chains, as observed by the peptide mapping technique [10]; 35 spots were common, whereas only three were distinctive. Furthermore, the specific determinant was unequivocally assigned to the Fc fragment (Fig. 2).

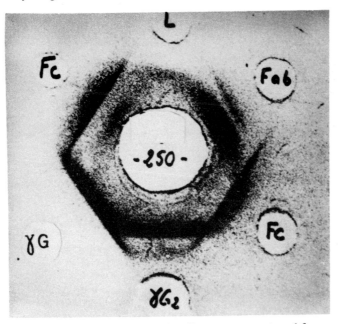

Figure 2. Immunodiffusion in agar of the different components and fragments: γG: pig γG immunoglobulin; γG2: pig γG2 immunoglobulin; L, Fab and Fc: light chains, Fab and Fc fragments from both sub-classes. 250-rabbit anti-whole pig serum. (Reproduced by permission of Recherches Vétérinaires.)

Pig γG immunoglobulins have been shown to be only slowly cleaved with papain [11]. Because of its more selective action, trypsin was utilized in our experiments, after the γG immunoglobulin molecules had been reduced and alkylated under such conditions as to cleave statistically three disulfide bonds. Alkylation was performed with [^{14}C] iodoacetamide. Hydrolysis was allowed to proceed for 40 min, and the complete reaction mixture was applied to a Sephadex G-100 column. The elution pattern is presented on Fig. 3. Six main peaks could be identified and, according to the evaluated size of the corresponding materials and to antigenic determinants as characterized by the Ouchterlony

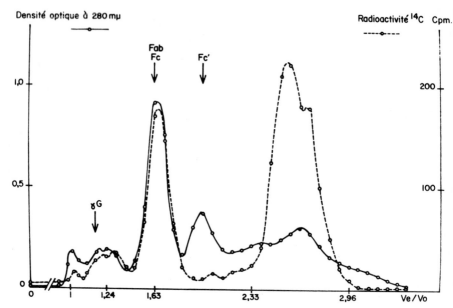

Figure 3. Separation on Sephadex G-100 of the products resulting from the cleavage by trypsin of pig γG immunoglobulin. $----$ O.D. at 280 mμ; $- - - - -$ radioactivity expressed in counts per minute. γG immunoglobulin was mildly reduced and alkylated with [14C]iodoacetamide prior to treatment with trypsin. (Reproduced by permission of Recherches Véterinaires.)

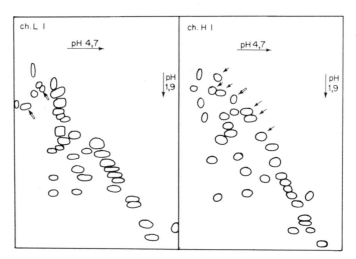

Figure 4. Two-dimensional high voltage electrophoresis of tryptic peptides from the light chains (left) and from the heavy chains (right). Arrows indicate peptides which were labelled with [14C]iodoacetamide (see text).

technique, were shown to consist by successive order of elution, of aggregates, intact γG immunoglobulin molecules, intermediate products of cleavage, presumably similar to those described by Nelson [12], Fab and Fc fragments, and peptides. Fc' fragment was shown to share antigenic determinants with the Fc fragment. As no radioactivity was found to be associated with the Fc' peak, this fragment is thought to represent most of the C-terminal half of the heavy chain. When tryptic hydrolysis was performed on the isolated γG2 class, a similar elution pattern was observed.

^{14}C-carboxymethylated peptides were located on the peptide maps (Fig. 4). Two peptides derived from the light chains were heavily labelled. This result is in good agreement with the existence of λ and π types of light chains in pig γG immunoglobulins, as described by Franĕk and Zorina [5]. One peptide identified on the map of the heavy chains was found to possess roughly the same level of radioactivity, as compared to that of the light chain peptides, and might therefore represent the sulphydryl-containing peptide involved in the inter-chain H-L linkage. Six more peptides were found to be ^{14}C-carboxymethylated to a lesser extent. Although differential solubilization of various peptides should be taken into account, this might indicate that sub-class heterogeneity of the heavy chains proceeds beyond the two components we have described.

ACKNOWLEDGEMENT

The present work was supported in part by a grant from the Communauté Economique Européenne. The authors express their gratitude to Mrs. F. Ville and Miss M. Nezonde for valuable technical assistance.

REFERENCES

1. Grey, H. M. and Kunkel, H. G., *J. exp. Med.* **120** (1964) 253.
2. Fahey, J. L., Wunderlich, J. and Mishell, R., *J. exp. Med.* **120** (1964) 223.
3. Benacerraf, B., Ovary, Z., Block, K. and Franklin, E. C., *J. exp. Med.* **117** (1963) 937.
4. Fougereau, M., *Annls. Biol. anim. Biochim. Biophys.* **6** (1966) 373.
5. Franĕk, F. and Zorina, O. M., *Colln. Czech. chem. Commun.* **32** (1967) 3229.
6. Rejnek, J., Kostka, J. and Trávníček, J., *Folia microbiol., Praha* **11** (1966) 173.
7. Kekwick, R. A., *Biochem. J.* **34** (1940) 1248.
8. Schwartz, J. H. and Edelman, G. M., *J. exp. Med.* **118** (1963) 41.
9. Metzger, J.-J. and Fougereau, M., *Rech. Vet.* **1** (1968) 37.
10. Metzger, J.-J. and Fougereau, M., *C. r. hebd. Seanc. Acad. Sci., Paris* **265** (1967) 724.
11. Hsiao, S. H. and Putnam, F. W., *J. biol. Chem.* **236** (1961) 122.
12. Nelson, C. A., *J. biol. Chem.* **239** (1964) 3727.

FEBS Symposium, Volume 15, 1969, pp. 193-198

Structural Characteristics of Pig Immunoglobulin π Chains

J. NOVOTNÝ, F. FRANĚK, B. KEIL and F. ŠORM

*Department of Protein Chemistry, Institute of Organic Chemistry
and Biochemistry, Czechoslovak Academy of Science, Prague, Czechoslovakia*

The π chains, which represent one of the types of pig immunoglobulin light chains, were first prepared from the S-sulpho derivative of pig immunoglobulin by Franěk and Zorina [1]. The light chains were separated from the heavy chains by gel filtration on Sephadex G-100 and fractionated by chromatography on SE-Sephadex at pH 3 in 8 M urea. Three types of chains, λ, π, and ρ were obtained. The λ and π chains differed in their mobility on starch gel electrophoresis, in their peptide maps, amino acid composition as well as N-terminal amino acid. The C-terminal tryptic peptide of the λ chains was found to

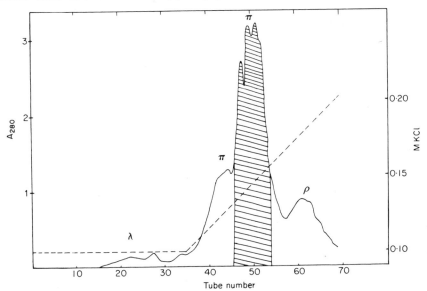

Figure 1. Rechromatography of π chains on SE-Sephadex C-25. The column (6 × 40 cm) was equilibrated with a buffer containing 0·005 M potassium formate and 8 M urea, the pH was adjusted with formic acid to 3·0. After applying the sample (2 g), the column was eluted with a linear gradient of potassium chloride in the buffer. Fraction volume was 30 ml. Solid curve—absorbance at 280 nm, dotted line—molarity of potassium chloride in the eluate.

193

correspond in its composition to the C-terminal peptide of human type L Bence-Jones proteins. On the other hand, the C-terminal tryptic peptide of the π chains differs considerably in the length and amino acid composition from analogous peptide derived from human type K Bence-Jones protein. Hence, the π chains were considered as a new structural type.

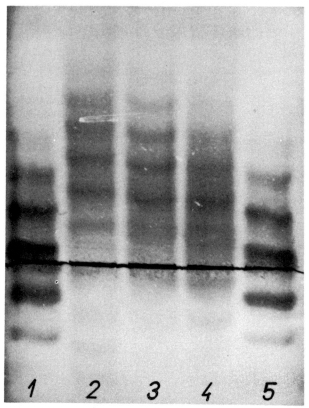

Figure 2. Starch gel electrophoresis at pH 8. The anode is at the top. The origin wells are visible in the lower part of the figure. 1,5: |λ chains, 2 to 4: samples of π chains of different degree of purity.

However, studies of Hood and co-workers [2] have shown that the peptide Asx-Glx-Cys-Glx-Ala found in pig immunoglobulin light chains could be the C-terminal peptide of κ-like chains, since there is a certain similarity with the C-terminal sequence Asn-Glu-Cys of mouse and rat κ chains. In this situation, more detailed characterization of π chains was highly desirable.

Light chains obtained by gel filtration of pig S-sulpho-γ G-immunoglobulin served as a starting material. The π chains were prepared from the light chain fraction by ion-exchange chromatography on SE-Sephadex, in formate buffer pH 3 in 8 M urea. To remove completely contamination with the λ chains, both ion-exchange chromatography and gel filtration were repeated.

The π chains represent a heterogeneous protein population (Fig. 1). This heterogeneity becomes most apparent when the chains are subjected to starch-gel electrophoresis in 8 M urea at pH 8 (Fig. 2). On the electropherograms, both λ chains and π chains yield a number of zones with equal spacings. Individual zones represent fractions which differ from each other by one unit of electric charge. The zones of π-chain preparations are shifted by a fraction of unit charge with respect to the λ chains. This behaviour can be accounted for by incomplete dissociation of histidine residues at pH 8. The molecule of the π chain contains

Table 1. Amino acid composition of pig π chains.

Cys	5·0	Gly	13·4
Lys	11·6	Ala	12·7
His	2·8	Val	17·5
Arg	7·3	Met	0·4
Asp	15·8	Ile	6·6
Thr	15·7	Leu	22·1
Ser	29·1	Tyr	8·5
Glu	23·0	Phe	8·9
Pro	13·3	Trp	1·9
		Total	215·6

The calculation of the number of individual amino acid residues was based on the assumed number of five cysteine residues, determined as cysteic acid.

The values of aspartic acid, serine, threonine and tyrosine were obtained by extrapolation to zero time of hydrolysis. The values of valine and isoleucine are those, determined in 72-h hydrolysates. Tryptophan was determined spectrophotometrically by the method of Edelhoch [5].

one histidine residue more than the molecule of the λ chain and this difference obviously causes the shift of zones.

Material for characterization and structure studies was provided by the protein from the main peak of the π chain (hatched area in Fig. 1). The peptide map of its tryptic digest showed that this material represents pure π chains, not contaminated with other types. The preparation has only one N-terminal group, alanine, in a yield of 0·7 mole per mole protein. Its amino acid composition is shown in Table 1. The molecular weight calculated from this amino acid composition (23,500) is in fair agreement with the molecular weight determined by the method of sedimentation equilibrium (25,000).

Special importance, as regards the structural characterization of the type of light chains, attaches to the determination of the amino acid sequence of their C-terminal invariant portion. Since the C-terminal pentapeptide has already been identified [1, 2], we decided to isolate this peptide from the tryptic digest of the π chains and to determine its complete amino acid sequence.

The peptide map of the tryptic digest (Fig. 3) shows two peptides of strongly acidic character. Peptide T1 remains at the origin during electrophoresis at pH 1·9, peptide T2 moves only a little towards the cathode. The amino acid

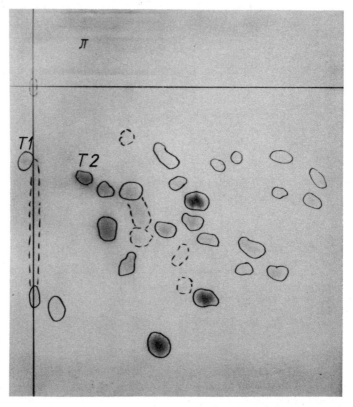

Figure 3. Peptide map of S-sulphonated π chains. Electrophoresis was carried out at pH 1·9. The origin is at top left corner. Horizontally electrophoresis, vertically chromatography (N-butanol:pyridine:acetic acid:water, 15:10:3:12). The anode is at the right.

sequence of these two peptides was determined by Edman-degradation combined with the dansyl technique (Fig. 4). Peptide T1 is obviously the C-terminal pentapeptide since it does not contain a basic amino acid. We found that it contains one cysteine residue, similar to the C-terminal peptides of all so-far studied light chains. Peptide T2 represents the C-terminal nonapeptide. It is the result of incomplete tryptic cleavage. When this peptide is subjected to additional tryptic digestion, it is cleaved to the tetrapeptide C-terminated with arginine and to the pentapeptide identical with peptide T1.

Special interest derives from a comparison of the amino acid sequence determined by us with the known C-terminal sequences of light chains of the κ type (Table 2). While the C-terminal tryptic pentapeptide of pig π chains does not bear too much resemblance to the C-terminal tryptic tripeptides of rabbit

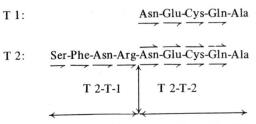

Figure 4 Determination of amino acid sequence of peptides T1 and T2. Sequence established by Edman-degradation. The amino acid sequence of the fragment T2-T-2 was determined in separate experiments, independent of the determination of the sequence of the whole peptide T2.

and human κ chains, a striking similarity has been found between C-terminal nonapeptide of pig π chains and C-terminal heptapeptide of mouse κ chains. This leads us to assume that the pig π chain represents, from the evolutionary aspect, an older form of the κ chains of mouse, rabbit or man. The C-terminal dipeptide is obviously unimportant functionally and was deleted during evolution. Evidently, the deletion of these two residues did not decrease the ability of light chains to combine with the heavy chains.

Table 2. Comparison of various C-terminal sequences of κ-like light chains.

		Reference
Pig:	-Ser-Phe-Asn-Arg-Asn-Glu-Cys-Gln-AlaOH	This paper
Mouse:	-Ser-Phe-Asn-Arg-Asn-Glu-CysOH	3,8
Man:	-Ser-Phe-Asn-Arg-Gly-Glu-CysOH	4,9,10
Rabbit:	-Ser-Phe-Asn-Arg-Gly-Asp-CysOH	2,6,7

At present it would be difficult to decide definitely whether the π chains should be classified as a separate light chain type or whether they should be considered as a member of the κ-chain family. Both these alternatives are essentially possible, depending on whether we consider the problem from the aspect of similarities or dissimilarities existing between the π chains and the κ chains. The identity of the amino acid sequence of penultimate tryptic peptides in the π chains and κ chains strongly suggests that the π chains should be put in the group of κ chains. This sequence is one of the most conservative and, at the same time, most characteristic of the K type.

Note added in proof. The assignment of the π chains to the κ chain family has been further supported by a recently published (Novotný, J. and Franěk, F., *FEBS Lett.* 2 (1968) 93) N-terminal sequence of the π chains. The sequence is closely related to the N-terminal sequence of mouse κ chains.

REFERENCES

1. Franěk, F. and Zorina, O. M., *Colln. Czech. chem. Commun.* 32 (1967) 3229.
2. Hood, L., Gray, W. R., Sanders, B. G. and Dreyer, W. J., *Cold Spring Harb. Symp. quant. Biol.* 32 (1967) 133.
3. Gray, W. R., Dreyer, W. J. and Hood, L., *Science, N.Y.* 155 (1967) 465.
4. Putnam, F. W., Titani, K. and Whitley, Jnr., E. J., *Proc. R. Soc.* Ser. B, 166 (1966) 124.
5. Edelhoch, H., *Biochemistry, N.Y.* 6 (1967) 1948.
6. Doolittle, R. F. and Astrin, K. H., *Science, N.Y.* 156 (1967) 1755.
7. Appella, E. and Perham, R. N., *Cold Spring Harb. Symp. quant. Biol.* 32 (1967) 37.
8. Perham, R. N., Appella, E. and Potter, M., *Science, N.Y.* 154 (1966) 391.
9. Hilschmann, N., *Hoppe-Seyler's Z. physiol. Chem.* 348 (1967) 1718.
10. Milstein, C., *Biochem. J.* 101 (1966) 338.

FEBS Symposium, Volume 15, 1969, pp. 199-204

Separation of Subfractions of Rabbit L Chains

M. LANCKMAN and G. de VRIES

*Laboratory of Animal Physiology and Laboratory of General
Biology, University of Brussels, Brussels, Belgium*

The study of sequences of L chains from pathological IgG has revealed the existence of subclasses corresponding to different structural genes in several mammalian species. In our attempt to determine if rabbit L chains are composed of subclasses, we have been led to the conclusion that two populations immunologically and structurally distinct are present.

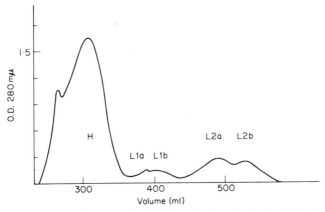

Figure 1. Separation of rabbit MRA-IgG (pooled) on Sephadex G-100 in 6 M urea, 0·05 M formic acid.

IgG from a commercial pool (Pentex) were mildly reduced by dithiothreitol and alkylated by iodoacetamide. In the conditions used, 4 to 5 disulphide bridges were opened. By gel filtration on Sephadex G-100 in 6 M urea, 0·05 M formic acid, L chains are resolved into the two main populations called L1 and L2 (Fig. 1) [1, 2]. Each of them consists of two subfractions L1a, L1b and L2a, L2b. The two main populations L1 and L2 appear to be unrelated antigens by immunodiffusion test using goat anti-L serum. The precipitation lines of L1 and L2 cross each other as shown in Fig. 2.

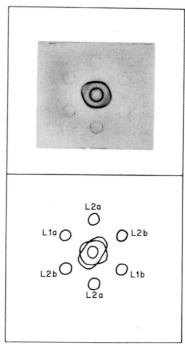

Figure 2. Immunodiffusion analysis of L chain subfractions when reacted with goat anti-L serum.

Table 1. Amino acid composition of L chain subfractions. Data expressed as moles of amino acid recovered per 22,500 g of L chains. The results were calculated for sets of three determinations. The error represents the double of the standard error and thus gives 95% of confidence to the mean.

	L1a	L1b	L2a	L2b
asp	17·5 ± 0·8	17·2 ± 0·3	19·6 ± 1·2	18·3 ± 0·8
thr	21·2 ± 0·4	20·7 ± 0·4	29·6 ± 0·7	29·1 ± 1·2
ser	26·6 ± 2·1	28·4 ± 0·05	22·0 ± 1·4	23·5 ± 2·2
glu	21·9 ± 1·2	22·3 ± 0·1	20·6 ± 0·9	21·0 ± 0·6
pro	15·3 ± 1·8	14·5 ± 0·7	11·7 ± 0·7	11·3 ± 1·3
gly	18·1 ± 1·2	19·3 ± 0·4	19·6 ± 0·8	20·1 ± 1·7
ala	14·9 ± 0·7	16·3 ± 0·5	16·3 ± 1·0	17·1 ± 0·6
val	16·6 ± 1·0	16·8 ± 0·4	20·1 ± 1·2	20·2 ± 1·1
ile	6·6 ± 0·4	6·9 ± 0·3	7·0 ± 0·2	7·3 ± 0·1
leu	15·0 ± 0·6	14·4 ± 0·2	10·7 ± 0·4	10·8 ± 0·1
tyr	8·3 ± 0·4	9·0 ± 0·8	10·2 ± 0·5	10·6 ± 0·6
phe	7·2 ± 0·2	6·9 ± 0·2	6·9 ± 0·2	6·9 ± 0·4
lys	10·4 ± 0·3	9·3 ± 0·3	8·8 ± 0·2	8·8 ± 0·3
his	3·5 ± 0·1	2·6 ± 0·6	1·3 ± 0·1	1·3 ± 0·2
arg	5·7 ± 0·1	5·0 ± 0·5	2·9 ± 0·5	3·2 ± 0·3

These findings were thought to indicate two immunologically-distinct groups differing in their primary structure. A comparison of the amino acid composition of the two main fractions effectively showed significant differences, especially for threonine, serine, proline, valine, leucine, histidine, and arginine. One finds very small differences between the subfractions of each group (Table 1).

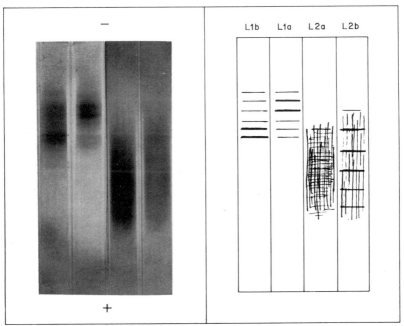

Figure 3. Electrophoretic patterns of L chain subfractions on polyacrylamide gel, pH 8·5.

Comparable results were obtained by disc electrophoresis on acrylamide gel at pH 8·5. Electrophoretic patterns of the L1 chains showed a separation into six components. In both L1a and L1b subfractions the same bands are found but the relative quantities of each component are different (Fig. 3). The L2 subfractions are characterized by a diffuse zone with some additional bands in the case of L2b.

The existence of two different L-chain populations led us to look for the presence of the allotypic specificities shared by each subfraction. The experiments described (Fig. 1) were made with a pool of IgG possessing the allotypic markers As4 and As5. Double diffusion experiments with the corresponding anti-allotypic sera show differences among the fractions. Both L2a and L2b give a strong reaction with anti-As4 sera. The quantity of immunological precipitate is very weak for the L1 fraction and could be due to contamination by L2. On

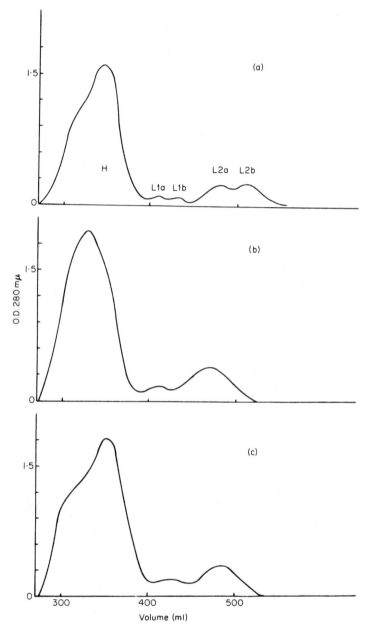

Figure 4. Separation of MRA-IgG from rabbits homozygous for the Ab locus, on Sephadex G-100, in 6 M urea, 0·05 M formic acid.
    (a) MRA-IgG from an Ab 4 rabbit;
    (b) MRA-IgG from an Ab 5 rabbit;
    (c) MRA-IgG from an Ab 6 rabbit.

the contrary, only L2a fraction gives a reaction with anti-As5 sera. This could suggest that only molecules corresponding to peak L2a are present in L chains obtained from IgG As5, or that other fractions could be present which gave no precipitin reaction. Therefore experiments were performed with IgG from homozygous rabbits [3].

L chains of As4 IgG shows the existence of four subfractions as L chains of pooled IgG (Fig. 4a). A precipitation reaction with anti-As4 sera is observed only for L2a and L2b fractions (Fig. 5). Radial diffusion experiments according to

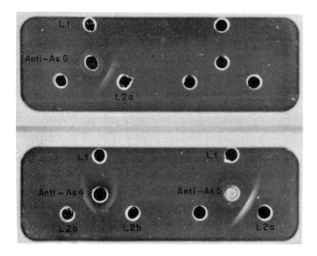

Figure 5. Immunodiffusion analysis of L chain subfractions from homozygous rabbit IgG, when reacted with the corresponding anti-allotypic sera. (In the lower photograph, the subfraction in the bottom left-hand corner should be labelled L2a not L2b.)

Heremans show that the amount of immunological precipitate is similar in both subfractions. In As5 IgG (Fig. 4b), the bulk of the L chains is in the L2a fraction; fraction L2b is absent. Fraction L2a only gives a precipitation reaction with anti-As5 sera. Similar results are obtained for IgG from homozygous As6 rabbits (Fig. 4c).

The results obtained show that L chains from rabbit IgG can be resolved into two immunologically and structurally distinct types like those of other mammalian species. The primary structure of both types are different, as shown by the amino acid composition. Each of them can be resolved into two slightly different subfractions. The distribution of subfractions is related to the nature of the allotypic markers of the L chains. For the As4 IgG, one observes always an additional population L2b with antigenic properties similar to those of L2a. It is interesting to note that the minor group L1 does not give a precipitation reaction with the corresponding anti-allotypic sera. This suggests that only one group of L chains possesses the known allotypic markers.

ACKNOWLEDGEMENT

This work was carried out under contract 007-61 ABIB between Euratom and the University of Brussels and it was supported by grants from the Fonds de la Recherche Fondamentale Collective. M. Lanckman is Aspirant du Fonds National de la Recherche Scientifique and G. de Vries is chercheur du Fonds National de la Recherche Fondamentale Collective.

REFERENCES

1. Lanckman, M., *Nature, Lond.* **210** (1966) 1379.
2. Zikán, J., Škárová, B. and Rejnek, J., *Folia microbiol., Praha* **12** (1967) 162.
3. de Vries, G. and Lanckman, M., *Archs. int. Physiol. Biochim.* in press.

FEBS Symposium, Volume 15, 1969, pp. 205-212

Separation of Rabbit L Chains and Localization of Allotypic Specificities

J. ZIKÁN and B. ŠKÁROVÁ*

*Institute of Microbiology, Czechoslovak Academy of Science,
Prague, Czechoslovakia*

The peptide chains of IgG are usually isolated in our laboratory by gel filtration on Sephadex G-100 in 6 M urea with 0·05 M formic acid [1]. In this case the partially S-sulphonated and S-carboxymethylated rabbit IgG separated in a rather unusual way. On the elution diagram the peak of H chains was followed by two peaks, instead of one peak which corresponds to L chains as observed with the other species [2, 3] (Fig. 1). These two fractions were designated as L_1 and L_2 chains. We have tried to characterize these chains by different chemical and immunological methods. The majority of these methods and materials have already been described [3, 4].

L_1 and L_2 chains were isolated both from the first and from the second fraction of rabbit IgG, which was resolved into these fractions by chromatography on DEAE Sephadex A-50 [5]. In both these fractions the ratio of the amounts of L_1 to L_2 chains was very similar. The content of L_1 chains amounted to about 38% of L_2 chains. In the purified antibodies, specific towards the dinitrophenyl group, we found 20% of L_1 chains only. Chromatography in 6 M guanidine HCl released 56% of chains which correspond to L_1. In the majority of cases we observed only one peak corresponding to L chains when using 1 M propionic acid. In the sequence 1 M propionic acid, 6 M urea with 0·05 M formic acid, 6 M guanidine HCl, the ability to dissociate partially split IgG was increased, however, the differences between the elution volumes of two compounds were decreased. In other words the slopes of the lines, corresponding to the plots of the logarithm of molecular weight versus elution volume, were decreased in that sequence. The elution volumes of L_1 and L_2 chains correspond to the molecular weights as shown in Table 1. The weight-average molecular weights were determined by sedimentation analysis [6] (Table 1). As the molecular weights of L_1 and L_2 chains were similar, it may be excluded that L_1 chains are aggregates of L_2 chains.

* Some of the sections of this work were done with the collaboration of Dr. J. Rejnek, Dr. J. Blažek, and Ing. O. Kotýnek.

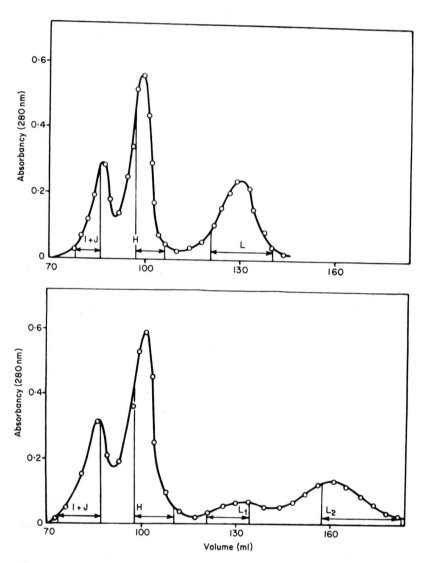

Figure 1. Upper: 10 mg S-sulphonated bovine IgG separated on a column of Sephadex G-100 (1·64 × 125 cm) in 6 M urea with 0·05 M formic acid. The collected fractions are designated by arrows.

Lower: A similar separation of S-sulphonated rabbit IgG.

N-terminal amino acids were determined by the dinitrophenyl [3] and dansyl techniques [7]. Dansyl amino acids were identified by thin layer chromatography with Kieselgel G/Merck in the solvent system isopropanol–toluene–ammonia (8:1:1). Chloroform–ethanol–ammonia (15:2:1) was used for the separation of glutamic and aspartic acids. N-terminal glutamic or aspartic acids were determined in different preparations of L_1 chains. N-terminal alanine was determined in L_2 chains. N-terminal amino acids from the second chain probably characterize its presence in preparations of the first one.

Table 1. Molecular weights of chains of rabbit IgG.

Substance	Molecular weight $\times 10^3$	Method
H_{SU}	58.9 ± 2.4	Ultracentrifuge (Yphantis) 6 M guanidine HCl
$L_{1\ SU}$	25.3 ± 1.8	
$L_{2\ SU}$	24.3 ± 1.6	
$L_{1\ SU}$	23.3	Ultracentrifuge (Yphantis) 6 M urea with 0.05 M formic acid
$L_{1\ SU}$	28	Sephadex G-100 6 M urea with
$L_{2\ SU}$	20	0.05 M formic acid
L_P	25	Sephadex G-100 1 M propionic acid

S S-sulphonated.
U isolated in 6 M urea with 0.5 M formic acid.
P isolated in 1 M propionic acid.

We found significant differences between the amino acid contents of L_1 and L_2 chains, especially with regard to the contents of threonine, serine, leucine, and proline, as shown in Table 2.

L_1 and L_2 chains were oxidized with performic acid [8] and their tryptic hydrolysates fractionated by paper electrophoresis in formic–acetic acid pH 1.9, and by paper chromatography in the other direction with butanol–acetic acid–pyridine–water (15:10:3:2). Detection was carried out with 0.2% ninhydrine solution in acetone. About one half of the peptides was common to these hydrolysates (Table 3). However, both hydrolysates differed considerably from those of the H chains.

Determination of disulphide bonds was carried out in 8 M guanidine HCl. SH-groups were titrated amperometrically with methylmercuric iodide after

Table 2. Amino acid content (moles/mole) in chains of rabbit IgG.

Amino acid	L_2 SU	L_1 SU
Asp	20·2	19·2
Thr	30	25·3
Ser	23·3	27
Glu	22·2	21·8
Pro	12·4	14
Gly	21·7	21·6
Ala	19	17·4
Val	22·7	21·8
Ile	8·3	7·7
Leu	12·5	15·2
Tyr	8·7	7·8
Phe	7·6	6·6
Lys	10·2	9·3
His	2·5	2·8
Arg	3·7	4·3

Molecular weight of chains is 24,000.
Hydrolysis time 22 h.
S S-sulphonated.
U isolated in 6 M urea with 0·05 M formic acid.

reduction with sulphite [9]. The total number of groups corresponding to half-cystines in S-sulpho chains were determined after reduction of S-sulpho groups with 0·5 M mercaptoethanol by titration of SH groups before and after the sulphite was added [3]. Oxidation and determination of cysteic acid were carried out according to Moore [10]. The results of the analyses of the groups mentioned above are shown in Table 4. The number of the disulphide bonds which were split was 7·3 by mercaptoethanol and 7·7 by oxidative sulphitolysis. L_1 chains had about 0·8 of disulphide bond while L_2 chains had about 2 disulphide bonds. We assumed that the tertiary structure of L_1 chains stabilized

Table 3. Peptide maps of chains of rabbit IgG.

Chains	Total number of main peptides	Common peptides		
		H_{SU}	L_1 SU	L_2 SU
H_{SU}	22	—	4	2
L_1 SU	21	4	—	10
L_2 SU	19	2	10	—

S S-sulphonated.
U isolated in 6 M urea with 0·05 M formic acid.

Table 4. Determination of some sulphur-containing residues in intact and modified IgG and its chains.

Substance	Disulphides in 1 mole	Disulphides in 10^5 g	SH groups in 1 mole (after reduction)	Cysteic acid in 1 mole (after oxidat.)
RGG	19·6	12·2		
SRGG	11·9	7·4		
CRGG	12·7	7·9		
H_{SU}	3·7	6·3	14·4	13·4
L_{1SU}	0·82 ± 0·02	3·24		6
L_{1SUU}	0·7	2·8	6·7	
$L_{2\ SU}$	1·75 ± 0·18	7·2	7·2	6·5
$L_{1\ CU}$	0·8	3·2		
$L_{2\ CU}$	2·4	9·9		5
$I + J_{SU}$		5·3	22·4 (in 10^5 g)	
$I + J_{SP}$		5·1		

C	S-carboxymethylated.
S	S-sulphonated
U	isolated in 6 M urea with 0·05 M formic acid.
P	isolated in 1 M propionic acid.
RGG	rabbit IgG.

Table 5. Inhibition of passive haemagglutination by chains of rabbit IgG.

Antiserum	H chains conc. μg per tube					L_1 chains conc. μg per tube					L_2 chains conc. μg per tube				
	0·25	1	3	5	10	0·25	1	3	5	10	0·25	1	3	5	10
Anti-Aa1		+	+	+	−	−	+	+	+	+	+	+	+	+	+	+
Anti-Aa2		+	+	−	−	−	+	+	+	+	+	+	+	+	+	+
Anti-Aa3		+	+	−	−	−	+	+	+	+	+	+	+	+	+	+
Anti-Ab4		+	+	+	+	+	+	+	−	−	−	+	+	+	+	−
Anti-Ab5		+	+	+	+	+	+	+	−	−	−	+	+	+	−	−
Anti-Ab6		+	+	+	+	+	+	+	−	−	−	+	+	+	+	+

+ haemagglutination.

− inhibition of haemagglutination.

by a lower number of disulphide bonds was more uncoiled in urea or in guanidine HCl solutions as compared to L_2 chains. The different shapes of L_1 and L_2 molecules probably accounts for their different behaviour on Sephadex G-100 columns in these solutions.

The behaviour of L_1 and L_2 chains was very different on starch gel electrophoresis in 8 M urea with 0·035 M glycine buffer pH 8·8 [11]. L_2 chains form unexpressive bands. On the contrary, L_1 chains form very clean-cut banding with a number of fractions exhibiting lower mobility than L_2 chains (Fig. 2).

On immunoelectrophoresis in agar gel the L_1 and L_2 chains had a similar mobility, different from the position of H chains. L_1 and L_2 chains gave the

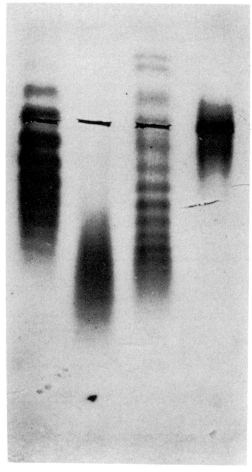

Figure 2. Starch gel electrophoresis in 0·035 M glycine buffer pH 8·8 with 8 M urea. From left to right: porcine L chains, rabbit L_2 chains, rabbit L_1 chains and rabbit H chains.

cross-reaction with duck or pig anti-L_2 and duck anti-L_1 serum. In the Ouchterlony diffusion test we observed the reaction of partial identity. L_1 and L_2 chains were not precipitated by duck or pig anti-H serum.

We used inhibition of passive haemagglutination for the determination of allotypic markers in the chains H, L_1 and L_2 [4]. The red cells coated by IgG were agglutinated by corresponding anti-allotypic marker serum. These reactions were inhibited by chains from the conjugated IgG (Table 5). H chains inhibited the precipitations with anti-Aa1, Aa2 and Aa3 serum. L_1 chains inhibited the

Table 6. Binding activity of chains of rabbit IgG.

Chains	Polarographic determination of bound ϵ DNP lys expressed by "r" at 10^{-5} molar ϵ DNP lys	Titre of agglutination of dinitrophenylated erythrocytes. Original concentrations of chains is $5 \cdot 6 \times 10^{-6}$ molar
H_{CP}	0·12	4
$H_{CP} + L_{CP}$	0·30	4
H_{CU}	0·12	16
$H_{CU} + L_{2CU}$	0·43	16
H_{SP}	0·033	32
$H_{SP} + L_{SP}$	0·206	32
H_{SU}	0·031	512
$H_{SU} + L_{2SU}$	0·48	512
$H_{SU} + L_{1SU}$	0·59	512

ϵ DNP lys, ϵ 2,4 dinitrophenyl-1-lysine.

$r = \dfrac{\text{molar concentration of bound } \epsilon \text{ DNP lys}}{\text{molar concentration of H chains}}$

C S-carboxymethylated.
S S-sulphonated.
U isolated in 6 M urea with 0·05 M formic acid.
P isolated in 1 M propionic acid.

precipitation with anti-Ab4, Ab5 and Ab6 serum. L_2 chains inhibited the precipitation with Ab4 and Ab5 serum only. Therefore L_2 chains did not contain, by this method, the L chain with Ab6 allotypic marker.

S-sulphonated and S-carboxymethylated chains were isolated also from the anti-dinitrophenyl antibodies [3] on Sephadex G-100 in 6 M urea with 0·05 M formic acid [1] and in 1 M propionic acid [12]. These antibodies consist of 80% of the first fraction resolved on DEAE Sephadex [5]. Both L_1 and L_2 chains increased the binding activity of H chains (Table 6). S-sulphonated H chains as determined in 1% solution of chains by means of polarographic method [13] had very low activity. On the contrary, the activity of S-carboxymethylated H chains was relatively high. The values of the association constant of H chains and their complex with L chains were of the same order as for native antibodies

(10^8mole^{-1} l). The binding activity was determined also by passive haemagglutination [14]. It was possible to use this method with S-sulphonated chains isolated in urea (Table 6). However, we did not observe the reactivation of H chains by L chains.

In conclusion, L_1 and L_2 chains correspond to fractions of L chains which have significant differences in structure. These chains partially do not carry the same allotypic determinants and play a similar role in the reactivation of H chains.

REFERENCES

1. Franěk, F. and Nezlin, R. S., *Folia microbiol., Praha* 8 (1963) 128.
2. Lanckman, M., *Nature, Lond.* 210 (1966) 1379.
3. Zikán, J., Škárová, B. and Rejnek, J., *Folia microbiol., Praha* 12 (1967) 162.
4. Škárová, B., Rejnek, J. and Kotýnek, O., *Folia microbiol., Praha* 13 (1968) 265.
5. Sela, M., Givol, D. and Mozes, E., *Biochim. biophys. Acta* 78 (1964) 649.
6. Yphantis, D. A., *Biochemistry, N.Y.* 3 (1964) 297.
7. Gray, W. R. and Hartley, B. S., *Biochem. J.* 89 (1963) 590.
8. Hirs, C. H. W., *J. biol. Chem.* 219 (1956) 611.
9. Leach, S. J., *Aust. J. Chem.* 13 (1960) 520.
10. Moore, S., *J. biol. Chem.* 238 (1963) 235.
11. Cohen, S. and Porter, R. R., *Biochem. J.* 90 (1964) 278.
12. Fleischman, J. B., Pain, R. H. and Porter, R. R., *Archs. Biochem. Biophys.* Suppl. 1 (1962) 174.
13. Zikán, J., *Colln. Czech. chem. Commun.* 31 (1966) 4260.
14. Zikán, J. and Šterzl, J., *Nature, Lond.* 214 (1967) 1225.

FEBS Symposium, Volume 15, 1969, pp. 213-219

The Relationship between the Papain Sensitivity of Human γG Globulins and their Heavy Chain Subclass

R. JEFFERIS* and D. R. STANWORTH

Department of Experimental Pathology, The Medical School, University, Birmingham, England

Normal human γG immunoglobulin has been shown to be comprised of two populations of molecules, which differ in their susceptibility to papain proteolysis in the absence of cysteine [1]. Incubation at 37°, for four hours, results in 65-70% of molecules being degraded to Fab and Fc fragments, whilst the remaining 30-35% can only be degraded on incubation with papain in the presence of cysteine. The homogeneous myeloma γG proteins have been shown to be either resistant or susceptible to papain proteolysis in the absence of cysteine [1, 2]. These studies have now been extended to a series of myeloma proteins of known heavy chain subclass; and, also, antigenic differences between the papain sensitive and resistant forms of normal and myeloma γG globulins have been detected using special antisera. A clear correlation between papain susceptibility and heavy chain subclass emerges.

Sephadex G-150 gel-filtration, following incubation of γG globulins with papain in the absence of cysteine, provides a convenient analytical and preparative technique for the study of papain susceptibility. The gel-filtration profiles of myeloma γG proteins of each heavy chain subclass following incubation with papain in the absence of cysteine are shown in Fig. 1. The finding that the γG2 and γG4 subclass proteins were resistant to proteolysis was confirmed with three γG2 and two γG4 samples. Similarly, that the γG1 and γG3 subclass proteins are susceptible to degradation under these conditions was confirmed with nine γG1 and two γG3 proteins. Papain susceptibility studies can thus be used to classify γG myeloma proteins as being of the γG1/γG3 or γG2/γG4 heavy chain subclass. Moreover, the γG2 and γG4 proteins can be further differentiated by their susceptibility to papain proteolysis in the presence of cysteine. A two hour incubation period results in the γG4 proteins being totally degraded to Fab and Fc fragments, whilst the γG2 proteins only undergo 10-20% degradation during this period of time.

Present address: Department of Chemistry, Revelle College, University of South California, San Diego, La Jolla.

The antigenic relationship between the papain-resistant fraction of normal human γG immunoglobulin and myeloma proteins of known heavy chain subclass has been investigated, using an antiserum specific for the papain-resistant fraction. Using the technique of Dvorak *et al.* [3], 100 μg of the papain-resistant fraction of normal human γG immunoglobulin was administered, in Freunds complete adjuvant, as two footpad injections. The animals were rendered tolerant to determinants shared between the resistant fraction and

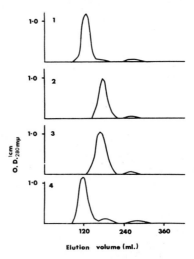

Figure 1. Sephadex G-150 gel-filtration patterns after 4 h incubation with papain in the absence of cysteine of (1) γG2, (2) γG1, (3) γG3, and (4) γG4 myeloma proteins.

the Fab and Fc fragments of the papain-sensitive fraction by simultaneous administration of 5 mg of the latter (1 ml of soluble protein solution) intravenously. At six weeks, an antiserum was obtained (A2 in Fig. 2) which reacted with the papain-resistant fraction and its Fc fragment obtained by digestion in the presence of cysteine, but not with the Fab or Fc fragments of the papain-sensitive fraction. Antigenic differences between the two forms are thus revealed, and this must be a reflection of structural differences within their Fc regions.

The Fab and Fc fragments of myeloma γG proteins of each heavy chain subclass were isolated by Sephadex G-150 gel-filtration following incubation with papain in the presence of cysteine. Immunoelectrophoresis of these Fab and Fc fragments, with development against a rabbit anti-human γG antiserum, showed all fragments to be antigenically active (Fig. 3). However, the antiserum specific for the papain-resistant form only gave precipitin arcs with the Fab and Fc fragments of the γG2 and γG4 proteins, the parent molecules of which were papain resistant.

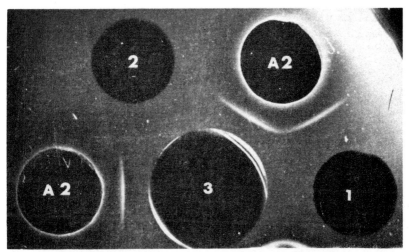

Figure 2. Gel diffusion precipitin analysis of papain-resistant human γG (1), the Fab and Fc fragments of papain-sensitive human γG (2) and whole human γG globulin (3) against guinea pig anti-serum A2. (Reproduced from *Nature, Lond.*, 1968, **219**, 646 by courtesy of Macmillan Ltd.)

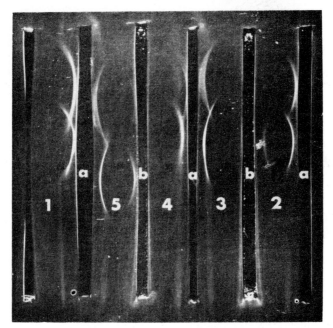

Figure 3. Immunoelectrophoretic patterns of the Fab and Fc fragments of normal human γG (1), γG2 (2), γG1 (3), γG3 (4), and γG4 (5) myeloma proteins developed against (a) rabbit anti-human γG globulin anti-serum and (b) guinea pig anti-serum A2.

Under the Porter [4] conditions of papain digestion, therefore, cysteine appears to act both as an enzyme activator and also as a reducing agent for the papain-resistant fraction, at least, effecting structural alterations which facilitate papain proteolysis.

The possibility of conformational differences within the Fc regions of the two forms accounting for their differing papain susceptibility was investigated by a parallel study of the papain susceptibility of the major pepsin cleavage fragments, $F(ab')_2$ of myeloma γG proteins. The 5 S, $F(ab')_2$, fragments of

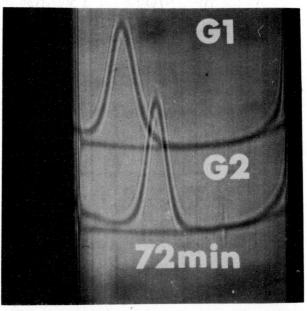

Figure 4. Analytical ultracentrifugal patterns (72 min at 59,780 r.p.m.) of the pepsin $F(ab')_2$ fragments of a γG1 (top) and a γG2 (bottom) myeloma protein after 7 h incubation with papain in the absence of cysteine.

myeloma proteins of each heavy chain subclass were incubated at $37°$ for a period of 7 h with papain in the absence of cysteine and the products examined in the analytical ultracentrifuge. As shown in Fig. 4 the pepsin $F(ab')_2$ fragment of the γG1 protein was further degraded by the papain treatment to yield 3·5 S fragments. However, the pepsin fragment of the γG2 protein remained undegraded, possessing an unchanged sedimentation coefficient of 5 S. Similarly the pepsin $F(ab')_2$ fragments derived from γG3 proteins were degraded by papain to Fab fragments, whereas the $F(ab')_2$ fragments from γG4 proteins remained resistant to this further degradation.

These results show that the differences in susceptibility of human γG globulins to cleavage by papain is not a manifestation of conformational differences within the Fc region but rather that it is a property of the $F(ab')_2$ regions of the molecules.

Reduction of a critical disulphide bridge with a resulting conformational change within the $F(ab')_2$ region of the papain-resistant form seems, therefore, to be a pre-requisite for papain cleavage. The inaccessibility of sites of papain cleavage, prior to rupture of this covalent bond, could be due to differences in amino acid sequence or to steric hindrance by a carbohydrate side chain. In relation to the latter possibility, the finding of Smyth and Utsumi [5] that in 35% of rabbit γG globulin molecules a second carbohydrate moiety (in addition to the major one located at amino acid residue 150, from the C terminus of the Fc) is present in the region at which initial papain cleavage takes place is particularly interesting.

Table 1. Carbohydrate analyses of several myeloma globulin fragments.

Myeloma γ G sample	Carbohydrate content
Ga (papain resistant)	
$\quad$ F(ab')₂ fragments	NIL
$\quad$ Fab fragments	NIL
$\quad$ Peptides	NIL
Ld (papain resistant)	
$\quad$ F(ab')₂ fragments	NIL
Ha (papain sensitive)	
$\quad$ F(ab')₂ fragments	NIL
$\quad$ Fab fragments	NIL

That a similar distribution of carbohydrate exists within human γG immunoglobulins was tested for by determination of the carbohydrate content of pepsin $F(ab')_2$ and papain Fab fragments. The $F(ab')_2$ fragments were reduced with dithioerythritol followed by "blocking" with ^{14}C-labelled sodium iodoacetate; and subsequent incubation with papain yielded Fab fragments and peptides from the "link" region. The results of this study are shown in Table 1; no carbohydrate was detected in any of the fragments or peptides. This finding agrees with that of Abel et al. [6], who studied myeloma proteins which had carbohydrate within the $F(ab')_2$ fragment but showed that it was not attached in the link region. Variability of carbohydrate content or location is not, therefore, the explanation of the variability in papain-sensitivity of human γG immunoglobulins.

Fingerprint analysis of the peptides liberated on papain digestion of the reduced and alkylated pepsin $F(ab')_2$ fragments are shown in Fig. 5. Peptide spots were checked for radioactivity by liquid scintillation counting. There are

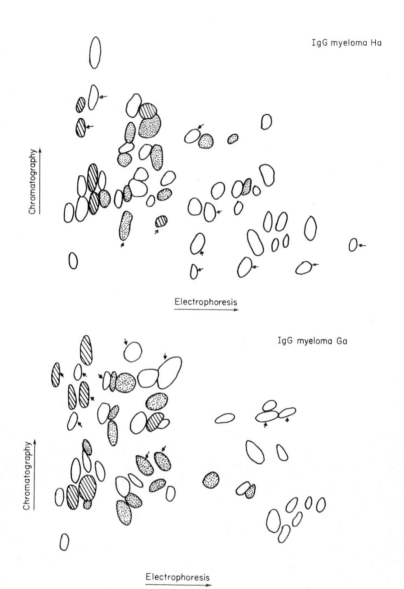

Figure 5. Fingerprint analysis of the "link" peptides of myeloma γG proteins Ha and Ga. Principal peptide differences are marked with an arrow; radioactive peptides are marked by diagonal stripes. Shaded spots were yellow or orange in the original print.

obvious differences in the number and distribution of both radioactive and non-radioactive peptides, indicating primary structural differences between the two myeloma proteins. Most interestingly, the papain-resistant protein yielded a larger number of radioactive peptides than the papain-sensitive one, reflecting a difference in the amount of cysteine present and therefore, presumably, in the number of disulphide bridges present.

ACKNOWLEDGEMENT

Dr. J. R. Clamp is thanked for performing the carbohydrate analyses.

REFERENCES

1. Gergely, J., Stanworth, D. R., Jefferis, R., Normansell, D. E., Henney, C. S. and Pardoe, G. I., *Immunochemistry* **4** (1967) 101.
2. Gergely, J., Medgyesi, G. A. and Stanworth, D. R., *Immunochemistry* **4** (1967) 369.
3. Dvorak, H. F., Billote, J. B., McCarthy, J. S. and Flax, M. H., *Immunology* **94** (1965) 966.
4. Porter, R. R., *Biochem. J.* **73** (1959) 119.
5. Smyth, D. S. and Utsumi, S., *Nature, Lond.* **216** (1967) 332.
6. Abel, C. A., Spiegelberg, H. L. and Grey, H. M., *Biochemistry, N.Y.* **7** (1968) 1271.

FEBS Symposium, Volume 15, 1969, pp. 221-225

Structural Factors Influencing the Varying Susceptibility to Papain Digestion of Immunoglobulin G Myeloma Proteins

J. GERGELY, G. A. MEDGYESI, M. PÁKH and É. PUSKÁS

Institute of Haematology, National Blood Center, Budapest, Hungary

In our previous investigations [1, 2], evidence was presented for the existence of two conformational forms of IgG in normal human serum, which differ in their behaviour when incubated with soluble papain in the absence of cysteine. Gel filtration through Sephadex G-100 of protein digests was employed to distinguish a papain-resistant form, digestible only in the presence of cysteine, from the products of digestion of a papain-sensitive form, digestible with papain in the absence of cysteine. IgG myeloma proteins have been found pre-dominantly either papain sensitive or papain resistant. It has been postulated that the difference between the papain-sensitive and papain-resistant IgG is one of molecular conformation within the Fc part of the molecules.

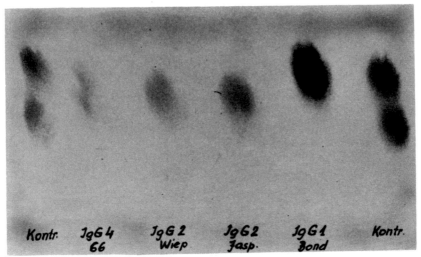

Figure 1. Thin layer gel-filtration (Sephadex G-150) of papain digests without cysteine of F(ab′)₂ fragments of papain-resistant globulins (66, Wiep, Jasp) and papain-susceptible (Bond) IgG myeloma proteins.
Control: papain-digest without cysteine of normal human IgG (digestion time 4 h).

In the present investigations the possible molecular basis for this varying susceptibility to papain digestion of IgG myeloma globulins was studied.

In our experiments we intended to answer the question as to whether the folded structure, responsible for the papain resistance, is recovered after peptic digestion at pH 4·2 and subsequent neutralization, or becomes ruptured by this procedure. $F(ab')_2$ fragments of five papain-sensitive and five papain-resistant IgG myeloma proteins were subjected to papain proteolysis. The results indicated the $F(ab')_2$ fragments to have a susceptibility essentially identical with that of the intact protein. Figure 1 demonstrates the thin layer gel-filtration on

Table 1. Papain susceptibility of IgG myeloma proteins.

Subclass	Cases	Papain sensitive	Papain resistant
IgG_1	9	8	1
IgG_2	4	–	4
IgG_3	2	2	–
IgG_4	2	–	2

Sephadex G-150 of $F(ab')_2$ fragments of one papain-sensitive and of three papain-resistant myeloma proteins. One can see that the $F(ab')_2$ fragments of the papain-resistant myeloma proteins remained undigested. These results point to the importance of the hinge region of the IgG molecule in developing the folded structure responsible for the papain resistance.

Further we studied the question as to whether there exists any correlation between papain susceptibility and H chain subclass of the myeloma proteins. The papain susceptibility of 40 IgG myeloma proteins has now been investigated in our laboratories, 15 of them being papain resistant, 25 papain sensitive.

In collaboration with H. H. Fudenberg and E. van Loghem, the H chain typing and typing for Gm factors were performed in 17 myeloma cases. Table 1 summarizes the results of these investigations. One can conclude that all the investigated myeloma proteins belonging to subclasses IgG2 and IgG4 are papain resistant, both IgG3 proteins are papain sensitive, and all the IgG1 proteins but one are papain sensitive as well. Figure 2 demonstrates the thin-layer chromatography of papain digests in the absence of cysteine of five myeloma proteins belonging to different subclasses. Figure 3 shows the result of papain digestion in the presence of cysteine of the same proteins. It is remarkable that IgG2 myeloma protein Wiepjes was practically undigested in the presence of cysteine; protein Jaspers from the same subclass, however, was almost completely digestible in the presence of cysteine. The former was negative for Gm(n), the latter, however, was Gm(n) positive.

These results point to a definite correlation between the papain susceptibility and H chain subclasses, but regarding the papain-resistant myeloma protein belonging to the IgG1 subclass and the different digestibility of the IgG2 proteins, we cannot exclude the possible role of other factors as well.

Studying the cysteine peptides derived from the hinge region of rabbit IgG, Smyth and Utsumi [3] suggested that the presence or absence of galactosamine in this region may influence the papain sensitivity of the molecule. As another possibility, we examined whether the heavy-light chain interaction has any

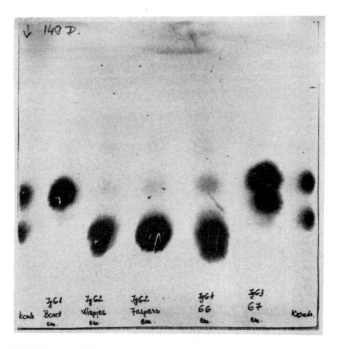

Figure 2. Thin layer gel-filtration (Sephadex G-150) of papain digests without cysteine of IgG myeloma proteins (digestion time 4 h).
Control: as in Figure 1.

influence on the papain sensitivity. To elucidate this point the papain sensitivity of IgG proteins recombined from isolated H and L chains was investigated.

The H and L chains of four papain-sensitive and four papain-resistant IgG myeloma globulins were isolated. Autologous and heterologous recombination of the chains was performed. The recombination was controlled by gel-filtration and immunoelectrophoresis. The recombined proteins were digested with papain in the absence of cysteine.

The papain sensitivity of a large fraction of recombined molecules was identical with that of the intact molecules when autologous H and L chains were

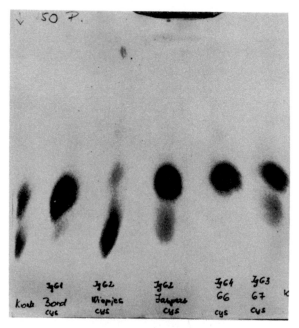

Figure 3. Thin layer gel-filtration (Sephadex G-150) of papain digests in the presence of 0·01 M cysteine of IgG myeloma proteins (digestion time 4 h).
Control: as in Figure 1.

Table 2. Papain sensitivity of recombined IgG molecules.

Protein	Recombined	molecule	Protein
Papain resistant			Papain sensitive
γ_2 K wi	wiH-szaL	wiL-szaH	sza γ_1 K
γ_4 L né	néH-szaL *	néL-szaH	sza γ_1 K
γ_1 K csö	csöH-szeL	csöL-szeH	sze γ_1 L
γ_4 L pr	prH-mlL	prL-mlH	ml γ_1 L
γ_4 L pr	prH-baL	prL-baH	ba γ_1 L

*The recombined *néH-szaL* papain resistant.

mixed. This means that the conformation responsible for the papain sensitivity or resistance was completely restored. According to the results of gel-filtration and immunoelectrophoresis, the recombination of H and L chains isolated from different myeloma proteins was successful in all cases. The recombination of H chains prepared from papain-resistant proteins with L chains of papain-sensitive proteins, or that of H chains of papain-sensitive with L chains of papain-resistant proteins, resulted only in one case in papain-resistant recombined molecules (Table 2).

These results point to two alternatives: (1) There exists the possibility that the primary structure of L chains, especially that of the variable part, influences the molecular conformation. (2) The complete restoration of the papain-resistant conformation may depend on the restoration of the disulfide bonds.

REFERENCES

1. Gergely, J., Stanworth, D. R., Jefferis, R., Normansell, D. E., Henney, C. S. and Pardoe, G. I., *Immunochemistry* **4** (1967) 101.
2. Gergely, J., Medgyesi, G. A. and Stanworth, D. R., *Immunochemistry* **4** (1967) 369.
3. Smyth, D. S. and Utsumi, S., *Nature, Lond.* **216** (1967) 332.

FEBS Symposium, Volume 15, 1969, pp. 227-232

The Reversible Conformational Transition of Polypeptide Chains of Human Immunoglobulin G During their Dissociation

A. Y. KULBERG, S. S. SHANIN and I. A. TARCHANOVA

Laboratory of Immunochemistry, The Gamaleya Institute of Epidemiology and Microbiology, Moscow, U.S.S.R.

This work was undertaken to study the conformational states of the human IgG polypeptide chains under conditions used for destruction of the quaternary structure of IgG.

It is well-known that the procedure for isolation of the IgG polypeptide chains consists of two stages: (1) the cleavage of the interchain disulphide bonds, and (2) the destruction of noncovalent interchain bonds either in the presence of monocarbonic acids or 6 M urea with 0·05 M formic acid.

As the cleavage of the IgG interchain bonds took place without addition of denaturating agents, it was probable that the interchain disulphide bonds were in the water environment. It was analysed by the investigation of the electron spin resonance spectra (ESR) of the reduced IgG treated by the maleimide derivate of the stable imidoxyl radical [1] which was used as the "spin label". This "spin label" specifically reacts with SH-groups at pH 6·3 according to the equation:

The reduction of IgG was performed with 0·1 M 2-mercaptoethanol.

The ESR spectra of the unbound "spin label" and "spin-labelled" protein (Fig. 1), both measured in saline, were alike except for some anisotropy of the signal of the protein-bound radical. From comparisons of the ESR spectra of "spin-labelled" protein in saline and after lyophilization (Fig. 1) it was evident that the IgG-bound radicals were in a relatively weak immobilization. These data

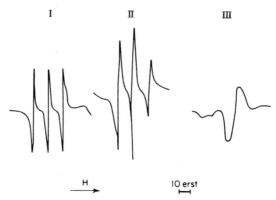

Figure 1. ESR Spectra of unbound "spin label" and "spin-labelled" IgG.
I—unbound "spin label" in saline,
II—"spin-labelled" IgG in saline,
III—"spin-labelled" IgG after lyophilization.

excluded the hydrophobic arrangement of the radicals connected to the IgG interchain disulphide bonds.

The effect of the carbonic acids used for the cleavage of the noncovalent bonds between the IgG polypeptide chains increased from acetic acid to butyric acid, as was shown by Porter [2]. This data and the possibility of dissociation of the reduced IgG in sodium decyl sulphate [3] led us to propose that the effect of the dissociating agents depended partially on the destruction of the inter and intra chain hydrophobic bonds.

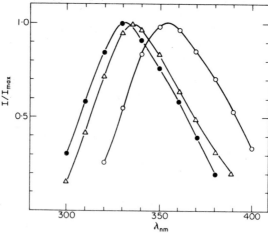

Figure 2. Spectra of fluorescence of tryptophan and IgG
○ tryptophan in saline
● tryptophan in dioxan
△ IgG in saline

For the estimation of these effects the state of the tryptophanyl residues of the IgG during the action of the dissociating agents was examined.

In the previous experiments it was found that most of the tryptophanyl residues of the IgG were in the hydrophobic environment as it could be seen at first from the comparisons of the fluorescent spectra of the IgG in saline and tryptophan in dioxan or in water solution respectively (Fig. 2). At the same

Table 1. The fluorescence maxima of IgG and accessibility of IgG tryptophanyl residues to NBS.

Solvent	Preparate	λ_{max}	$\dfrac{E^o_{275}}{E^{oxid}_{275}}$	After dialysis λ_{max} [a]	$\dfrac{E^o_{275}}{E^{oxid}_{275}}$ [b]
0·15 M saline	unreduced	335	–	335	–
	reduced	335	–	335	–
1 M glycine buffer pH 2·5	unreduced	335	1·3	334	1·3
	reduced	337	1·4	336	1·4
1 M propionic	unreduced	340	1·75	336	1·4
	reduced	340	2·0	337	–
6 M urea with 0·05 M formic acid	unreduced	350	2·4	337	1·5
	reduced	350	2·3	337	–

a: against saline
b: against 1 M glycine buffer pH 2·5

time, the ineffectivity of oxidation of the tryptophanyl residues by N-bromsuccinimide (NBS) [4] could be considered as the result of masking of the tryptophanyl residues in the hydrophobic regions of the IgG molecule.

The red shift of the fluorescence maximum of IgG was observed by investigation of the unreduced IgG in 1 M propionic acid (Table 1). This change was more pronounced after reduction of the IgG by 0·1 M 2-mercaptoethanol. The maximum of fluorescence of the unreduced and reduced IgG in 6 M urea with 0·05 M formic acid approached that for free tryptophan in water.

After removal of the dissociating agents by dialysis against saline, the fluorescent maxima reverted to the original values (Table 1).

In the same order, the propionic acid and 6 M urea with formic acid increased the susceptibility of the IgG tryptophanyl residues to oxidation by NBS (Table 1). (The calculations were performed on the basis of extinction coefficients for the original and oxidized IgG at 275 nm). The reversibility of this effect was established for the unreduced IgG after dialysis of protein against 1 M glycine buffer pH 2·5.

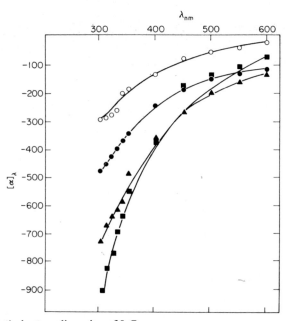

Figure 3. Optical rotary dispersion of IgG
     o in saline
     ● in 1 M glycine buffer pH 2·5
     ▲ in 1 M propionic acid pH 2·5
     ■ in 6 M urea with 0·05 M formic acid

The red shift of the fluorescence spectra, and the enhanced effects of the NBS on the tryptophanyl residues in the presence of dissociating agents, which could be considered as the increase in hydration of the IgG tryptophanyl residues, correlated with the enhancement of negative levorotation of the unreduced IgG in the same solvents. The optical rotary dispersion patterns are presented in Fig. 3.

There are two hypotheses for the explanation of the data presented above. It is probable that most of the IgG tryptophanyl residues were in the "contact sites" of the heavy and light chains in the hydrophobic environment. In the presence of dissociating agents the noncovalent bonds between chains were cleaved and the water penetrated into interchain space. According to other hypotheses the arrangement of the tryptophanyl residues is more diffuse, and the hydration of the hydrophobic zone of the IgG molecule in the presence of dissociating agents was the result of change of the original conformation of the IgG polypeptide chains.

To test these hypotheses we analysed the fluorescent spectra of the heavy and light chains isolated according to the method of Fleischman [5].

Table 2. The fluorescence of isolated chains and accessibility of isolated chain tryptophanyl residues to NBS.

Solvent	Preparation	λ_{max}	$\dfrac{E^{\circ}_{275}}{E^{oxid}_{275}}$	λ_{max} After dialysis against saline
0·15 M saline	H chain	336	—	336
	L chain	341	—	341
1 M glycine	H chain	336	1·7	336
buffer pH 2·5	L chain	—	1·4	—
1 M propionic	H chain	344	2·3	336
acid pH 2·5	L chain	346	1·8	341
6 M urea with 0·05 M	H chain	350	2·3	335
formic acid	L chain	351	1·8	340

The fluorescence maxima of the heavy chain in propionic acid and in the solvent-containing urea were comparable with that of unreduced IgG in the same solvents (Table 2). In saline the fluorescence spectrum of the heavy chain did not differ from that of the original IgG. On the contrary, the light chain tryptophanyl residues were more hydrated in saline, as can be seen from the fluorescence spectrum.

The analysis of the fluorescence properties of the isolated chains indicates a reversible conformational transition of the heavy chains during their isolation. A more hydrated state of the light chain tryptophanyl residues may be attributed to their localization in the "contact site" of the chain.

In spite of similarities of the fluorescence spectra of the isolated heavy chain and the original IgG, it is probable that the conformational state of the isolated heavy chains differs from that in whole IgG molecule. Thus, the tryptophanyl residues of the heavy chain are more accessible to oxidation by NBS in glycine buffer pH 2·5 (Table 2). The differences of the conformational states of isolated heavy chain and original IgG molecule were established also by the optical rotatory dispersion technique [6].

REFERENCES

1. Griffith, O. H., Cornell, D. N. and McConnel, H. M., *J. chem. Phys.* **43** (1965) 2909.
2. Porter, R. R., *in* "Symposium of Basic Problems of Neoplastic Diseases" (edited by A. Gelhorn and E. Hirschberg), Columbia University Press, New York (1962) p. 177.
3. Utsumi, S. and Karush, F., *Biochemistry, N.Y.* **3** (1964) 1329.
4. Tarchanova, I. A. and Kulberg, A. J., *Proc. med. Chem.* (Russian), **8** (1962) 163.
5. Fleischman, J. B., Pain, R. H. and Porter, R. R., *Archs Biochem. Biophys.* **Suppl. 1** (1962) 174.
6. Dorrington, K. J., Zarlengo, M. H. and Tanford, C., *Proc. natn. Acad. Sci. U.S.A.* **59** (1967) 996.

Author Index

Numbers in parentheses are reference numbers and are included to assist in locating references. Numbers in *italics* refer to the page on which the reference is listed.

A

Abaturov, L. V., 122(24), *131*
Abel, C. A., 217(6), *219*
Adler, F. L., 2(5), *11*
Alescio-Zonta, L., 58(20), 63(20), *73,* 100(35), *103*
Anderson, J. S., 95(15), *103*
Appella, E., 29(26), *40,* 59(39), 61(39), 63(39), 70(59), *74,* 95(13), *103,* 197(7, 8), *198*
Armentrout, S. A., 94(11), *103,* 117(13), 118(13), *131*
Askonas, B. A., 94(6), 97(6, 27), 98(27), 99(6, 27, 32, 33), 100(6), 102(44), *102, 103, 104,* 106(7, 8, 9), 107(19, 20, 23, 24, 25), 108(26, 28), 109(26), 110(25, 28), 111(9, 25), *116,* 117(4), *130*
Astrin, K. H., 197(6), *198*
Attardi, G., 105(2), *115,* 152(36, 37), *167*
Avogadro, L., 43(4), 45(4), *55*
Avrameas, S., 86(17), *91*
Awdeh, Z. L., 102(44), *104,* 106(7, 8), *116*

B

Baglioni, C., 58(20), 61(36), 63(20), *73, 74,* 97(24, 25, 28), 98(24, 25), 99(24, 25, 28), 100(28, 35), *103*
Barnikol, H. U., 59(32), 62(32), 65(32), *74,* 80(14), *81*
Beale, G. H., 152(41), 159(41), *167*
Becker, M. J., 94(7), 100(7), *102*
Benacerraf, B., 94(10), *103,* 117(15), 118(15), *131,* 187(3), *191*
Bennett, J. C., 55(23), *56,* 58(27), *73*

Bennich, H., 83(6), 84(6), 86(14), 89(6), *91*
Berggård, I., 83(7), 84(7), 90(7), *91*
Bernier, G. M., 22(9), 24(9), *40,* 83(8), 84(8), 90(8), *91,* 134(13), 150(24), *167*
Beutler, E., 150(29), *167*
Biegel, A. A., 134(17), *167*
Billingham, R. E., 133(12), *166*
Billote, J. B., 214(3), *219*
Bishop, J., 117(3), *130*
Black, J. A., 101(42), *104*
Block, K., 187(3), *191*
Bloth, B., 84(13), *91*
Boyse, E. A., 152(42), 159(42), *167*
Braun, W., 152(33), *167*
Braunitzer, G., 66(48), 67(50), *74*
Breinl, F., 1(1), *11*
Brenneman, L., 75(4), *81*
Brenner, S., 55(24), *56,* 58(22), *73*
Breuninger-Peck, E., 134(20), *167*
Brown, E. S., 2(3), *11*
Buckley, C. E., 83(5), 89(5), *91*
Burnet, F. M., 7(20), 8(22), *12*

C

Callan, H. G., 72(62), *74*
Campana, T., 97(25), 98(25), 99(25), *103*
Campbell, P. N., 117(1), *130*
Carbonara, A., 58(20), 63(20), *73*
Cebra, J. J., 17(18, 19), 19(18, 19), *19,* 38(39, 40), *41,* 44(13), *55,* 105(4), *116,* 134(13), 150(24), *167,* 179(19), *182*
Ceppellini, R., 9(27b), 11(27b), *12*
Cheng, H. F., 2(3), *11*
Chesebro, B., 84(13), *91*

233

Advances in

THE STUDY OF BEHAVIOR

VOLUME 17

Advances in
THE STUDY OF
BEHAVIOR

Edited by

JAY S. ROSENBLATT
Institute of Animal Behavior
Rutgers University
Newark, New Jersey

COLIN BEER
Institute of Animal Behavior
Rutgers University
Newark, New Jersey

MARIE-CLAIRE BUSNEL
UER Biomédicale
Groupe Génétique et Comportements
Faculté de Médecine Paris V
Paris, France

PETER J. B. SLATER
Department of Zoology and Marine Biology
University of St. Andrews
Fife, Scotland

VOLUME 17
1987

ACADEMIC PRESS, INC.
Harcourt Brace Jovanovich, Publishers

Orlando   San Diego   New York   Austin
Boston   London   Sydney   Tokyo   Toronto

ACADEMIC PRESS, INC.
Orlando, Florida 32887

United Kingdom Edition published by
ACADEMIC PRESS INC. (LONDON) LTD.
24–28 Oval Road, London NW1 7DX

LIBRARY OF CONGRESS CATALOG CARD NUMBER: 64-8031

ISBN 0–12–004517–6 (alk. paper)

PRINTED IN THE UNITED STATES OF AMERICA

87 88 89 90   9 8 7 6 5 4 3 2 1

Contents

The Dwarf Mongoose: A Study of Behavior and Social Structure
in Relation to Ecology in a Small, Social Carnivore

O. ANNE E. RASA

Ontogenetic Development of Behavior: The Cricket
Visual World

RAYMOND CAMPAN, GUY BEUGNON,
AND MICHEL LAMBIN

Preface

The aim of *Advances in the Study of Behavior* is to serve the increasing number of scientists who are engaged in the study of animal behavior by presenting their theoretical ideas and research to their colleagues and to those in neighboring fields. Since its inception in 1965, this publication has not changed its aim to serve ". . . as a contribution to the development of cooperation and communication among scientists in our field." We acknowledge that in the interim new vigor has been given to traditional fields of animal behavior by their coalescence with closely related fields and by the closer relationship that now exists between those studying animal and human subjects. Scientists studying animal behavior now range from ecologists to evolutionary biologists, geneticists, endocrinologists, ethologists, comparative and developmental psychobiologists, and those doing research in the neurosciences. As the task of developing cooperation and communication among scientists whose skills and concepts necessarily differ in accordance with the diversity of phenomena that they study has become more difficult, the need to do so has become greater. The editors and publisher of *Advances in the Study of Behavior* will continue to provide the means to meet this need by publishing critical reviews, by inviting extended presentations of significant research programs, by encouraging the writing of theoretical syntheses and reformulations of persistent problems, and by highlighting especially penetrating research that introduces important new concepts.

Receptive Competencies of Language-Trained Animals

Louis M. Herman

DEPARTMENT OF PSYCHOLOGY AND
KEWALO BASIN MARINE MAMMAL LABORATORY
UNIVERSITY OF HAWAII, HONOLULU, HAWAII 96814

I. Introduction

Two major themes appear among the recent critiques of the attempts to teach languages to great apes: (1) whether apes can use the symbols (words) of a language as true surrogates for the objects and events they reference, including objects and events remote in time or space, and (2) whether apes can construct or understand sentences by using combinations of words as information. The first theme, recently pursued most vigorously by Savage-Rumbaugh and colleagues (e.g., Savage-Rumbaugh et al., 1980b, 1983), addresses the semantic aspect of language—the meaning and reference of words and phrases. The second theme, identified recently with Terrace and colleagues (e.g., Terrace et al., 1979), addresses the syntactic aspect—the information that is added to the string of words comprising a sentence by the structure of the string, such as the ordering of the words. In human languages, it is most often necessary to account for both the semantic and the syntactic components of a sentence to interpret a sentence correctly. Semantics and syntax have been described as the "indispensable core attributes of any human language" (Paivio and Begg, 1981, p. 25).

The contention of the Savage-Rumbaugh group is that the use of symbols by apes to name objects or to make requests for foods or other desirables is not of itself evidence that the symbols function as surrogates for objects and events, as do words in human languages. Careful analysis of the majority of the work with apes reveals that the symbols used are often constrained to limited contexts and are principally a learned means for obtaining a desired outcome. Typically, the words are not used to "refer" (cf. Terrace, 1985) but with special training may eventually take on that function (Savage-Rumbaugh and Rumbaugh, 1978).

The syntactic issue, as raised in the review by Terrace et al. (1979) (also see Ristau and Robbins, 1982), asked whether the language produced by apes was grammatical, showing evidence of the use of structure, such as word order, as

1

information. Or, as the question was put directly by Terrace *et al.* in the title of their 1979 paper, "Can an Ape Create a Sentence?" It was acknowledged that apes occasionally generated long strings of words but that successive words added little or no information, being mainly repetitions, synonyms, or the like, without elaboration or expansion of meaning. For example, Terrace *et al.* described one sequence produced by Nim, the chimp they tutored in sign language. To request an orange, Nim produced the following 16 signs: "give orange me give eat orange me eat orange give me eat orange give me you." Nim probably did get the orange.

In other cases of apparently well-formed word sequences produced by apes additional problems were cited by Terrace *et al.* (1979) and in other reviews (e.g., Bronowski and Bellugi, 1970; Fodor *et al.*, 1974; Petitto and Seidenberg, 1979; Ristau and Robbins, 1982; Savage-Rumbaugh *et al.*, 1980a; Seidenberg and Petitto, 1979, 1981; Terrace, 1979a; Terrace *et al.*, 1981). These problems included insufficiencies or deficiencies in the reporting of data; the presence of context cues to guide responding, prompts, or other paralinguistic cues from the trainers that may have led the ape into a prescribed series of signs; the probable underreporting of examples that did not conform to a grammatical sequence; the practice in some cases of deleting "extraneous" or redundant signs in reports of the sequences produced by the apes; and the overinterpretation of a string of signs or unique combination of words produced by the apes. Thus, when the chimp Washoe signed "water bird" on seeing a swan in a lake for the first time, did she create a novel combination of words and thereby name the swan, or was she simply giving two independent signs "WATER——BIRD?" These criticisms cast grave doubt on the evidence for sentence-processing abilities of apes and, by implication, on all of the claimed linguistic skills of these animals.

II. Language Production versus Language Comprehension

Work with apes has emphasized language production, rather than comprehension. Humans, of course, both produce language and understand it. As noted by Savage-Rumbaugh and colleagues (Savage-Rumbaugh *et al.*, 1980a, 1983), by Seidenberg and Petitto (1979), and by others, the unfortunate assumption was made in much of the work with apes that production implied comprehension. Premack, who studied the chimp Sarah and other chimps, using an artificial language in which words were represented by plastic chips (Premack, 1971, 1976), recognized that production and comprehension may evolve as separate systems, in child or chimpanzee. Although Premack carried out a number of studies of comprehension, shortcomings in methodology and data reporting limited the strength of the conclusions that could be drawn from the work (R. A. Gardner and Gardner, 1978; Ristau and Robbins, 1982; Savage-Rumbaugh *et al.*, 1980a; Terrace, 1979a). Premack's work on receptive competencies, as well as that of other researchers teaching languages to apes, is reviewed in Section III.

There is evidence for an asymmetry of comprehension and production in the development and maintenance of language in humans. During early childhood, comprehension generally precedes and exceeds production (Fraser *et al.*, 1963; Ingram, 1974), although there may be exceptions (Chapman, 1974; Chapman and Miller, 1975; also see the review in Bloom, 1974). Production may involve more complex processes than does comprehension (Bloom, 1974; Schiefelbusch, 1974), giving support to the notion that the two systems, though mutually dependent, are somewhat separate.

Some separation of the systems may remain at adulthood, as suggested by the specificity of some aphasic disorders. Difficulties in speaking (expressive aphasia) generally involve lesions in anterior areas—Broca's area or other regions of the frontal lobe—while difficulties in comprehension (receptive aphasia) involve lesions in posterior areas, particularly Wernicke's area (see the review in Paivio and Begg, 1981, p. 367). Similarly, syntax and semantics may be subserved by different areas: syntactic functions by anterior structures and semantic functions by posterior structures (Caramazza and Berndt, 1978).

In studying children's language, it has proven fruitful to analyze production and comprehension separately when assessing linguistic competency (e.g., Fraser *et al.*, 1963; Ingram, 1974). Tests of comprehension have been particularly useful in the analysis of the grammatical competency of normally developing children (Chapman and Miller, 1975; Churchill, 1978; Strohner and Nelson, 1974) and in demonstrating language competencies in nonverbal or preverbal children (Curtiss, 1977; Ingram, 1974; Itard, 1932). Seidenberg and Petitto (1979) commented that in view of the attention given to comprehension in work with children it was puzzling that so little attention was given to comprehension in work with apes.

Focus on receptive competencies of animals (or children) has several advantages. The situation in which comprehension is tested can be described, controlled, and repeated, and objective, quantitative measures of performance can be obtained. Given the extensive problems in method, assessment, and interpretation of the results of the productive language studies with apes, it is strategic at this juncture to emphasize receptive competencies. Theoretically, if production and comprehension involve separate or only partially overlapping systems in animals, then there may be inherent limitations in one system which are not present in the other. Consequently, although it is imperative to study both systems eventually, a current emphasis on comprehension provides a needed balance to the extensive work on production and contributes toward a better understanding of the capabilities and limitations of animals in languagelike tasks.

In this article, I review what is known of the receptive competencies of animals in languagelike tasks. The emphasis is on the extensive work with apes as well as the recent work with marine mammals, including my own studies of bottle-nosed dolphins.

III. RECEPTIVE COMPETENCIES OF LANGUAGE-TRAINED APES

A. SIGN LANGUAGE PROJECTS

Sign language projects (e.g., B. T. Gardner and Gardner, 1971, 1979; R. A. Gardner and Gardner, 1969; Miles, 1983; Patterson, 1978a,b; Terrace, 1979b) have given little attention to receptive competencies. Generally, data from these studies are insufficient for judging the degree to which apes understand the signs of their trainers. The Gardners (B. T. Gardner and Gardner, 1975), in fact, disavowed the importance of receptive vocabulary, stating that for assessing the linguistic ability of the chimp Washoe "our practice is to list items of expressive vocabulary only" (p. 248). They go on to say that "to include items of receptive vocabulary [in the list of expressive vocabulary] we would have to add several score or several hundred additional items, depending on the standards of evidence that one would impose on the data" (p. 248). Further, the Gardners take exception to forced-choice tests of receptive competencies, claiming that "productive tests are methodologically more sound" (p. 256). This claim runs counter to the extensive criticisms leveled against the methods of productive tests.

It is unfortunate that the Gardners did not test and document the receptive vocabulary of Washoe or of other chimps they studied, as this might have made for meaningful comparisons between productive and receptive abilities, enabled the assessment of sentence understanding, and possibly blunted those criticisms that tended to summarily dismiss their work as failing to provide convincing evidence for any language competencies in apes. The only test of receptive ability systematically applied to signing chimps by the Gardners was the ability to answer *wh-* questions appropriately (B. T. Gardner and Gardner, 1975, 1979). Responses of the chimps Washoe, Pili, Tatu, and Moja to questions such as *Who that? What you want? Where Susan?* were tested. A limitation of these tests, pointed out by Seidenberg and Petitto (1979, 1981), was the policy of scoring replies as correct if they were from the appropriate grammatical category, such as nouns as answers to *what* questions and locatives as answers to *where* questions. This scoring criterion is adequate for assessing mastery of a question *form* (Brown, 1968), but allows for semantically inappropriate answers. Since the Gardners provided only examples of the replies of the chimps, it is difficult to judge the degree to which the chimps understood the content as well as the form of the question. Understanding of form was itself quite variable within and among chimps, ranging from a low of 12% correct categorizations to a high of 100%.

Despite the Gardners' caveat against forced-choice receptive tests, Patterson (Patterson, 1978b; Patterson and Linden, 1981) administered a standard children's forced-choice test of receptive skill (*Assessment of Children's Language Comprehension Test*) to the gorilla Koko. Koko's task was to look at a card containing multiple drawings representing objects, attributes, or relationships among objects and point to a particular drawing in response to verbal or signed words or both. The first 10 cards of the set tested understanding of single words (vocabulary) and the remaining 30 tested understanding of phrases, for example, "point to the bird above the house." The phrases were at three levels of difficulty, corresponding to the number of "critical elements" (two, three, or four) referred to by the phrase (e.g., three in the above example: *bird, above,* and *house*). Koko's performance ranged from 72% correct responses for the 50 vocabulary items (five items per card) to 30–70% correct for phrases (chance accounting for 20–25%, depending on the number of alternatives on the cards). The combination of sign plus voice yielded somewhat better scores than did either alone, and there were no differences between sign-only versus voice-only testing. Patterson claimed that Koko performed significantly better than chance, but summed binomial distribution tests that I applied to her data show that this was true only for the vocabulary test and for three of the nine conditions using phrases (three levels of critical elements × three replications: sign plus voice, sign only, and voice only). An additional limitation on the findings is the replication over language conditions. Although Patterson provided no information on how these replications were carried out, it appears that Koko went through the 30 phrase cards three times; therefore, her performance during the second and third replications might have benefited from the previous replication(s). Terrace *et al.* (1981) noted that the lack of detail in Patterson's reports makes it difficult to attribute Koko's performance to true comprehension, as opposed to learning sets, rote drilling, social cueing (which Patterson seems to have controlled for), or the like. Petitto and Seidenberg (1979), in an article devoted primarily to an evaluation of Patterson's (1978a) study, did not comment on Patterson's forced-choice tests (which might not have been available to them at the time of publication). However, these authors stressed that the simultaneous use of gestures and spoken English during normal social interactions with Koko made it difficult to assess Koko's understanding of the primary language medium—gestural signs. They also cautioned that Koko's performance might have been guided by paralinguistic cues such as body movements or pointing, a criticism that has been leveled against all of the signing projects. In fairness to Patterson, her findings of equivalent performance on comprehension of single vocabulary items with either gesture or voice cues are given increased credence by recent work by Savage-Rumbaugh *et al.* (1985), who reported that the pygmy chimpanzee Kanzi understands some spoken English words, though no specific training for this was given (see Section III,C) (also see the related report by Fouts *et al.*, 1976). Nevertheless, Patterson's work as a whole continues to suffer from a spareness of objective assessment.

Fouts *et al.* (1976; described in Fouts, 1978) reported understanding by the chimp Ally of signed commands to select one of five objects and deliver it to one of five locations. Fouts (1978) stated that some of the commands were novel, obtained by vocabulary substitutions at the object and location positions of the sequence of signs. The use of imperatives for testing comprehension is an important, objective procedure and was used in our work with dolphins (see Section IV). Unfortunately, the report by Fouts (1978) failed to provide details of the training and testing methods, or of the results, so that some of the reservations noted for Patterson's work apply here as well.

Fouts, like the Gardners, suggested that the receptive skills of the apes he tutored were extensive. A similar claim was made for Nim, the ape tutored by Terrace and colleagues (e.g., Terrace, 1979b). Seidenberg and Petitto (1981) commented that while extensive receptive vocabularies were *claimed* for the chimps Ally and Nim—approximately 130 Ameslan signs for Ally (Fouts *et al.*, 1978) and 199 signs for Nim (Terrace *et al.*, 1985)—no formal tests were ever reported.

B. ARTIFICIAL LANGUAGE PROJECTS

1. Premack Project

Projects by Premack (1971, 1976) and by Rumbaugh and associates (Rumbaugh, 1977) with artificial languages focused to varying degrees on receptive competency. The most extensive attempt to quantify sentence comprehension in apes was that by Premack (1976). The chimps Sarah, Peony, and Elizabeth were tutored in a system in which plastic symbols of arbitrary shape and color were used to represent objects, properties, and actions within an artificial language. Sentences could be constructed, by the experimenter or by the chimp, by arranging the symbols in a linear array on a board. In early tests, the chimps failed to transfer spontaneously between production and comprehension. For example, although the chimps could write "Give apple" or "Give banana" to request those specific foods and also understood the sentences "Take ball" and "Take block" in the receptive mode, they showed no immediate understanding of the novel constructions "Take apple" or "Take banana." After brief, specific training in transfer from production to comprehension or vice versa, the apes were able to pass new transfer tests.

Premack also carried out extensive studies of the apes' answers to questions. Like similar work described for the Gardners, answers to questions are a measure of receptive competency. In Premack's studies, a symbol for an interrogative particle was introduced as a straightforward extension of an already familiar "same–different" paradigm—for example, *A ? A,* where the possible answers are "same" or "different." The interrogative particle continued to be used in this form as well as in other question forms that were implicit *wh-* questions. For example, "A ? A" was glossed by Premack as "*What* is A to A?", while the symbol string "A same ?" (for which the correct answer is *A*) was glossed as "*What* is A the same as?". The task of the chimp was to substitute one of the available symbols for the question symbol.

Using symbols meaning "same" or "different," Premack generated additional Yes–No question forms; for example, "A *same* A ?" was glossed as "Is A the same as A?" Symbols meaning Yes and No were available as answers. In the earlier work, the items compared in the question need not have names (only their physical identities were at issue). In later work, questions consisting solely of linguistic elements were constructed, such as "? color-of apple," a string consisting of three symbols to be answered by choosing one of two available color symbols. Another example is "Round ? ball," to be answered by substituting the symbol for "color-of," "shape-of," or "name-of" for the question symbol. Premack reported high levels of performance in response to most of these types of questions.

Several grammatical categories of words were taught to the apes in the comprehension mode or by intermixing the production and comprehension modes. These included negation (e.g., "*No* Sarah honey bread take"), the demonstrative (e.g., "Sarah insert *this*" versus "Sarah insert *that*"), quantifiers ("Sarah take *some*"), and the preposition "on" ("A *on* B"). Some structurally novel sentences were also taught in the comprehension mode (e.g., "Sarah take red dish," as derived from the previously taught atomic sentences "Sarah take red" and "Sarah take dish"). Nonetheless, these demonstrations, as well as additional tests of comprehension (or production) skill presented by Premack, have been criticized on a number of grounds that, in sum, moderate any strong conclusions about receptive competencies. The Gardners (R. A. Gardner and Gardner, 1978) commented on the sparsity of Trial-1 data in Premack's reports of transfer and argued that because chimps are capable of rapid intra-problem learning, without Trial-1 data it is unclear whether or not there was any *inter*-problem learning. The Gardners' contention is supported, for example, by examination of Table 6.2 in Premack (1976, pp. 120–121). The table reports "noun contrast" testing of the understanding of new combinations of object and action terms. Trial-1 results are available for only eight of 22 new combinations tested.

Terrace (1979a), as well as Savage-Rumbaugh *et al.* (1980a), provided extensive critiques of Premack's work that need not be repeated in detail here. In brief, however, contextual constraints present during Premack's experiments could have guided the apes' responses. Problems of a given type were clustered within a testing session, the number of alternative choices available for response was usually limited to two, and in many cases the problems might have been solved by nonlinguistic means. For example, the symbols for "Mary," "give," and "Sarah" were used repeatedly within a session in imperative strings such as "Sarah give Mary X." Alternative, contrasting symbols were not available during a session (e.g., alternative trainer names). Sarah, therefore, need not have made any semantic interpretation of the symbols "Mary," "give," and "Sarah" and could have simply responded to X as in an associative naming exercise by, for example, giving an apple if X was "apple."

Because of the attention given in this paper to competencies for processing syntactic information, it is worthwhile to consider Premack's evidence for this ability in apes. This evidence occurs in several contexts in Premack's work. One involves the ability to demonstrate an understanding of the relationships among nonadjacent words in ordered strings. For example, in the string "Sarah apple pail banana dish insert," an instruction to Sarah to insert the apple in the pail and the banana in the dish, "insert" is not adjacent to "apple" or "banana" but nevertheless directs the action to be taken toward these fruits. Sarah's ability to carry out such instructions suggests, therefore, that she can interpret the hierarchical structure of these sentences. Again, however, there are limitations to any conclusions since, for sentences of the type listed, the only objects available to Sarah were the two listed in the sentence, and sentences of the stated type were clustered within a training session. Therefore, if Sarah understood that the problem at hand was that of "insertion," she need not attend to the word "insert." Also, as soon as she placed the first object in the correct receptacle, which would reveal some understanding of those two words and their relationship, the further operation on the remaining objects could be determined by default. That is, only one object and one receptacle remain.

Syntactic processing demands also occurred in a prepositional form that permitted the construction of semantically contrasting sentences of the form "A on B" versus "B on A," where A and B were names of objects or names of the colors of cards. The task of the chimps Sarah, Peony, and Elizabeth was to place the first-named object or first-named color on top of the second. Sarah learned the task with a fixed set of colors to a level of 75% correct responses, and then passed a single transfer test to a new pair of colors at the 80% level (eight of ten correct responses). The other two apes worked with objects rather than colored cards. Elizabeth required fairly extensive training to learn the problem, but then passed a single transfer test (nine of ten correct responses). Similar results were obtained for Peony. Later, Premack demonstrated that the chimps paid attention to both the A and B names, by providing three alternatives rather than only two. Performance declined to 70%, but was still well above chance.

Semantically contrasting sentences provide a powerful vehicle for testing syntactic processing ability and, together with other tests of sensitivity to word order, have been used to show that children may be surprisingly slow to develop receptive competency in processing syntactic information (C. Chomsky, 1969; de Villiers and de Villiers, 1973; Horgan, 1980; Wetstone and Friedlander, 1973). Premack's results appear to show that the apes were able to understand, to a reasonably proficient level, the role of word order, as revealed by their responses to semantically contrasting sentences. However, the contextual constraints noted earlier, the lack of Trial-1 data on most transfer tests, the comparatively few transfer tests given, and the fact that transfer tests immediately followed training (thereby the problem to be solved was largely predetermined) again limit the conclusions. Additionally, as noted by Terrace (1979a), there was no contrasting preposition, for example, "under" as well as "on." Therefore, "on" was redundant in the context given and it is not clear that any semantic interpretation was given to that word by the chimps.[1] Nevertheless, Premack's approach in these studies was well founded conceptually. It is unfortunate, therefore, that the methodological flaws limiting the conclusions were not anticipated and eliminated.

A briefly reported study by Muncer and Ettlinger (1981) used the contrasting prepositions "behind" and "in" to describe relations between two objects, for example, "apple in bag" versus "apple behind bag." Both production tests (using signs to describe an observed relation) and comprehension tests (observing signs given by the trainer to select among three different object relations) were given to the single chimpanzee subject. While the study hints that a chimpanzee trained in sign language might understand how word order changed meaning (for example, the difference between "bag in box" versus "box in bag"), the description of methods and data are too sparse to make confident judgments of ability. It appears that, during testing, only relational sentences were given, so that all problems involved some comparison among two objects; the particular errors made were not given in detail; and there were many more "behind" sequences than "in" sequences, although the exact numbers of each were not reported by the authors. Furthermore, it appears that only one semantically reversible sequence could be formed with "in" (the reversible sequence named above) but relatively many could be formed with "behind." Hence, responses would be expected to be biased toward "behind," obviating any clear test of the ability to deal with contrasting prepositions.

2. Projects by Savage-Rumbaugh and Rumbaugh

Savage-Rumbaugh and colleagues (Savage-Rumbaugh and Rumbaugh, 1978; Savage-Rumbaugh et al., 1980a, 1983) have shown that comprehension does not automatically flow from the production of symbols. Savage-Rumbaugh et al.

---

[1]Premack (1971, p. 214) implied that training for "under" and "beside" was underway, but, to my knowledge, no reports of the results of that training have ever appeared.

(1980a) stressed that receptive competency was never established in the chimps Washoe, Lana, or Nim, the animals studied, respectively, by the Gardners, by Rumbaugh and associates, and by Terrace and associates.

However, Savage-Rumbaugh *et al.* (1983) discussed the findings of an early study of Lana's receptive competency (Essok *et al.,* 1977) and concluded that receptive competency was a multidimensional skill that might appear in some guises but not others. In the Essok *et al.* study, Lana was able to answer questions successfully about the name of an object of a specified color or about the color of a named object. In both cases, either three or six objects were present simultaneously. To carry out the task, Lana had to search among the displayed objects for the named object or the named color and then, using her lexigram keyboard, provide the correct symbols (object name and object color) for her response. Yet, Lana was *not* able to respond successfully in what appeared to be a simpler task, giving a named object in response to an imperative "Give *X*." Rather than giving the requested object reliably, Lana offered a sequence of objects until she arrived at the correct response. Although Savage-Rumbaugh *et al.* (1983) stated that Lana carried out the object/color tasks with no prior receptive training for the task, the procedures of Essok *et al.* (1977) suggest that the final level of competency was attained through a series of experiments or training steps. Lana first learned to give the name or color of a photographed object of a set of six possible objects of six possible colors (correction trials were given following errors), then to give the colors of novel real objects displayed one at a time, then to give either the name or color of three different objects displayed simultaneously, and finally to give the names of six different objects displayed simultaneously. Hence, it appears that the terminal receptive skill was accomplished through a reasonably designed series of steps that trained Lana in the task requirements. In contrast to this sequenced training, Savage-Rumbaugh *et al.* (1983) stated in regard to Lana's failure to give the object requested, "None of Lana's training prior to the time she was asked to give objects required that she act directly on objects" (p. 474). That receptive competency requires at least some degree of training should be anticipated and should no more be at issue than the ready acceptance of the training necessary for productive competency (but see Section III,C for a discussion of findings with a pygmy chimpanzee).

The receptive competencies of children may also not emerge spontaneously. Rice (1980), as described by Savage-Rumbaugh *et al.* (1983), carried out a study in which young children (ages 2–3 to 3–4) were given object/color tasks similar to those given to Lana. Children who did not spontaneously sort objects on the basis of color required extensive training to attach color names to colored objects. Some children, even after this training, could not give the experimenter an object of a named color (e.g., giving red in response to "Give me the red one"), and thus failed that test of receptive competency.

Receptive competency (as well as productive competency) was made an explicit part of the training regimen applied to the chimps Sherman and Austin (Savage-Rumbaugh, 1981; Savage-Rumbaugh and Rumbaugh, 1978; Savage-Rumbaugh *et al.*, 1983). Sherman and Austin were routinely asked to search for, retrieve, or give objects named by the trainer. The contexts in which this was done were varied and included one ape making requests of another ape, as well as trainer-to-ape communication. The trainer entered requests on a keyboard that contained visual symbols ("lexigrams") for various objects and actions. The trainer and her keyboard were not visible to the apes. The apes "read" the trainer's requests on a projector system that displayed the keyed lexigrams. (A keyboard was also available to the apes for requests or for symbolic responses.) In the Savage-Rumbaugh and Rumbaugh (1978) study, the apes provided any of six tools in response to two-word lexigram commands by the trainer, such as "Give key." Each ape was 90% correct in a blind test consisting of the six possible requests replicated five times for a total of 30 trials. In ape-to-ape communication, comprehension performance was even higher: 97%. Considerable practice occurred prior to and during these tests and the results of any first-trial transfer tests to new objects were not given. Moreover, the tests appeared to be clustered, providing a strong context cue to the nature of the response desired. For example, if as it appears, all 30 trials of the receptive test were given together, the word "Give" was redundant, the problem could be identified by the context, and only the tool name need be attended to. Hence, sentence understanding was not tested.

A later study (Savage-Rumbaugh, 1981) investigated the ability of Sherman, Austin, and Lana to categorize any of 16 items as tools or foods. Blind tests of the chimps' responses to requests for these 16 items, plus 10–15 additional items, were also given, following the procedures of Savage-Rumbaugh and Rumbaugh (1978). Some of the items were used in training while the remainder were test objects (including some photographs of objects) introduced at successively later stages of practice. Sherman's ability to deliver the requested object was usually 90% or better over successive days; Austin's performance was more variable, generally between 80 and 90% correct. Lana, who received relatively little training on this task, most often scored between 70 and 85% correct responses. Lana's receptive scores were below her scores on labeling tests (naming the object shown to her) or on requesting tests (asking for an object by pressing a lexigram symbol), with the same objects used on all tests. In contrast, Sherman and Austin each showed a proficiency in reception equal to that for labeling and requesting. The co-occurrence of training for labeling, requesting, and receptive skills used with Sherman and Austin probably accounts for the equivalent proficiencies. In contrast, Lana was trained in the receptive task only after having had extensive experience with labeling and requesting tasks. These results again underscore that receptive competency may not emerge spontaneously or fully through simple exposure to productive tasks.

Recent work with a young captive-born pygmy chimpanzee (*Pan paniscus*) named Kanzi (Savage-Rumbaugh *et al.*, 1985) holds promise of establishing levels of language competency not seen with common chimpanzees (*Pan troglodytes*), the species used in all other work on language learning by chimps. The pygmy chimpanzee, unlike the common chimpanzee, spontaneously accompanies gestures with vocalizations and spontaneously points at objects (Savage-Rumbaugh, 1984b; also see Woodruff and Premack, 1979). The latter behavior is reminiscent of the indicative pointing in young children that presages the emergence of the one-word stage of language (Bates, 1976; Savage-Rumbaugh *et al.*, 1983). The current work with Kanzi employs a mechanical keyboard like that used by Sherman and Austin, as well as a portable, folding posterboard containing printed lexigram symbols. Reportedly, Kanzi presses or points to lexigram symbols to make spontaneous references to objects in his environment as well as to make requests. No formal training was given in the use of the keyboard; Kanzi apparently learned its use through observation of his mother during her specific training in the use of a keyboard. The mother was taught to make requests through the keyboard for food, blankets, trips outdoors, grooming, or tickling. However, her performance on the keyboard was reported as marginal, inferior to that displayed by Sherman and Austin.

Kanzi's observations of his mother continued from the age of 6 months to $2\frac{1}{2}$ years, when his mother was temporarily removed from the study area for 4 months. Shortly afterward, Kanzi began approaching the keyboard spontaneously and pressing specific food keys or keys denoting a play object, such as a ball. On noting these behaviors, the investigators decided against implementing formal training on use of the keyboard in favor of allowing Kanzi to develop that facility on his own. Savage-Rumbaugh *et al.* (1983) reported that during their daily walks with Kanzi through the 55-acre woods in which he resided, Kanzi spontaneously pressed keys "to direct attention to places and things that are not visible or to activities in which he and others are not currently engaged" (p. 658). This was in contrast to the findings with Sherman and Austin, who revealed an ability to refer to absent objects only after specific training was given and not earlier than the age of 5.

Kanzi's documented vocabulary appears to consist of about 42 words, of which 28 are the names of food or drinks. Although the authors discuss Kanzi's use of two- and three-word "combinations," these appear to be combinations of symbols with gestures, such as keying the symbol for "chase" and then pointing at an individual or individuals. As the authors note, these combinations are not to be taken as sentences.

Sherman and Austin repeatedly failed to demonstrate an understanding of spoken English in blind tests. Kanzi, in contrast, correctly selected from among three alternatives the photograph of any of 39 different objects vocally named by the experimenter. Kanzi similarly selected 56 of 57 photographs requested through *lexigrams* by the experimenter.

The work with Kanzi is still at an early stage but, hopefully, more formal tests will be incorporated into Kanzi's regimen that will permit detailed, objective comparison of production and comprehension, examination of the referential quality of the symbols used by Kanzi, and assessment of any grammatical capacities that may emerge.

C. REFERENCE

Throughout her work, Savage-Rumbaugh's emphasis has been on the word, rather than the sentence, and on whether and how a symbol used by an ape may take on the deeper, representational properties of a word as used by a human (Savage-Rumbaugh, 1981, 1984a; Savage-Rumbaugh and Rumbaugh, 1978; Savage-Rumbaugh et al., 1980b). According to her analyses, symbolic representation does not come easily for the ape, and may only occur under training procedures that emphasize the functional use of the symbols ''to convey or specify actions and goals that are not known to all parties in advance of the use of the symbols'' (Savage-Rumbaugh, 1984a, p. 292). The result of these procedures, according to Savage-Rumbaugh, is the development of true symbolization, in which symbols come to be understood as surrogates for the things referenced. This emergence of ''reference'' is distinguished from the simple, contextually appropriate use of signs by apes to obtain desired rewards, such as food or tickling. The distinction, therefore, is between the limited, pragmatic application of a symbol and the more generalized or abstract use.

Abstraction is a relative property; the use of a symbol may be partially pragmatic, partially abstract, and the level of abstractness may also vary. Judgments of the degree of abstractness of symbol understanding are difficult but several partially overlapping criteria can be identified as guides: the interchangeable use of symbols in production and comprehension tasks, as was emphasized in the work with Sherman and Austin; whether the symbol use generalizes to various exemplars of the referent; whether the animal can use the learned symbols in new contexts or perhaps even create a context to enable symbol use; and whether the referents need be present for the symbol to be used appropriately. None of these criteria, in isolation, uniquely indexes symbolic representation or reference. Additional criteria could probably be stated (cf. Savage-Rumbaugh et al., 1983), but those listed appear to be the main ones considered in the animal language literature.

The generalization criterion is met if symbols extend to a class or a category, rather than being tied to a single exemplar. In her work with apes, Savage-Rumbaugh has shown that tool and food words are represented categorically as well as individually (Savage-Rumbaugh et al., 1980b). The Gardners (R. A. Gardner and Gardner, 1984) have carried out controlled tests of naming skills of chimps, using photographs of objects. Their sign language-trained chimps could apply the correct label to various exemplars of objects in the majority of cases: Performance scores among four chimps on naming exemplars for as many as 32 different objects ranged from 54 to 88% correct, with all values greatly exceeding chance. Savage-Rumbaugh *et al.* (1983) have cautioned, however, that labeling tests like those of the Gardners are insufficient to distinguish between associative naming and referential naming.

There appear to have been few formal tests of the ability of apes to use symbols learned in one context in a different context or to create contexts to make an action possible. Premack and Premack (1983, p. 116) described one situation in which Sarah manipulated objects in order to make her use of a symbol appropriate. When given a sentence such as "Red on green ?" ("Is red on green?"), refering to the relationship of two colored cards, Sarah not infrequently (30% of the occasions) altered the relationship to make it possible for her to answer Yes rather than No.

The ability to make or understand references to objects or events that are remote in space or time constitutes a major test of reference. This is the "prolongation of reference" (Bronowski and Bellugi, 1970) or "displacement feature" of human language (Hockett, 1960). Terrace (1984a) stressed the importance of assessing the ability of language-trained animals "to refer to things which are not present" as well as "to exchange information about objects that are not in view" (p. 200). Bees show this ability in informing nestmates through their "dances" of the direction, distance, and abundance of a food source (von Frisch, 1967; Gould, 1976), or of the characteristics of a cavity that may be suitable for a new nest site (Seeley, 1977). However, the ability seems restricted to events of biological relevance for the species and to symbols that are the conventions of the species. What is of interest for the animal language work is the ability to refer to objects or events of no natural biological relevance for the species and to make these references through arbitrary, learned symbolic systems (Herman and Forestell, 1985). Ristau and Robbins (1982) cite as evidence for the understanding of references to arbitrary remote objects the chimp Sarah's ability to answer questions about an object with only the symbol for that object present (Premack, 1976). Sarah, for example, could select the correct color for a food item (e.g., apple or banana) with only the symbol for that food present; the symbol was not the color of the food.

References to remote objects occurred during the interactions between the chimps Sherman and Austin in the tool using studies mentioned earlier (Savage-Rumbaugh and Rumbaugh, 1978), as well as by the pygmy chimpanzee Kanzi during his walks though the 55-acre woods. The tools requested by Sherman or Austin of the other ape were not visible to the requester. More recently, Savage-Rumbaugh *et al.* (1983) have shown that Sherman and Austin can indicate, through use of the lexigram symbols on a keyboard, which one of a variety of specific foods they desired, although no food was immediately present. The indicated food was then in fact selected by them from among a table full of different foods located in an adjoining room.

D. SUMMARY

The sign language studies have largely ignored receptive competency as an empirical or theoretical issue. The few tests of receptive skill, as given by the Gardners, Fouts, Patterson, or Muncer and Ettlinger, were sparingly reported. Nevertheless, all of the investigators commenting on receptive competency expressed confidence in the skills of their subjects.

Premack (1976) carried out explicit studies of comprehension using an artificial language in which plastic symbols represented objects, actions, properties, and relations. The studies were extensive and touched on many issues relevant to an assessment of receptive competencies. The conclusions that can be drawn are limited, however, by inadequacies in methods and data reporting. Nevertheless, the trends of much of the data suggest impressive receptive competencies, especially for the chimpanzee Sarah.

The studies with Sherman and Austin have shown semantic comprehension of a limited set of words used in tool- or food-getting and -sharing tasks, including the ability to understand references to objects not immediately present (as did some of the studies with Sarah by Premack). Sentence comprehension was not emphasized or studied, so there are no data on which to base judgments of abilities to process syntactic information. The ongoing work with the pygmy chimpanzee Kanzi appears to reveal semantic comprehension of a vocabulary of some 40–60 lexigram symbols or spoken English words. Together with reports from Patterson (1978a,b) and Fouts et al. (1976a), the data from Kanzi suggest that artificial receptive languages based on either visual or acoustic symbols might be used successfully by apes. No evidence for the processing of syntactic information by Kanzi has yet been reported, and additional formal tests and analyses of Kanzi's semantic skills are needed.

In their work with Kanzi, Savage-Rumbaugh et al. (1985) have placed a great deal of emphasis on comprehension, a theme recurrent in this paper. These authors speculate: "If Kanzi, though unable to speak, is learning English simply by hearing it spoken around him it is possible that the capacity to comprehend speech phylogenetically precedes the capacity to produce speech" (p. 664).

Thus, emerging evidence, together with selective portions of older data, may yet reveal an asymmetry in productive and receptive competencies of apes that opens new questions about the languagelike skills of animals.

IV. RECEPTIVE COMPETENCIES OF LANGUAGE-TRAINED DOLPHINS

In our work with dolphins (Herman, 1980, 1986; Herman and Forestell, 1985; Herman *et al.*, 1984), we have emphasized comprehension from the start, posing the question raised by Terrace and colleagues somewhat differently, namely: "Can a dolphin *understand* a sentence?"

A. SENTENCE FORMS

Specifically, we examined the ability of dolphins to understand imperative and interrogative sentences expressed within artificial acoustic or gestural languages. Imperative sentences directed the dolphins to take named actions relative to named objects and their named modifiers. Comprehension was measured by the accuracy and reliability in carrying out the imperatives, as a function of the number of words in the sentence, the type and complexity of syntactic rule that governed word combinations, and whether the language medium was acoustic or visual (gestural).

Because many sentences could be constructed, each a unique instruction, we could ask both about reliability in responding to familiar sentences and about the ability to understand novel sentences—sentences that were well-formed grammatically, and meaningful, but which had not been given to the dolphins previously.

Interrogative sentences posed binary questions about the presence or absence in the dolphins' tank of specific objects referenced symbolically. For example, in response to BALL QUESTION (glossed as "Is there a ball [in the tank]?"), the dolphin could, in effect, reply Yes or No by pressing one of two paddles. Thus, this "reporting" procedure tested the dolphin's knowledge of the physical contents of its immediate world and its understanding of references to absent objects as well as to objects that were present. An important aspect of semantic comprehension is addressed by this procedure: Can symbols come to function as surrogates for their referents (or, more precisely, for the mental representations of those referents)?

B. DESCRIPTION OF THE LANGUAGES

Two young female bottle-nosed dolphins (*Tursiops truncatus*), housed together in a large seawater tank, were tutored in the artificial languages. One dolphin, Phoenix, was specialized in the acoustic language in which words were computer-generated sounds broadcast into the tank through an underwater speaker. The sounds were mainly whistlelike in character and 1 second or less in duration. The second dolphin, Akeakamai (Ake, for short), was specialized in the gestural language in which words were the movements of a trainer's arms and hands, as in sign languages. We did not attempt to use an existing sign language but instead created our own "dolphinized" version.

Each language was composed of a vocabulary and a set of syntactic rules governing how the categories of vocabulary could be sequentially ordered to form grammatical sentences. The vocabulary, 35–40 words, overlapped greatly (though not entirely) across the two languages and referred to objects in the dolphins' tank world (e.g., CHANNEL, GATE, PERSON, SPEAKER, BALL, HOOP), to actions that could be taken to those objects (e.g., TOSS, [go] OVER, [go] UNDER, FETCH, [put] IN), and to modifiers of object location (SUR-FACE, BOTTOM) or direction (RIGHT, LEFT). The dolphins were the agents of all imperative sentences and each sentence began with the dolphin's acoustic name (PHOENIX or AKE) broadcast through the underwater speaker. PHOE-NIX and AKE also were object names that could direct one dolphin to take an action to the other. For example, the sentence PHOENIX AKE UNDER directs Phoenix to swim under Ake.

Additionally, there were control and function words including YES, NO, ERASE (a word which cancels previous words in the sentence), and QUES-TION. If a dolphin completed an instruction correctly, she heard a three-word acoustic string: YES (dolphin name) FISH. Only the dolphin whose name was inserted in the string responded by returning to her station for a fish reward and contact with her trainer. If the dolphin was incorrect, she heard only her name calling her back to station. NO was rarely used since it had but one meaning, "wrong" (unlike the dolphins' names, which were used in several positive contexts), and not uncommonly caused emotional responding, such as flinging a pipe out of the tank.

The syntactic rules were the same across the two languages for the simpler, *nonrelational* sentences, but differed markedly for the more complex, *relational* sentences. The rules for nonrelational imperative sentences were: Object names precede action names and modifiers precede the object modified. Either two- or three-word sentences could be constructed. For example, the sentence PIPE TAIL-TOUCH instructs the dolphin to touch any pipe with her tail flukes, while RIGHT PIPE TAIL-TOUCH instructs her to touch only the pipe to her right (and not the one to her left). When modifiers were used in a sentence, there were always one or more contrasting pairs of objects of the same name available for response.

Relational sentences were three or more words in length and described a relationship between two named objects—taking one object to another (FETCH) or putting one object in or on another object (IN). For Phoenix, trained in the acoustic language, a straightforward linear left-to-right grammar was used in which the object to be manipulated (grammatically, the direct object of the sentence) was stated first, and the destination (grammatically, the indirect object) last. The relational term FETCH or IN was sandwiched between the two object names. In Ake's inverse grammar the destination was stated first, then the object to be manipulated, and finally the relational term. The two different grammars were chosen to investigate whether different types of syntactic rules could be learned and, particularly, whether the rule need be linear. In the linear grammar, the order of appearance of words and the order in which responses to those words must be executed were the same. In principle, the dolphin could respond word by word as in a simple linear chain of responses. In practice, successive words often appeared before the dolphin could begin or complete its responses to prior words. Nevertheless, for surer assessment of sentence-processing abilities, it would be desirable if word-by-word responding were precluded. This was done through the inverse grammar used with Ake. Here, the order in which words appeared was not the same as the order in which responses to those words were to be executed. Consequently, the dolphin must receive the entire instruction before the required sequence of responses can be correctly interpreted. Consider, for example, the five sentences HOOP OVER, HOOP QUESTION, HOOP BALL FETCH, HOOP BALL IN, and HOOP BALL ERASE. All begin with HOOP but the response to HOOP cannot be determined until the second word occurs, or even the third. In the first sentence, the dolphin is instructed to jump over the hoop; in the second, she is asked whether a hoop is present in the tank, but not to respond to it; in the third and fourth sentences, HOOP is the indirect object—the destination of BALL—but whether HOOP functions as a simple terminus for BALL or as a receptacle for it is determined by the third word, FETCH or IN; and, in the last sentence, no action at all is to be taken to HOOP (or BALL), since ERASE cancels all prior words. Hence, an ability to perform accurately with the inverse grammar cannot be explained as a simple linear chain of responses, with each successive word controlling each successive response.

Within each language, the relational rules permitted construction of semantically contrasting sentences by reordering of words. An example in Phoenix's language is FRISBEE FETCH SURFBOARD contrasted with SURFBOARD FETCH FRISBEE. The first sentence requires Phoenix to transport the frisbee to the surfboard while the second requires her to take the surfboard to the frisbee. An ability to respond correctly to semantically contrasting pairs or groups of sentences (there can be more than two contrasts for sentences of more than three words) indicates that the dolphin is attending not only to the particular words in the sentence but to their ordering.

Relational sentences of four or five words in length are constructed by adding modifiers to the name of the object manipulated, the name of the destination, or both. Semantic contrasts can be formed not only by changing the ordering of object names, as in the above example, but by changing the ordering or assignment of modifier names. In Ake's language, for example, the sentences WATER RIGHT BASKET FETCH and RIGHT WATER BASKET FETCH are semantic contrasts (WATER refers to a stream of water entering the tank from a suspended hose, not to the ambient in which the dolphins live). The first sentence requires AKE to take the basket that is to her right (and not the one that is to her left) to any stream of water. The second sentence requires Ake to take a basket to the stream of water that was to her right when she received the instruction; the dolphin may in fact have to go to her left to retrieve a basket, but then must return to the water stream that *was* to her right rather than simply continuing toward the closer one that was to her left. As with all sentences, the instructions are given while the dolphin is at her station facing the trainer.

In summary, I want to emphasize that although the vocabulary is limited in size, it is not vocabulary size that is important but the ability to combine and recombine words to form new meanings (cf. Bronowski and Bellugi, 1970; Hockett, 1960). Using the syntactic rules currently available, well over 1000 unique imperative sentences of two to five words in length can be constructed in each language, each sentence requiring a unique sequence of responses by the dolphins.

Interrogative sentences have thus far been limited to two-word questions asking whether a named object is present or absent in the tank. Responses to interrogatives are discussed in Section IV,F.

C.   SENTENCE UNDERSTANDING

1.   Novel Sentences

It is generally held that the ability of humans to understand and generate novel sentences reflects their tacit knowledge of the grammar of their language. The ease with which humans handle this task is surprising enough that Chomsky termed it a "mysterious ability" (N. Chomsky, 1972, p. 100). In principle, tacit knowledge by the dolphins of the miniature grammar of their artificial languages should make accurate responses to novel sentences possible; conversely, accurate responses imply such knowledge, given that other means allowing for accurate responding are excluded. These other means include nonlinguistic social cues, experimenter bias, context cues, and symbol sequence cues. Our testing procedures guarded against these artifacts, many of which have proven troublesome in the ape language work. Trainers wore opaque goggles that prevented the dolphin from using eye gaze cues from the trainer and also prevented the trainer from observing the responses of the dolphins or noting the momentary position of objects which floated freely about the tanks, driven by wind and current. A "blind" observer having no prior knowledge of the sentence given the dolphin watched the response and labeled it using the language system. If the label corresponded to the sentence given, the dolphin was scored as correct. To control for context cues, sentences of various syntactic forms were intermixed during a session according to a preplanned schedule such that there was no way to predict the next sentence in the list or to benefit from prior sentences. This was true not only for sentence types but for the words used across or within sentences. Further details of these controls are given by Herman *et al.* (1984).

Symbol sequence cues are familiar, redundant stock phrases that enable one to produce or understand a sentence without necessarily understanding all of the words in that sentence. For example, the chimp Lana could successfully complete the sentence "Please machine give piece of X" without understanding any of the first five words (Savage-Rumbaugh *et al.*, 1980a). The same is true for some of the stock phrases used in training the chimp Sarah (Premack, 1976). The point is that, to demonstrate sentence understanding, the language used should entail word sequences in which context alone cannot govern understanding, and in which no word is redundant and an understanding of all words is necessary for a correct interpretation of the sentence. This was the case for the artificial languages given to the dolphins. There were no context cues and no stock phrases in the sense outlined for the ape studies. The exact word that followed another word could not be determined in advance, and no word could be deleted without changing the meaning of the sentence or making it anomalous. Performance on the novel sentences given to the dolphins was therefore a strong measure of sentence understanding.

a. Types of Novelty. Responses to two types of novelty were studied: (1) lexical novelty, defined as the insertion of new words into the syntactic slots of a familiar syntactic form, and (2) structural novelty, defined as the creation of new syntactic forms. Consider, for example, the syntactic frame Object + Relational Term + Object, which directs Phoenix to take the first named object to the second or to put the first named object in or on the second. Thus, HOOP FETCH SURFBOARD directs Phoenix to take the hoop to the surfboard, while HOOP IN SURFBOARD directs her to put the hoop *on* the surfboard. Many different sentences can be formed by changing one or both object names and/or by changing the relational term. Any sentence so created that has not been given to the dolphin previously constitutes a lexically novel sentence. A large number of lexically novel sentences were given to the dolphins and their responses were studied in detail.

Now, suppose we create a new syntactic variant by adding a modifier before the first object name: Modifier + Object + Relational Term + Object, and for the first time give a sentence using this new frame, e.g., BOTTOM HOOP FETCH SURFBOARD ("take the hoop lying on the tank bottom to the surfboard"). This is an instance of a structurally novel sentence. Both the initial performance with this new sentence form as well as performance on subsequent tests is of interest. Several different types of structurally novel sentences were given to the dolphins. Structurally novel sentences allow one to evaluate whether the dolphins can understand sentence forms for which there was no specific training.

b.   Scoring Criteria and Performance on Lexically Novel Sentences.   In assessing performance, two types of scoring criteria are relevant. One, a strict criterion, measures whether the response was wholly correct—whether all words of the sentence given, as well as the structure of the sentence, were interpreted correctly. For example, if in response to the five-word sentence BOTTOM PIPE FETCH SURFACE NET ("take the pipe on the tank bottom to the net that is floating") the dolphin takes the bottom pipe to the *bottom* net, a sentence error is scored, although four of the five words were interpreted correctly and the main intent of the imperative as given by its structure was understood. The second criterion focuses on the understanding of the major intent of the sentence by looking at the number of words responded to incorrectly in each sentence scored as incorrect by the strict criterion.

c.   Performance Using the Strict Criterion.   Phoenix responded *wholly* correctly to 138 (66.7%) of 207 lexically novel sentences given to her over an approximately 3-year period, and Ake responded correctly to 220 (59.1%) of 372 lexically novel sentences given to her during the same period. Chance levels of performance were 4% or less, depending on the sentence type (Herman *et al.*, 1984).

Performance on these novel sentences can also be judged against performance on familiar sentences during the same 3-year period; familiar sentences were given to a dolphin at least once previously, but in most cases many times previously. For meaningful comparisons, the proportion of familiar sentences of each syntactic form was adjusted statistically to reflect the proportions given during novel-sentence testing. This resulted in a lowering of performance levels on familiar sentences from that actually observed, since the more complex, longer, and hence more difficult sentences occurred relatively more frequently during novel-sentence testing than during familiar-sentence testing. The resulting adjusted performance levels on familiar sentences were 75.5% correct responses for Phoenix and 75.3% correct responses for Ake, for the more than 22,000 sentences that each was given during the 3-year period (an average of about 25 sentences per day for a 300-day year). As might be expected, there was a significant facilitating effect of sentence familiarity for each dolphin [X^2 (1) ≥ 8.5, $p < .01$], amounting to 8–16 percentage points.

d.   Understanding of Major Intent of Imperative.   Figure 1 summarizes performance using the second scoring criterion. For Ake, single errors predominated, regardless of sentence type or length: 118 (78%) of the 152 novel sentences scored as incorrect by the strict criterion contained only a single word-error. In addition to the five sentence types shown in Fig. 1, Ake was given two novel five-word relational sentences, the only ones of this type given. She made a single word-error on one sentence and two word-errors on the second sentence.

For Phoenix, single errors were the most frequent for all but the last two sentence forms illustrated in Fig. 1, both of which involved modified indirect objects. Nevertheless, of the total of 69 novel sentences scored as incorrect using

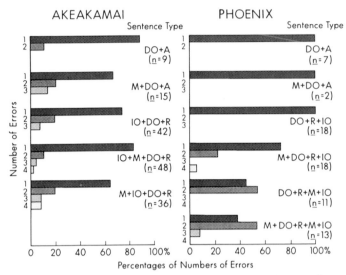

FIG. 1. The percentage of novel sentences to which one, two, three, or four errors were made, for each dolphin and for each sentence type. For example, for the three-word sentence form IO + DO + R in Ake's language, there were a total of 42 novel sentences responded to incorrectly by the strict criterion (see text). Of these, 31 (74%) contained only one semantic error, 8 (19%) contained two errors, and 3 (7%) contained three errors, where a semantic error is an incorrect response to a semantic element, such as selecting an object other than that specified by the DO term or the IO term or taking the wrong action. Semantic element key: M, modifier; DO, direct object; IO, indirect object; A, action (nonrelational term); R, relational term. Relational sentences are expressed in an "inverse" grammar for the dolphin Akeakamai (Ake) and in a "linear" grammar for Phoenix.

the strict criterion, 60 (87%) contained only a single word-error. For both dolphins, the most common error occurred during relational sentences and consisted of taking the correct object (the direct object of the sentence) to the wrong destination (the indirect object). Errors involving the destination were 3.5 times (Phoenix) or 4.4 times (Ake) more frequent than errors involving the object to be manipulated.

For Phoenix, her modifiers (SURFACE and BOTTOM) were an additional frequent source of error, yielding 19% error, despite what would seem to be a meaningful ecological dimension for an aquatic animal. In contrast, RIGHT and LEFT, the modifiers in Ake's vocabulary, were surprisingly easy, producing less than 5% error.

  e. *Categorization of Errors.*   Overall, the second error criterion reveals that in most cases the main intent of a sentence was understood and that errors tended to be limited to misprocessing of a single word, either because of a semantic confusion at the time of coding or possibly because of some forgetting at the time of response. The errors to objects were not random but fell into a pattern suggestive of a categorization of objects based on their transportability. There were those objects that could be carried by the dolphins such as BALL or FRISBEE and those that could not, such as the other dolphin, permanent tank fixtures like GATE and WINDOW, or the underwater speaker (SPEAKER) that was temporarily affixed to the side of the tank during testing sessions. Transportable objects were much more difficult as destinations than were nontransportable objects; for Ake, errors were more than twice as frequent when the destination was a transportable object than when it was a nontransportable object, and for Phoenix errors were more than four times as frequent. Moreover, for both dolphins, the destination errors were predominantly within the same category (transportable or nontransportable object) as the target object specified by the sentence: 22 (79%) of 28 destination errors made by Phoenix were within the same category as the target, as were 72 (71%) of the 102 destination errors made by Ake. Both distributions departed significantly from chance [X^2 (1) $\geq$ 15.4, p < .001]. Thus, information about the category of a destination object might be retained in memory although the specific exemplar chosen was mistaken.

f. Performance on Structurally Novel Sentences. One type of structural novelty given to the dolphins consisted of four-word sentences that for the first time used a modifier term in a relational sentence, as in PERSON LEFT FRISBEE FETCH, an instruction to Ake to take the frisbee on her left to a person. Ake was given two structurally novel sentences of this type, the one with the modifier attached to the direct object in the above example, and the second with it attached to the indirect object (RIGHT WATER BASKET FETCH, meaning take a basket to the stream of water to your right). Ake responded correctly in both instances. Over a subsequent 4-month period, she was given a total of 69 different exemplars of these new structural forms and responded correctly (by the strict criterion) to 44 (64%). Phoenix was given one structurally novel four-word sentence (FRISBEE FETCH BOTTOM HOOP), to which she responded correctly. She then responded wholly correctly to 17 (63%) of 27 additional exemplars of this form over the next 4-month interval. The percentages for both dolphins were similar to those obtained for all novel sentences given them, as reviewed in Section IV,C,1,c above.

A second type of structural novelty was a new sentence form linking the action term FETCH with the term THROUGH, OVER, or UNDER to form the sentences FRISBEE FETCH THROUGH HOOP, FRISBEE FETCH OVER HOOP, and FRISBEE FETCH UNDER HOOP. The first sentence is an instruction to Phoenix to carry the frisbee *through* the hoop, the second *over* the hoop, and the third *under* the hoop. These sentences contrast with the familiar sentence form FRISBEE FETCH HOOP, meaning take the frisbee *to* the hoop. Phoenix responded correctly to her initial trial with the new sentence form (FRISBEE FETCH UNDER HOOP). Repeated probes of these three variants were given intermittently over a 3-month period for a total of 436 probes. Phoenix responded wholly correctly to 231, or 53%.

A third form of structural novelty employed conjoined sentences that linked two Object + Action sentences into a single instruction, as in PIPE TAIL-TOUCH PIPE OVER (in response, Phoenix swam to the pipe, touched it with her tail flukes, and then jumped over it). A total of 15 such conjoined sentences were given Phoenix as probes, without any specific training or reinforcement history. The probes were given over a several week period, with each probe interspersed among sentences of familiar form. Phoenix carried out both indicated actions in 11 of the 15 cases. She completed only one action in three of the remaining cases, and carried out what appeared to be an integrated response in the fourth case, by inverting herself in response to UNDER, her typical posture for going under an object, and then touching the designated object (a basket) with her tail, in response to TAIL-TOUCH. In principle, conjoined sentences allow one to extend sentence length indefinitely, as in the recursive features characterizing natural languages. In practice, however, memory limitations impose performance constraints for both natural and artificial languages if sentence length grows appreciably with little or no redundancy in content.

A final form of structural novelty given consisted of syntactically anomalous sentences (ungrammatical sentences) given without any training or instruction (Herman *et al.*, 1983). Of immediate interest here were those anomalies that violated the learned syntactic rules by preceding or following a legitimate Object + Action string with an object or an action term. Examples are SPEAKER ⟨PERSON PEC-TOUCH⟩, SPIT ⟨BASKET UNDER⟩, ⟨FRISBEE TAIL-TOUCH⟩ PIPE, and ⟨BASKET MOUTH⟩ SPIT, where the embedded Object + Action string is shown in brackets. All of these sentences have no meaning in their entirety within the artificial languages constructed. The question then was, Would the dolphins detect and act on the embedded Object + Action string, or reject the sentence as a whole by not responding, or possibly revise it by lexical substitutions for the anomalous terms? For Ake, acting on the embedded string while ignoring the extraneous word was the most common response. She was given ten anomalies of the four types described above and responded solely to the embedded Object + Action string in eight cases. For example, given the string SPEAKER ⟨PERSON PEC-TOUCH⟩ she ignored the underwater speaker and swam to the person and touched her with the pectoral fin. When given ⟨FRISBEE TAIL-TOUCH⟩ PIPE she touched the frisbee with her tail flukes and ignored the pipe. In the two cases which were the exception, both Object + ⟨Object + Action⟩ strings, Ake took the second-named object to the first, as in a relational sentence. In the inverse grammar used with Ake, two object names in succession occur only in relational sentences. At the time of this particular test, FETCH was the only permissible concluding term after two successive object words, and hence was redundant and often not attended to.

Phoenix was considerably less responsive to the embedded string with the ten similar anomalies given to her. She responded solely to the embedded string in two cases, and possibly also in a third for which the underwater action component was difficult to see. She gave conjoined responses in another two cases, both ⟨Object + Action⟩ + Action sequences (e.g., going over and then under a person in response to PERSON OVER UNDER), and swam through the gate and then jumped over the surfboard in response to SURFBOARD OVER GATE. In the remaining four cases she responded by substituting other objects or actions for one or two but not all three of the specified words. Thus, some lexical substitution as well as some responding to embedded strings characterized Phoenix's performance. Neither dolphin rejected a string entirely, although rejection did occur in response to some lexical anomalies, as discussed in Section IV,3,A.

2. Syntactic Understanding

The responses to structurally novel sentences revealed an understanding of the learned syntactic rules sufficient for an interpretation of extensions to those rules or even exceptions to the rules. Additional evidence for understanding of the word-order rules comes from the low reversal-error rate in response to relational sentences. A reversal error occurs when the object to be transported and the destination are reversed—for example, a hoop is taken to a frisbee rather than a frisbee to a hoop. If there were frequent reversal errors, it would indicate that the words themselves were being processed but their arrangement was not. Since the structure for relational sentences for the two dolphins was different—the destination occurs last in the relational sentences given to Phoenix and first for those given to Ake—any effect of a particular word order can be studied. Furthermore, if we restrict our data to lexically novel relational sentences, any potential effect of sentence familiarity on reversal error is eliminated. The data show the following: Ake never made a reversal error within the 286 novel relational sentences given to her, and Phoenix made only one reversal error among the 168 novel relational sentences she received. These data underscore the ability of both dolphins to take account of the sequences in which words appeared when ordering their responses to the referents of those words.

Among the types of anomalies given to the dolphins (Herman *et al.*, 1983) were two-word sentences in which the normal Object + Action word order was changed to Action + Object, e.g., WATER PEC-TOUCH was changed to PEC-TOUCH WATER. Each dolphin was given six anomalies of this type and, with only one exception for each dolphin, the normal Object + Action string was not reconstructed in a dolphin's response. Instead, the action term was carried out to an arbitrary object. For example, in response to PEC-TOUCH WATER, Ake touched a hoop with her pectoral fin. These responses suggested that action terms were sentence endings for both dolphins, as stated by their word-order rules. Words following an action term were generally ignored, although there were exceptions in some of the structurally novel sentences given to the dolphins.

The responses of the dolphins to these various sentences evidences their attention to word order, and their dependence on word order for organizing their responses. In English, and in many other languages, word order is a major vehicle for conveying syntactic information and guides the interpretation and responses of the listener.

3. Semantic Comprehension

a. Understanding of the Limits of the Lexicon. An interesting facet of human cognition is our knowledge of the contents of our personal knowledge— our "metaknowledge." Thus, we can often say immediately whether or not we know a fact or can define a word, without retrieving that fact or giving the definition. Does metaknowledge apply at all to the dolphins' understanding of their artificial languages? One way to judge this is to test the dolphins' understanding of the limits of their lexicon. Herman *et al.,* (1983) presented Phoenix and Ake with lexical anomalies consisting of properly structured ("well-formed") sentences containing one or more nonsense words. For example, the two-word Object + Action sentence WATER X was given to Ake, where X is a gesture not in Ake's vocabulary. Ake rejected this sentence by making no response other than remaining at her station and "staring" at her trainer. She similarly rejected an additional seven of the 21 lexically anomalous strings she was given. Phoenix rejected 11 of her 23 anomalous strings. Phoenix's rejections sometimes included swimming to the object designated by a real word and then doing nothing further, as well as simply remaining at her station.

Substitution responses also occurred in which a real object or action was substituted for the nonsense word. For both dolphins, it was more compelling to substitute a real object for a nonsense object term than a real action for a nonsense action term. Thus, WATER X produced no response, but Y TOSS resulted in Ake tossing her frisbee, where Y is a nonsense gesture different from X. These results may mirror the tendency, noted earlier, for the dolphins to regard an action term as a sentence terminator, responding only when an action term appears (and not usually volunteering an action). Young children, like dolphins, tend to be affected by the position of a nonsense word in an imperative sentence (Shipley *et al.,* 1969). Children, unlike dolphins, are most disrupted by a nonsense word in the initial position of an imperative sentence.

Overall, the responses of the dolphins to these lexical anomalies indicate an awareness of the limits of their lexicon and, correspondingly, an awareness that symbols require referents.

b. Rejecting Semantic Anomalies. Semantic anomalies were grammatical sentences that did not make sense or could not be carried out. The dolphins' responses to semantic anomalies tended to reveal their understanding of the semantic limits of grammatical strings. This was most apparent in the case of semantically anomalous "fetch" strings. Here, the dolphins were requested to take nontransportable objects to some destination. Examples are WINDOW FETCH GATE in Phoenix's language and PIPE PHOENIX FETCH in Ake's language. The first sentence asks Phoenix to take the immovable underwater window to the gate in the tank; the second sentence asks Ake to transport the unwilling Phoenix to a pipe. Phoenix's responses were either to substitute a transportable object for the one that could not be carried, or to use the named transportable *destination* object as the object of transport. Thus, she took a *hoop* to the gate in response to WINDOW FETCH GATE and took the hoop to the frisbee in response to WINDOW FETCH HOOP. Ake either refused to respond at all to the anomalous sentence or, like Phoenix, substituted a transportable object for the anomalous one. In response to PIPE PHOENIX FETCH, Ake started away from her station on seeing the sign for pipe, but then returned on seeing the sign for Phoenix. That Phoenix and Ake's substitution or rejection responses were not simply an unwillingness to carry out the instructions of unfamiliar strings was shown by the results for novel sentence testing (Section IV,C,1), in which responses to grammatical *and* meaningful, but unfamiliar, sentences were carried out immediately.

All in all, the responses to these semantic anomalies revealed that both dolphins knew the semantic boundaries of their world, as it was represented within their respective languages.

   c.   Object Generalization.   Throughout the course of our studies, many exemplars of objects have been used as a natural consequence of breakage of old exemplars and construction of new examples or because of the special requirements of a new study. A number of instances were described in Herman *et al.* (1984) and need not be repeated here. The new exemplars were readily accepted in almost all cases, showing that the symbols of the languages generalized beyond the training materials to classes or categories of objects or events. To obtain some quantitative data, we recently carried out a brief study with Ake in which four novel exemplars were introduced for each of six object names: HOOP, PIPE, BASKET, BALL, FRISBEE, and WATER. Responses to the novel exemplars were tested by giving a two-word sentence, e.g., HOOP OVER, and observing whether the new hoop was indeed chosen. At each testing session, two novel exemplars, each having a different name, were present in the tank along with seven to nine familiar objects all having object names different from the novel exemplars and from each other. The two novel exemplars were referred to once each, during a session consisting of 24 sentences altogether. These two probes appeared at unpredictable locations in the sequence of sentences. A blind observer labeled all responses. Of the total of 24 probes given over all sessions, Ake responded correctly to 19 (79.2%). Two of the errors were to PIPE exemplars, two to WATER exemplars, and one to a BALL exemplar. Thus, no name failed to show generalization, giving evidence of transfer of a name to new exemplars of the class of object referenced.

   d.   Context Generalization.   Context generalization entails extending the responses trained in one context to different contexts. Context variations included the frequent use of different trainers, haphazard distribution of objects in the tank, different numbers of paired objects (paired objects allowed for the use of modifiers), and unpredictable sequences of sentences. Within their home tanks, instructions to the dolphins were given with the trainer stationed at any arbitrary location around the periphery of the tanks, in the shallow channel connecting the tanks, at one of the underwater windows, or even in the water itself, with no effect on performance. A study described by Herman (1986) tested specifically for effects of variation in location of objects and of the dolphin Ake. Objects were located in the same tank as Ake, in the opposite tank, or divided between tanks. This produced six unique conditions representing all two-way combinations of dolphin in Tank A or Tank B and objects in Tank A, Tank B, or both. Ake's accuracy in responding to two-word sentences measured her ability to understand references to objects whose locations varied considerably and which were often at a considerable distance from the dolphin and hidden from her view. The results were that performance was equally good (95–97% correct responses) whether the objects were in the same tank as the dolphin, the opposite tank, or divided between them.

There were two occasions when the dolphins were temporarily moved to new facilities while repairs were made on their home tanks. The new tanks and their surroundings were very different from the home environment as well as from each other. Although we could not test Phoenix's performance at the temporary facilities because sound generation equipment was not available there, we were able to work with Ake using her sign language. Ake showed no hesitation in responding to the gestural signs in the new locations. The accuracy of her responses were equal to those at her home tank, and included new object generalizations as well. For example, she immediately responded to a waterfall entering the tank at one of the temporary facilities when WATER was used in a sentence for the first time at that new location. In her home tank WATER referred to a thin stream flowing from an ordinary garden hose.

   e. Extensions of Action Understanding.   Extensions involve novel variations in the form or context of responses to action words. Included here are occasions when the dolphins "rearranged reality" to make it possible to carry out the requested action. As an example, the wind frequently blew floating objects against the sides of the open-air tanks. If requested to leap over one of those objects, the dolphins first carefully moved the object away from the tank walls and then leaped over it. No training was given for this behavior; it originated with the dolphins. Another example occurred when Phoenix was given the sentence BOTTOM HOOP THROUGH for the first time. The hoop was lying flat on the tank bottom. Using her rostrum (beak), Phoenix raised one edge of the hoop until it was poised vertically, and then darted through. Ake, when later tested in the same way as Phoenix, also spontaneously raised the hoop off the tank bottom and swam through (Ake was simply given the sentence HOOP

THROUGH since BOTTOM is not in her language). Phoenix, when asked to toss a frisbee lying on the bottom (BOTTOM FRISBEE TOSS), brought the frisbee to the surface and tossed it in the air, the only medium in which it could be satisfactorily tossed (and observed by the trainers). All of these spontaneous behaviors continue to be performed in the original manner by the dolphins.

In several cases of what appeared to us, *a priori*, to be semantic anomalies, the dolphins in fact carried out interesting interpretations of action terms. Each dolphin "tossed" the stream of water in response to WATER TOSS by moving her head rapidly through the stream in a manner similar to that used for tossing a frisbee, ball, or some other floating object. Also, Phoenix made an admirable effort to toss the heavy, fixed gate in response to GATE TOSS and succeeded in raising it upward slightly.

There was also evidence that the dolphins understood the goal of an action response. This was most apparent during responses to relational sentences. Here, the dolphins carefully "defined" the intended destination object. If the destination object was in a cluster of objects, the dolphins separated them to isolate the destination. They did this by pushing and shoving the object being transported against the intended destination until it was separated from the cluster, and then ceasing to push or shove. They also corrected their trajectories if overshooting an intended destination. If, in response to SURFBOARD FETCH FRISBEE, the surfboard glided past the frisbee, Phoenix brought it back until it rested in place, touching the frisbee. Or, if pushing a floating person to an underwater window, in response to PERSON FETCH WINDOW, Phoenix maneuvered the person around other objects in the way of the window until the person was stationary at the window. Either dolphin would persist in a response until it was accomplished. Putting a frisbee on top of a surfboard in response to SURFBOARD FRISBEE IN was difficult, as the frisbee tended to roll off. Yet Ake placed it again and again, carefully, until it finally held in place. Then she would back away from the surfboard as if to signify that the response was completed.

Other examples could be given, but those described are sufficient to illustrate the broad, and appropriate, interpretation given to action terms by the dolphins.

D.   PRODUCING SYMBOLS: OBJECT LABELING ("NAMING")

Richards *et al.* (1984) described the training of the dolphin Ake for mimicry of computer-generated sounds and for use of the imitated sounds as labels for real-world objects. Among other goals, the study provided modest parallels with the productive vocabulary tests given to chimpanzees (e.g., R. A. Gardner and Gardner, 1984).

Ake's initial task was to listen to a "model" sound broadcast through an underwater speaker and to produce an imitation of that sound vocally. A hydrophone located adjacent to the speaker detected all sounds and transmitted them to an oscilloscope, where they were displayed visually as a frequency-versus-time graph. A trained observer, watching the visual display, made immediate judgments of the accuracy of the imitation by comparing it with the model. If the imitation was a good copy, Ake heard the Yes sound through the underwater speaker; otherwise, she heard her acoustic name calling her to return to the mimicry station. Ake's vocal accuracy improved rapidly for most model sounds, and in many cases her copy became almost indistinguishable from the model. She was able to extend her trained mimicry ability to the imitation of new model sounds, in many cases providing good copies on her first attempt. She faithfully copied a variety of sound parameters including frequency, frequency shift, pulse characteristics, and amplitude variation.

During subsequent training, the elicitation of several of Ake's vocal imitations was transferred from model sounds as stimuli to real-world objects shown her. In fact, some of the model sounds successfully imitated by Ake were the names of objects in Phoenix's acoustic language. These included BALL, HOOP, PIPE, PERSON, and FRISBEE. If one of these objects was shown to Ake she was required to give its vocal name. Transfer from the model sound to the real object as elicitor was achieved by displaying the object just before the model sound was heard and then inserting probe trials consisting of the object alone. The ratio of probe trials to sound-cued trials was increased over successive sessions as Ake's facility in the task improved.

Once transfer was complete for each of the five listed objects, a naming test was given in which the five objects were presented 33 or 34 times each, in a random sequence. The observer judging the vocal responses had no knowledge of which object was being shown to Ake. Ake produced the correct vocalization for 152 (91.0%) of the 167 test trials. Her errors were restricted to name confusions between FRISBEE and PERSON, the two most similarly sounding names.

Among mammals other than humans, vocal mimicry has been experimentally verified thus far only for the bottle-nosed dolphin. However, some of the other marine mammals may also have an ability for vocal mimicry, judging by the spontaneous mimicry of a few human speech sounds reported for a harbor seal (*Phoca vitulina*), formerly in captivity at the New England Aquarium but now deceased (D. Wartzog, personal communication), and for a beluga whale (*Delphinapterus leucas*) in captivity at the Naval Ocean Systems Center in San Diego (Ridgway *et al.*, 1985). The evolution of vocal mimicry in animals may reflect the advantages of defining and maintaining social relations with one's own species or subgroup at a distance, especially in the absence of visual contact (e.g., Andrew, 1962; Nottebohm, 1972). In dolphins, vocal imitation may function referentially to establish contact with a particular individual, to direct attention of an individual, or to refer to that individual by imitating that individual's typical "signature" whistle (Tyack, 1986). Such functions meet with Bruner's (1983) view of the development of reference in children: "The problem of how reference develops can . . . be restated as the problem of how people manage and direct each other's attention by linguistic means'' (p. 68). Bruner goes on to suggest that in the young child, patterned sounds may accompany, and eventually replace, ostensive referential gestures. Dolphins, of course, have little capability for producing gestures. Reference, if it develops, may involve sounds from the beginning.

The degree to which a capability for vocal mimicry generalizes to arbitrary situations and arbitrary sounds may index the cognitive flexibility of the species (Richards, 1986). Richards stressed that rapid formation of a generalized concept of mimicry, as was demonstrated by Ake, may be a key criterion for distinguishing between versatile motor control of vocalizations that allow for a variety of sounds to be imitated and versatile cognitive abilities that allow for the understanding and use of the *concept* of mimicry. Applying learned vocal labels to arbitrary objects can be cognitively demanding as well as indicative of the flexibility of the mimicry system. Although the vocal labeling of three types of predators has been observed in vervet monkeys (Seyfarth *et al.,* 1980), this appears to involve learned associations rather than learned vocalizations, since infant vervets possess the different alarm calls but use them less selectively than do adults (Seyfarth and Cheney, 1980). In contrast, an African grey parrot learned to use human speech sounds to label arbitrary objects shown it (Pepperberg, 1981), a task more comparable to that of the dolphin. While the number of objects labeled by the dolphin was less than that of the parrot and far less than the number of gestural labels used by chimps (R. A. Gardner and Gardner, 1984), the training time given to the dolphin Ake in this task was not as extensive as that for the other species, nor were the sounds chosen as labels as distinct as one would like in working toward increased repertoire size (Richards, 1986).

The findings on vocal labeling show that the same objects that were the targets for Ake's action responses when she was given gestural symbols were themselves effective as stimuli for eliciting vocal responses. However, no attempt was made to map the production of unique vocal labels onto unique consequences— all successful productions yielded the same end result: fish. Judging from the findings of Savage-Rumbaugh and Rumbaugh (1978) with chimpanzees, different outcomes may enhance the referential quality of symbols, so that eventually they serve as surrogates for real-world objects. Given the limited context in which Ake produced her vocal labels, the labels may not have acquired a level of meaning beyond that of simple, learned associates of the objects.

The vocal repertoire of the dolphin could probably be extended beyond that demonstrated in the Richards *et al.* (1984) study. However, before vocalizations could be employed usefully as pragmatic communication tools for human–dolphin exchanges in structured artificial situations, sizable technological problems would have to be overcome to allow for the rapid discrimination of a large repertoire of dolphin-produced sounds by humans (or by computers). Consequently, other means for symbol production by the dolphins, such as the use of keyboards, may be more feasible.

E. SENTENCE MEMORY

The level of understanding of references to objects can be studied in many ways. One way is to give an imperative with all removable named objects absent from the tank. After a delay, multiple objects can be introduced at once to test the dolphin's ability to carry out the prior instruction. This procedure tests the dolphin's ability to remember a sentence, but it also measures an important aspect of semantic comprehension: the ability to understand symbolic references to things not immediately present, as in the "displacement" feature of the human language concept discussed earlier in Section III,C. As was the case with the studies of apes, our interest was in the ability to understand references to objects of no natural relevance, as given through arbitrary symbolic systems.

The sentence-memory tests given to the dolphins and the results can be summarized briefly. In an initial study with both dolphins, seven objects were introduced at once immediately after an Object + Action sentence referring to one of those objects was completed (0 sec delay). Altogether, 43 two-word sentences were given to each dolphin, and each responded correctly to 35 (81.4%). In a subsequent study with the dolphin Ake, delays after the Object + Action sentence were 0, 7.5, 15, or 30 sec. There was also a control condition in which the objects were introduced just *prior* to the start of signing. Each delay and the control condition were tested 15 times in a counterbalanced order, for a total of 75 trials together. Ake correctly responded to 68 (90.6%) of the 75 sentences. Five of the seven errors were at the 30-sec delay (66.7% correct); there was one error each at the 7.5- and 15-sec delays.

These results showed an understanding of semantic references to absent objects, and also revealed that there was relatively little loss of memory for the sentences given, within the limits of the delays tested. Because the responses to the sentences given were delayed—the entire sentence, of necessity, stored in memory—the studies additionally addressed the issue raised earlier in Section IV,B of whether the understanding of sentences must proceed on a word-by-word basis, such that the response to one word is carried out before the second word can be effectively processed. Clearly, this was not necessary. On some occasions, in fact, one could see the intended action to the referenced object being "rehearsed" overtly during the delay interval. For example, if given a sentence such as BALL UNDER or BALL PEC-TOUCH, Ake might carry out anticipatory responses during the delay interval, swimming on her back, which is her method of going under an object, or holding her pectoral fin straight out from her body as she does when touching an object with that fin. When multiple objects were later flung into the tank simultaneously from the four quadrants, Ake swam rapidly about the tank conducting a visual in-air search for the high, floating ball. On sighting it, she typically accelerated toward it and carried out the rehearsed response. Rehearsals did not always occur for these actions, and in the case of some of the other actions, no obvious rehearsal was seen.

F. The Interrogative Form

The interrogative form was used in "reporting" tasks given to the dolphin Ake (Herman and Forestell, 1985). The reporting tasks, like the sentence memory procedures, test the ability to understand symbolic references to absent objects. For example, the interrogative BALL QUESTION, given gesturally to Ake, asks whether a ball is present in the tank. Ake can respond No by pressing a paddle to her left or Yes by pressing a paddle to her right. Alternatively, if given an imperative, such as BALL TOSS, the dolphin can carry out the requested behavior if the object is indeed present, or respond on the No paddle to indicate that the object is absent (or that the requested action cannot be carried out).

Herman and Forestell studied three forms of reporting. The first form (Experiment 1) occurred in the context of the studies of responses to anomalous sentences (Herman et al., 1983), and examined the spontaneous, untutored responses of the dolphins to three sentences referring to absent objects. Each of these sentences was inserted into a block of 16 additional sentences referring to objects that were present, such that there was no way for the dolphin to know in advance that reference to an absent object would be made. In response to two of the three sentences, each dolphin made long, fruitless searches of the tank (30 sec or more) and then returned spontaneously to her instruction station. For the third sentence, each dolphin made an unusually slow response to an object that was present, before returning to her station. The long searches and the spontaneous return to station were not seen in response to other forms of anomaly, suggesting, therefore, that the dolphins were, in effect, "reporting" the absence of the referenced object.

Experiment 2, carried out with Ake only, provided a means for her to report explicitly that a referenced object was absent, in contrast to the implicit form of report in Experiment 1. The procedures of Experiment 1 were continued, except that a No paddle was introduced. Ake could press this paddle to report the absence of a referenced object. A total of 97 "probe" sentences referring to absent objects were inserted among 594 sentences referring to objects that were present. Ake correctly reported the absence for 84 (86.6%) of the probes after a mean search time of 15 sec. For the remaining 13 (13.4%) probes she falsely responded to some object that was present, after a mean search time of only 7 sec. The short search times suggested that the false reports may have resulted mainly from false coding of the sign for the object. The 13.4% error rate was, in fact, only slightly above the object-confusion rate of 12.6% occurring among the 594 sentences referring to objects that were present.

False-negative reports were rare (7.6%). These were reports that objects actually present were absent. Overall, then, the results of Experiment 2 gave evidence of an impressive ability to report the absence of an object referenced symbolically in a two-word Object + Action imperative.

Experiment 3 investigated Ake's ability to report *either* absence or presence of an object. A gestural sign for QUESTION was introduced for this experiment, as was a second paddle, called the Yes paddle. Ake was shown one to three objects as they were flung into the tank behind her. She was then given either an Object + Action imperative or an Object + Question interrogative. If the referenced object was present in the tank, Ake was required either to carry out the named action to that object if given an imperative or to press the Yes paddle if given an interrogative. If the referenced object was absent, then the required response was to press the No paddle, regardless of whether the sentence was an imperative or an interrogative.

Overall, Ake responded correctly to 264 (81.5%) of 324 imperative or interrogative sentences given her. She responded Yes (79.6%) and No (76.9%) correctly about equally often and carried out the imperative correctly on 95 (88.0%) of 108 trials. The imperative and interrogative forms were easily differentiated, as measured by the complete restriction of responses to the Yes and No paddles when given the interrogative form, and by the proper execution of action responses when given imperatives referring to an object that was present.

The long search times for absent objects in Experiment 2 indicated that Ake expected all objects to be present, and was not relying on a mental inventory of changes in the number of objects present or in the particular objects present. In contrast, during Experiment 3, she appeared to be maintaining, updating, and relying on a mental inventory for deciding on the presence or absence of referenced objects. Evidence for this was the performance differences obtained as a function of the number of objects placed in the tank at each trial. With one object present, Ake's responses were 90.7% correct; with two, 82.4% correct; and with three, only 71.3% correct. In comparison, performance during Experiment 2 was unaffected by the number of objects in the tank. An additional indication that Ake was relying on searching her mental inventory during Experiment 3 was the U-shaped, serial-position curve obtained for the three-object case as a function of order of introduction of the objects. Performance was best when the last object introduced was referenced (83% correct responses), next best for the first object (75%), and worst for the middle object (50%), with the chance level of performance estimated as 26%. Hence, both primacy and recency effects occurred, as is the case for many human memory studies (e.g., Murdock, 1962) as well as for some animal memory studies (Wright *et al.,* 1984). This was the first occasion, however, that primacy effects have been observed in a study of dolphin short-term memory, although recency effects have been reported previously (Thompson and Herman, 1977).

Maintaining and updating a mental inventory apparently was strategic during Experiment 3, because only a limited number of objects were present and because the objects were removed after each trial and a new set presented at the succeeding trial. The difference in performance between Experiments 2 and 3 (superior performance during Experiment 2) makes it clear that an environmental search was generally superior to a memory search, although obviously more effortful, especially as the number of objects present increases. However, that both strategies were used successfully (and appropriately) by Ake is a mark of adaptive cognitive flexibility.

The overall results of the reporting studies demonstrated Ake's ability to understand symbolic references to absent objects as well as to ones that were present. In reporting absence, Ake may be said to have shown an understanding, at a pragmatic level, if not an abstract one, that absence is information. Hearst and colleagues (Hearst, 1984; Newman *et al.*, 1980) have suggested that animals may be selected more for monitoring the occurrence of events than for noting their absence. Our results show, however, that absence can be a meaningful event for an animal—in this case, the absence of arbitrary real-world objects of no natural relevance for the dolphin. Reports of absence were made either spontaneously or through arbitrary, learned responses.

In the artificial language used with Ake, the interrogative form is distinguished from the imperative by the terminal word, either QUESTION or an action term (e.g, OVER), and not, as in English, by a change in word order. Nevertheless, the interrogative contributes to the assessment of the dolphin's ability to understand sentences, particularly the ability to interpret the grammatical function of earlier words in a sentence on the basis of succeeding words. Earlier, we noted that in the imperative form of Ake's gestural language the grammatical function of a word could not be reliably assigned until succeeding words appeared. With the addition of the interrogative form, it was no longer only the function of the initial word that could not be determined but the sentence form itself. Accuracy in responding to contrasting interrogative and imperative forms is thus a further indicant that the entire sequence of words was accounted for in interpreting a sentence and organizing a response.

G. AUDITORY VERSUS VISUAL PROCESSING AND SOME LIMITATIONS

Given the demonstrated auditory capabilities and specializations of the bottle-nosed dolphin (Herman, 1980), it was not unexpected that Phoenix would develop some facility within her acoustic language medium. The extensive capabilities of Ake with the visually based gestural language were surprising, however. Many animal species show limitations in the processing of symbolic or arbitrary complex information through secondary sensory modalities—modalities other than those used as the primary interface with the natural world. For example, the auditory and visual sensory systems are both well developed in the cebus monkey (*Cebus apella*). This species (as well as most other primates) is generally regarded as a visual specialist. The cebus monkey has little difficulty with visual matching tasks but immense difficulty with auditory matching (D'Amato, 1973; D'Amato and Salmon, 1984). Similarly, hearing and vision are both well developed in the dolphin, but this animal's remarkable range of hearing, its echolocation abilities, and the visual limitations of the underwater world mark it as an auditory specialist. The dolphin easily learns auditory matching, but has greater difficulty with visual matching under most conditions (see reviews in Herman, 1980, 1986).

Thus, the reasons for success with the visual medium in the current language studies are unclear. One possibility is that the use of gestures early in training predisposed Ake to attend to information in the visual modality. D'Amato and Colombo (1985) have recently reported the first success in teaching auditory matching to some cebus monkeys. The successful monkeys were those whose first training experiences (prior to the D'Amato–Colombo study) were with auditory materials. D'Amato and Colombo proposed that this early experience may have directed attention to auditory materials. That this type of early experience may not suffice as an explanation for the dolphins is suggested by our recent success in teaching visual delayed matching to Phoenix, the animal specialized in the *auditory* language (Hovancik *et al.*, 1985). Phoenix's early training experience was mainly with auditory materials, although she was exposed to some gestures as well. Possibly, the language training helped Phoenix to attend to visual materials through the requirement to respond to the visual referents of her auditory symbols (such as the named floating objects in her tank).

Another possibility for Ake's good performance in the visual medium lies in the nature of the visual symbols used. Gestures are, in effect, visual temporal patterns. Movements of the arms and hands trace out a pattern over time. Sounds, likewise, are temporal patterns, the pattern identified by the structure of the sound components (pitch, rhythm, etc.) over time. Dolphins, given their auditory world and auditory specializations, may be especially proficient in the recognition of auditory temporal patterns, a capability that may generalize readily across modalities. That the recognition of auditory temporal patterns is a specialization not found in all mammals is suggested by the failure of cebus monkeys to recognize tunes (D'Amato and Salmon, 1984).

Regardless of which explanation for the dolphins' good visual performance proves correct, a major conclusion from the results with Phoenix and Ake is that the languagelike skills demonstrated are general and largely independent of sensory modality. This independence was most apparent during the earlier years of our studies but, paradoxically, the acoustic medium, rather than the visual, has recently shown some limitations.

Throughout most of the course of study of Phoenix and Ake, both have shown idiosyncratic limitations in performance, but with overall performance remaining more or less comparable. Each dolphin developed some enduring object confusions. For Phoenix, BALL and FRISBEE were never reliably resolved, although much effort was expended in training the discrimination. Ake has no problem in differentiating between BALL and FRISBEE, but has difficulty with SPEAKER versus PANEL, words that are easily discriminated by Phoenix. Other examples could be given, but these demonstrate the general finding that while object confusion was common to both dolphins, the particular confusions were not. The confusion appears to be between some attributes of the objects themselves, including how the objects may function, rather than between the symbols for the objects. Changing the symbols, for example, changing the sound for FRISBEE in Phoenix's acoustic language, did not resolve the confusion.

More puzzling is that while Ake's overall performance on comprehension of imperatives has remained remarkably stable over the years, Phoenix's has not, and in fact has shown a decline recently. The decline is counterintuitive to what one might expect, given the auditory specializations of the dolphin. Phoenix's annual performance level on imperative sentences (overall percentage of correct responses, using the strict performance criterion) was 84% in 1981, 88% in 1982, 84% in 1983, 73% in 1984, and 68% in 1985. The decline in 1984 and 1985 occurred in all categories of sentences and for all semantic elements. In contrast, during each year of that same 5-year period from 1981 through 1985, Ake's overall performance on imperatives remained between 82 and 89% correct. The low end occurred during 1984 and the high end during 1982 and again during 1985. It is difficult to isolate reasons for the decline in Phoenix's performance relative to that of Ake from among several possibilities: different animals, different grammars (for relational sentences), and different social links for the source of language information given the dolphin. Also, it may be that Phoenix has undergone some general type of intellectual decline over the years that accounts for her lowered performance. This is unlikely, however, given the relative youth of Phoenix, currently a young adult having only recently experienced her first estrus cycle. Phoenix, in fact, is the same age as Ake, who is also recently postpubescent. Moreover, Phoenix has shown exceptional facility in learning new visual delayed-matching tests first given during 1985. Her performance on these tests was better than 90% correct after delays as long as 20 sec, and better than 80% correct at delays of 40 sec (Hovancik et al., 1985).

Possibly, Phoenix has undergone a motivational decline relative to Ake, but again supporting evidence is weak. Phoenix continues to participate eagerly in the daily testing sessions, as does Ake; the testing regimens are similar for the two animals. If the problem was traceable to motivation, random performance errors should emerge as a result of inattention to stimuli. Instead, error patterns and semantic confusions remain much the same as they were during the earlier years of better performance. Also, Phoenix's motivation during her visual matching tests is high, evidenced not only by her high levels of performance but by her patience during the long delay intervals and absence of negative emotional responding.

The different grammars for the two languages—a linear grammar for Phoenix and an inverse grammar for Ake—seem unlikely sources of the difference in current performance levels of Phoenix and Ake. Phoenix's grammar is clearly simpler. Her performance on relational sentences was consistently superior to that of Ake from 1981 through 1984, and declined marginally below Ake's only during 1985.

Finally, do the performance differences relate to social factors? Ake's gestural sentences come directly from her trainer, with whom she interacts socially in many different ways. Although Phoenix also interacts socially with her trainer, her acoustic sentences come from the impersonal underwater speaker located away from the trainer. Language is a social phenomenon in human use, but it is not clear why the noted social difference between Ake's and Phoenix's languages should manifest itself as a performance difference only after several years.

At this juncture, then, we are left without a satisfactory explanation for Phoenix's decline in performance, but with several interesting hypotheses that can be tested in later research.

H.   CRITICISMS OF THE DOLPHIN STUDIES

The dolphin studies, which began in 1979 after the bulk of the criticisms of the ape language work were published, were designed to minimize or avoid the reported methodological shortcomings of that work (see Section IV,C,1 for examples of experimental controls we used). Additionally, because of their focus on comprehension, the studies of the dolphin were easily repeatable and capable of objective and reliable scoring. As a consequence, the results of these studies, as summarized in this paper and reported in detail elsewhere (Herman, 1980, 1986; Herman and Forestell, 1985; Herman et al., 1984; Richards et al., 1984), appear to have withstood the methodological scrutiny of the scientific community. However, one might still contest interpretations of the work or some of its conceptual bases, as has been done recently by Premack (1985, 1986)[2] in his discussion of the "animal language controversy."

_____

[2] In a quirk of publishing, these two references are identical in content, word for word, except for a very few additional paragraphs inserted here and there in the 1986 work. Quotations from Premack's work appearing here are taken from the 1986 version.

Premack acknowledges, begrudgingly it seems, the methodological advance of the dolphin studies (Premack, 1986, p. 25), but treats the overall work in a dismissive way. Throughout Premack's 1986 book, descriptions and comments on the dolphin work are intermixed with expositions on the performances of Sarah and other apes given language training by Premack. At the same time, little or no attention is given to the work of the several other investigators having studied ape language competencies, even when the work is of obvious relevance to the topic being discussed. For example, in his section entitled "What Is a Word?" Premack considered how words may function for chimpanzees, what mental representations these words may have, and whether words learned in the production mode transfer to the comprehension mode or vice versa. These are the same issues considered at length by Savage-Rumbaugh and colleagues in an extensive series of studies (e.g., Savage-Rumbaugh, 1981, 1984a; Savage-Rumbaugh *et al.,* 1983), many of which were reviewed earlier in Section III,B of this paper. Premack, however, makes no mention of *any* work by Savage-Rumbaugh in the 1985 version of his paper, and in the 1986 version provides only a brief synopsis of an early study (Savage-Rumbaugh and Rumbaugh, 1978). This omission is troublesome, since some of the data by Savage-Rumbaugh seem at odds with that reported by Premack—for example, the difficulty of transfer from production to comprehension as reported by Savage-Rumbaugh versus the relative ease reported by Premack. In the least, these differences need to be acknowledged, and resolved if possible.

Premack also ignores, in both the 1985 and 1986 versions (and, to my knowledge, in any other of his publications), the critical paper by Terrace (1979a) commenting on the methodology and conclusions of Premack's major empirical work on ape language competencies (Premack, 1976). However, in the 1985/1986 papers Premack continues to draw essentially the same conclusions about the apes' performances as in his 1976 article. These and other selective omissions of work commenting critically on his findings (e.g., R. A. Gardner and Gardner, 1978; Ristau and Robbins, 1982; Savage-Rumbaugh *et al.,* 1980a) may mislead the uninformed reader into concluding that Premack's findings have been accepted without question. For the informed reader, the omissions dilute the impact of Premack's frequently incisive presentations of linguistic and cognitive theory.

Premack's comments on the dolphin work are restricted to selected portions of the materials presented in Herman *et al.* (1984). Not included, or given at best minimal consideration, were a number of topics important to the assessment of the competencies of the dolphins within their artificial languages: for example, the unique processing requirements of the structurally different relational sentences given to the two dolphins, the different media used (visual versus acoustic), the responses to anomalous sentences, the demonstrated vocal mimicry and vocal labeling abilities, and the ability to report on the absence of a named object. An appreciation of performance in these areas is necessary for reaching conclusions about the types and levels of receptive competencies of the dolphins.

Within the limitations of the materials selected by Premack, the main themes he pursues in criticism of Herman *et al.* (1984) appear to be the following:

1. *Can terms developed for analyses of human language be used when assessing animal language competencies?* Premack (1986) contends that in the work of Herman *et al.* "portentous terms are applied to inappropriate referents, falsely conferring on the dolphin those capacities demonstrated thus far only in the human" (p. 26). The portentous terms he refers to include "word," "sentence," "syntax," and "semantics." The same terms can be found sprinkled liberally throughout Premack's own work (e.g., Premack, 1971, 1976, 1986), both in reference to the kinds of problems he provided the apes and to the resulting responses of these animals. Other even more portentous terms appear: for example, "demonstrative pronoun," "demonstrative adjective," "nominative phrase," "accusative phrase" (Premack, 1976, pp. 320–321). Moreover, despite his admonition, cited above, that certain linguistic capacities have been "demonstrated thus far only in the human," Premack (1986) confers on Sarah and his other apes some of those same capacities he reserves for humans (and denies for the dolphins). Regarding sentence-processing abilities, for example, Premack (1986) states unequivocally, "not only gifted apes but also quite ordinary ones can 'create sentences' " (p. 28).

In fact, all workers investigating animal language competencies have found it convenient to use "portentous" linguistic terms (those listed, or others). While it is often difficult to give definitions to these terms that express all of their meaning and reference, they are in common use in many fields concerned with language or languagelike processes and enable the worker to relate his methods and findings to a vast body of literature on language. In this way, the terms serve a heuristic function, as a model or metaphor of conceptual richness within which to examine and evaluate animal performance.

Consider, for example, the linguistic terms "displacement" and "recursion," used by Premack (1976) to discuss certain aspects of Sarah's performances, and by us to conceptualize some performances of the dolphins. Hockett (1960) included the concept of displacement within his list of "design features" of human language, defining it as the ability to refer to objects remote in space or time. He found it quite acceptable, though, to include as an instance of displacement the performance of a bee communicating the location of a food source to its nestmates, leaving open the question of how the case for the bee might differ quantitatively or qualitatively from the characteristics of displacement references in human language use. Hockett (1960, p. 415) noted that "an increasing capacity for internal storage clearly has to accompany any radical increase in displacement."

In our discussion of the dolphins' understanding of references to absent objects and their ability to report such absence, we stated that the results of those studies offered "a first approximation to the displacement characteristic of human language (Hockett, 1960)" (Herman *et al.*, 1984, p. 184). Premack (1986, p. 25), considering only our sentence-memory tests (see Section IV,C), and not our tests of the ability to report the absence of named objects, takes issue with this use of the term displacement. Premack (1976, pp. 204–205), however, paralleling the earlier comment of Hockett, offers this appraisal: "Displacement is merely a special outcome or symptom of a general mnemonic capacity and can be expected whenever the memory capacity of the species reaches a certain level." In fact, as I discussed earlier, the sentence-memory tests addressed several issues: mnemonic capacity, the ability to understand symbolic references to absent objects, and whether sentence understanding necessarily proceeds on a word-by-word basis.

The issues in the present case, then, do not involve the use of the term displacement per se, but ask whether the communication system, be it human language or some other form of animal communication, allows for references to objects or events remote in space or time, whether the users of that system understand such references, and the range of displacement activity that can be demonstrated. It is clear that the dolphins of our studies understood references to absent objects, especially in view of the findings of Herman and Forestell (1985). The limitations of such understanding remain to be studied in more complex paradigms than those used thus far; yet, it is the availability of the concept of displacement that impels us to look further and that provides a conceptual guide to the interpretation of our results and to the development of new studies that may examine other dimensions of this skill, as Premack himself suggests we ought to do.

The term "recursion" occurred in Herman *et al.* (1984) in discussion of the ability of the dolphin Phoenix to understand two conjoined sentences. Our study of this ability was motivated by a desire to know whether Phoenix might understand such new sentence forms without specific training (see Section IV,C,1,f). The concept of recursion offered a framework within which to develop our procedures and assess Phoenix's performance. As used in human linguistic analyses, recursion refers to that property of human language that allows for the construction of sentences of increasing (even infinite) length by, for example, embedding clauses within a sentence. We chose, again as a first approximation, to study conjunction, one of several forms of recursion. It is ironic that Premack elected to dispute such use, since in his 1976 work he states: "Both Sarah and the other female chimps use conjunction, which, along with nominalization and relativization, is a major recursive form" (Premack, 1976, p. 321). Premack then goes on to describe how Sarah joined two sentences together to make a request for two objects (e.g., "Mary give Sarah apple banana" as derived from the atomic sentences "Mary give Sarah apple" and "Mary give Sarah ba-nana").

Finally, Premack exaggerates our actual, and cautious, use of some terms and on one occasion misrepresents our use. He states: "Herman *et al.* attributed to the dolphin a finite-state grammar; thereafter, they speak freely of 'syntactic categories,' 'semantic proposition,' 'lexical component,' 'syntactic rules,' and the like" (Premack, 1986, p. 15). In fact, nowhere do we attribute a finite-state grammar to the dolphin. The only place that the term "finite-state grammar" appears in our 1984 text of 90 pages is in the statistical appendix where that grammatical model is used, *for convenience,* to evaluate the probabilities of a dolphin responding to a sentence correctly by chance alone, and again in one paragraph of the text referring to that appendix. The text reference occurs 30 pages into the paper, well after the other terms noted by Premack are introduced.

2. *Is comprehension a useful approach to the study of animal language compe-tencies?* According to Premack (1986), "Herman *et al.* have not yet arranged for the dolphin to produce language, and they would make a virtue of this weakness, claiming unusual advantages for comprehension. One might grant part of the claim if they would acknowledge that, however great the virtues of comprehen-sion, adding the study of production does not detract from them" (p. 17). Granted, of course. The conclusion of our 1984 paper states: "Expanded re-search with the dolphin is needed . . . including the ability for productive lan-guage and the limitations on productive language relative to receptive language" (Herman *et al.,* 1984, p. 210). Premack goes one step further, however, and claims that there are several telling aspects of language that cannot be addressed by comprehension alone—displacement and recursion, for example, which are topics already dealt with and which can, as we have seen, lend themselves to study through comprehension.

Premack also suggests that self-description and description of others cannot be studied through comprehension. It is not clear what Premack really means by this: that one cannot devise an experiment that will test such description through comprehension approaches or that a dolphin could not describe itself or others. The latter is an empirical question if the former task can be devised. In fact, to devise a relevant comprehension task is easy. Through a series of answers to binary Yes/No questions, we in effect elicited from the dolphin a report (descrip-tion) of the contents of its tank world (see Section IV,F). One could, in theory, similarly elicit reports about others or of oneself. We have not yet attempted this, but such tasks could take the form of asking one dolphin about the state or actions of the other (or of a trainer), or asking it about its own state or actions. For descriptions of the other, we might ask: "Is Phoenix in the channel?" (a question to Ake) or "Did Phoenix jump over the ball?". For self-description, the ques-tions need only be rephrased as "Are you in the channel?" or "Did you jump over the ball?".

Premack calls the imperatives we gave to the dolphins "motor commands," and then argues that little can be learned about language from responses to motor commands (by "motor command," Premack apparently means that the dolphin is instructed to carry out some action with its own body, such as jumping over a ball). There are at least two problems with Premack's contention. One is that not all would agree with his basic premise about the limitations of motor commands. Lieberman (1985), for example, attempts to show that motor behaviors and the neural mechanisms controlling these behaviors were the evolutionarily necessary preadaptations for the emergence of syntax. Presumably, motor programs, like syntax, consist of rules for hierarchical organization and sequential ordering. In fairness, Premack offers arguments against Lieberman's position.

Second, the bulk of the imperatives given to the dolphins were *not* motor commands in Premack's sense (nor, of course, were the interrogatives, which are not considered at all by Premack). Instead, the majority of imperatives were in the form of relational sentences that directed the dolphin to *construct* a relationship between two objects—taking one object to another or putting one object in or on another. Relational sentences of these types are particularly useful for demonstrating sensitivity to the influence of word order on meaning (such as the difference in meaning between SURFBOARD FRISBEE FETCH and FRISBEE SURFBOARD FETCH in Ake's inverse grammar) and for showing how the dolphin organizes its response when the grammatical function of a word cannot be assigned by word order alone (see Section IV,F). Premack (1976) in fact freely makes use of functionally similar relational sentences to test for understanding of the role of word order in sentences given to his apes, such as "(put) red on green" versus "(put) green on red" (see Section III,B).

In summary, comprehension has proven itself a useful tool for analyses of language competencies of animals (and children) and allows for the examination of the subject's responses to both the functional and structural aspects of the language system used. Again, this is not to imply that the study of language production (if properly executed) cannot also address these issues and provide expansions to findings derived from comprehension studies.

3. *How shall we describe the concepts that an animal deals with in a language-learning paradigm?* The syntactic rules for the artificial languages given to the dolphins were stated in terms of the concepts of "object," "property," and "action" (see, for example, Section IV,B). Premack (1986, p. 16) writes: "What is most notable about these rules, quite apart from their simplicity, is that they are framed in terms of categories that owe nothing to linguistics. . . . Object, property, and action do not derive from linguistic theory but have one foot in common sense and another in psychology. . . . An individual knowing nothing of 'word' or 'sentence' could walk through the world and point to examples of object, action, and property." Premack goes on to describe three sets of categories, with the first set consisting of objects, properties, and actions

(the "neutral" set), the second consisting of concepts such as agent, action, and recipient (the "semantic" set), and the third consisting of concepts such as noun phrase and verb phrase (the "syntactic" set). He then states, with little equivocation, "The best available evidence suggests the following: the 'neutral' set will be found in all mammals, even perhaps all vertebrates; the semantic set to at least some degree in all primates (but in well-developed form only in humans); and the syntactic set in humans alone" (p. 17). Quite apart from the fact that we are left wondering exactly what is "the best available evidence" of which Premack speaks, in banning certain of the taxa from the more "advanced" categories, Premack reveals a species chauvinism that harkens back to the comparative psychology of the 1950s and 1960s when it was fashionable to search for tasks that might be solved by primates alone, mammals alone, vertebrates alone, etc. Few, if any, of these tasks, when appropriately engineered for the species under study, were in fact found to reliably separate the taxa. As Premack himself acknowledges: "The study of learning has steadfastly refused to disclose interesting systematic differences among species" (Premack, 1986, p. 39).

Nevertheless, it is not the ability of the dolphins to "point to" objects, properties, or actions that interest us, but the ability to understand relationships among these concepts as expressed though arbitrary symbols and combinatorial rules (that were different for the two dolphins). It is one matter for an animal to detect an object, judge it large, or note that it is moving away, and another to be able to interpret the relationship among objects, properties, and actions on the basis of symbolic references and combinatorial rules. In interpreting relationships, the animal is, in effect, operating in the domain of the semantic set proposed by Premack.

A major *raison d'etre* for language would seem to be to describe or refer to relationships among the objects, properties, and actions of one's world (or their representations in one's mind). At this stage of study we have learned that dolphins can interpret or even construct at least simple relationships of these types within their tank world, as governed by the meanings of symbols and their grammatical relations. In short, the concepts of object, property, and action have proven very useful for examination of language competencies of animals. "Object," "property," and "action" are the explicit materials we use in teaching language to children or animals (we do not teach semantic or syntactic concepts explicitly) and that is why we find these terms replete throughout the animal language literature, including the work of Premack (e.g., Premack, 1971, 1976).

4. *Is object generalization a key finding of the dolphin work?* Premack erects a straw man by claiming that we have proposed object generalization as a major feature of our language demonstrations. He then states: "It is not clear why they [Herman *et al.*] favor this position. There is nothing demanding about the object classes they use, and surely there is no mammal that could not discriminate among them" (Premack, 1986, p. 26). Compare Premack's claim with our actual posi-

tion: "Two forms of semantic generalization were identified in this study. One was the extension of an object word learned with respect to one exemplar . . . to other exemplars of that class. The second was the extension of an action word, learned with respect to a particular object, or within a limited context, to other objects or contexts. Both types of semantic generalization were shown by both dolphins, but the second type—the generalization of an action word—is perhaps the more interesting of the two" (Herman *et al.*, 1984, p. 178). Nowhere do we attribute anything special linguistically to object generalization; we stress only what was of *empirical* importance—that the words taught applied to classes of objects and not to particular training exemplars. More disturbing is the omission by Premack of mention of action generalization (or, for that matter, context generalization), especially the spontaneous behavior of the dolphins in manipulating objects to make it possible to perform the requested action on those objects, such as lifting a hoop off the tank bottom in order to swim through it (see Section IV,C,3,e). I also noted the dolphins' propensity for clarifying their responses, for example, by separating the destination object on arrival from other objects nearby. These behaviors go beyond the boundaries of what is normally subsumed by "generalization" and might be better thought of as revealing the animal's understanding of the *concept* implied by the action term—an understanding of "fetchingness" or "throughness," for example.

5. *How shall we view the understanding of novel sentences?* Premack states that producing novel sentences is a weak use of language (in contrast, he offers "conversation" as a strong use). He then dismisses the dolphins' understanding of novel sentences as follows: "The distinctive feature of dolphin performance may appear to be that of transfer. Trained to associate, say, stick with fetch and ball with touch, the animal applies fetch to ball and touch to stick. But transfer per se does not distinguish this from any other case of learning. Any animal trained to fetch one object or touch another will fetch or touch objects different from those on which it was trained. Similarly, an individual trained to fetch or touch objects signalled by distinctive stimuli ('words') will respond to other objects signaled by the 'words' associated with them" (Premack, 1986, p. 34).

Premack thus treats the process of producing (or understanding) unique *combinations* of words cavalierly, brushing aside that "mysterious ability" referred to by N. Chomsky (1972). For the dolphins, the understanding of lexically novel relational sentences involved attention not only to objects signaled by words but to the semantic category of the words (as object, property, or action) and their temporal ordering. In some cases, relationships among nonadjacent words had to be taken into account to interpret a sentence correctly. Premack (1986) was, in fact, concerned enough with the question of temporal-order processing to devote half a chapter to the topic. He noted that temporal-order processing was considered a key, even unique, human skill by many prominent investigators into language and learning—Charles Hockett, George Miller, and Donald Hebb, among others—and then showed that Sarah was able to process temporal-order information. Premack readily acknowledges that the work of Herman *et al.* showed temporal-order processing by dolphins. Premack's purpose, however, was not to show that chimps and dolphins belonged to an exclusive processing club chaired by humans, but that temporal-order processing was not a uniquely human property or a sufficient ingredient for the emergence of natural language skill. I find no problem with that view, nor with Premack's invocation of special "hard-wired" language circuits in the human species that are lacking in other animals. However, Premack stops short of the important corollary of that stance: Does the absence of hard-wiring exclude all competency in language (metaphorically, would a dolphin claim that if you lack hard-wired tail flukes, moving through the water isn't swimming)? What does the animal language learning work tell us about the degree of control over language exerted by hard-wiring, or about the components of language that are available (unavailable) without hard-wiring?

Premack's equating (lexical) novelty with transfer also ignores the data on structural novelty and the recognition of anomalous sentence forms. Both apes (Premack, 1976, p. 322) and dolphins have shown an understanding of some types of structurally novel sentences. The understanding by apes would be difficult to view as simply "transfer," nor did Premack (1976) attempt to do so. The same is true for the understanding shown by dolphins.

In rejecting a semantically anomalous sentence, such as refusing to take the immovable gate in the tank to a hoop, refusing to respond at all to a lexical anomaly, or acting only on the grammatical component within a larger syntactic anomaly, the dolphin revealed that its "transfer" could not be characterized as simple generalized responses, executed by rote. Instead, the data suggested that the dolphin casts a semantic interpretation on the sentence as a whole before acting on that sentence fully.

6. *Is the "animal language controversy" politics or science (or both)?* In the final analysis, Premack (1985, 1986) leaves us with mixed feelings: appreciation for insightful, stimulating theoretical discussions and disappointment in the selective omission of relevant data or the misinterpretation of some data presented. The data omissions may indict Premack's historical view of the animal language controversy as embedded in politics (in political contests, there is only one winner; the other participants are "opponents" to be overcome, rather than contributors to a common fund of ideas and knowledge on which all draw). If this seems a strange or even unkind interpretation, consider Premack's own words. According to Premack (1986, p. 2), the animal language controversy arose on the East Coast, which "gave it all of the stigmata of that intellectual locale" (p. 3). On the East Coast, Premack states, "intellectual disputes rapidly become political contests, and the number of adherents, the location of adherents in academic hierarchy, dialectical skill, connections with media, representation at international meetings—in short, power- -play a role surprising to the outsider" (p. 2).

Premack contrasts this regional climate with the Midwest of his academic roots, where "intellectual disputes are settled on intrinsic grounds . . . the struggle is not one for power and arguments come close to being settled in terms of the positivistic ideal" (p. 2). These views are more revealing of an unfortunate scientific chauvinism than of historical, geopolitical truths about "the animal language controversy." With such views, Premack's new work is in many respects a continuation of that controversy, rather than a remedy for its future.

I. SUMMARY

Extensive receptive competencies were demonstrated within the medium of the artificial languages used. New sentences of a variety of familiar syntactic forms were often understood immediately; in many cases, understanding required the processing of both semantic and syntactic information. Errors in responding were most often limited to one word of a multiword sentence, such as arriving at the incorrect destination with the correct object. Such errors, however, tended to preserve the major intent of the sentence. New syntactic categories or sentence forms were generally understood immediately. Ake, especially, was able to extract and respond to the meaningful segments of otherwise ungrammatical (anomalous) sentences.

The understanding of words included an ability to respond to novel exemplars of an object word, to respond appropriately in new contexts, and to rearrange cricumstances to make it possible to carry out a required action. The limits of the lexicon were understood, demonstrated by refusals to respond to grammatical sentences containing a nonsense word. References to objects not immediately present were understood in sentence-memory tests in which sentences were given with the referenced object, as well as all other removable objects, temporarily absent. An interrogative sentence form taught to Ake was used to question her about the presence or absence in her tank of specific named objects. Ake reported either presence or absence successfully by responding on the appropriate paddle of a pair. Within the same context, Ake could distinguish the imperative from the interrogative, by taking an appropriate action if an imperative made reference to an object that was present or by responding on a paddle if given an interrogative. Ake was also proficient at signifying "absent" by a paddle press if given an imperative referring to an absent object.

Finally, Ake was able to apply vocal labels to any of five objects shown her, a trained extension of her native ability to mimic sounds, including arbitrary, computer-produced sounds.

Comprehension was not limited to either the auditory or the visual modality. Phoenix was specialized in the auditory language and Ake in the visual language; the two dolphins showed comparable levels of proficiency with their languages for the first 3–4 years of training. Recently, Phoenix, but not Ake, has shown some declines in performance, despite the extensive auditory capabilities of dolphins. The reasons for the decline are unclear at the present time.

V. RECEPTIVE COMPETENCIES IN SEA LIONS

Using procedures modeled after those applied to dolphins (Herman, 1980; Herman *et al.*, 1984), Schusterman and Krieger (1984) studied comprehension of an artificial gestural language by two California sea lions (*Zalophus californianus*). California sea lions are commonly used as the trained "seals" of circuses and oceanariums, and are relatively large-brained mammals. Brain/body weights for females are 277 g/40–68 kg, on the average (S. Ridgway, personal communication, November 1984), compared with 325 g/44 kg average brain/body weights for female common chimpanzees (Jerison, 1973). Sea lions have been the subjects of several early studies of learning and sensory processes (reviewed in Schusterman, 1968, 1981). Vision is well developed in this species.

To test for sentence comprehension in sea lions, Schusterman and Krieger gave the pair they studied two- or three-word gestural strings constructed as Object + Action or Modifier + Object + Action. Different modifier sets were used for the two sea lions—BLACK, WHITE, and GREY for one animal (Rocky) and WATER and LAND for the second (Bucky). The first set refers to the color of a named object, while the second indicates its location. In one series of tests, responses to familiar two-word sentences were 96% correct ($n = 854$) for Rocky and 90% correct ($n = 600$) for Bucky, when choices of objects were made from among six alternatives, on the average, and either five or six actions. The exact number of unique sentences given is not provided by the authors but appears to be on the order of 50 two-word sentences.

Object names were understood regardless of the physical orientation of the referenced familiar object. However, when new exemplars were introduced, performance decreased significantly in most cases for both animals. With subsequent experience with multiple exemplars, performance improved to previous levels.

Rocky's responses to three-word sentences were 90% correct ($n = 384$) when only two modifiers were in his vocabulary (BLACK and WHITE) and 87% correct ($n = 574$) after the third modifier (GREY) was introduced. There were perhaps 100–150 different three-word sentences among these numbers. Training of Rocky on a second modifier set (LARGE and SMALL) was reported as "in progress," with initial levels of performance at about 74% correct responses. Training of Bucky on modifiers (LAND or WATER) was also reported to be in progress, with performance for 280 trials at 86%. These are all impressive levels of performance. Schusterman and Krieger used controls for nonlinguistic cueing similar to those used by Herman *et al.* (1984), including requiring trainers to wear opaque goggles when signing (to guard against eye gaze cues) and having the responses of the sea lions scored by observers other than the trainer or session supervisor. The obtained results therefore evidence an understanding of the semantic components of the sentences constructed.

In more recent work (Schusterman, 1984), the two sets of modifiers used with Rocky have been combined to form four-word sentences, such as LARGE GREY BALL OVER or WHITE SMALL CAR UNDER. The two categories of modifiers may be used in either sequence and, reportedly, are responded to appropriately regardless of order. The deliberate use of word order to modulate meaning was not explored by either Schusterman and Krieger or Schusterman, so that syntactic processing ability could not be studied. Work is reportedly under-way, however, on training for the understanding of relational sentences similar to those used by Herman *et al.* (1984). This will provide an opportunity to assess syntactic processing abilities. The overall results of Schusterman's studies, within the limits of the issues he has addressed thus far, parallel the findings with dolphins and give promise that the techniques used for measuring receptive competencies can be extended to other animals as well, including apes.

VI. Conclusions

A. Receptive Competencies

The work with marine mammals—bottle-nosed dolphins and California sea lions—was carried out under controlled testing procedures that emphasized the development of receptive skills within the framework of artificial gestural or acoustic languages. The results showed that these animals could learn to make correct interpretations of ordered strings of symbols, or sentences, that often contained both semantic and syntactic information. The work with great apes—chimpanzees, gorillas, or orangutans—has in large part proceeded on a different path that has either emphasized productive skill (while ignoring receptive abilities) or has been mainly focused on the semantic comprehension and use of single words, the referential attribute explored at length in the work of Savage-Rumbaugh and colleagues. Evidence is lacking or weak that the apes have used sequential order to produce information through strings of words, conclusions that are nearly unanimous among those having reviewed the language work in detail in recent years (e.g., Ristau and Robbins, 1982; Savage-Rumbaugh *et al.*, 1980a; Terrace *et al.*, 1979).

Portions of Premack's (1971, 1976) work deal with comprehension of sentences and include strings in which word order plays a role in producing meaning. Sarah, Premack's star chimpanzee pupil, was exposed to a variety of tests of understanding, with results that suggest that chimpanzees have considerable ability to process both semantic and syntactic information in the receptive mode. Personally, I do not doubt this. However, confidence in Premack's own conclusions is tempered by the weaknesses in his procedures and analyses, as highlighted in several reviews of his work (e.g., Terrace, 1979a; Savage-Rumbaugh et al., 1980a). One might be more supportive of Premack's conclusions were there data from other research with apes to bolster his claims, yet the opposite is sometimes true. For example, where Premack claims that comprehension proceeds, with a little help, from production, or vice versa, others find linking the two to be fraught with difficulty (e.g., Savage-Rumbaugh et al., 1980a, 1983). Also, Premack too often ignores the work of other researchers into ape language competencies, even when that work may support his findings. Thus, in the area of reference, in which Premack's work is particularly strong, he fails to make contact with the relevant empirical work of Savage-Rumbaugh.

Producing sequential-order information is certainly within the capabilities of many animals, at least within simple, nonlexical contexts. Pigeons have learned to respond to four simultaneously presented colors in a fixed sequence, regardless of the physical ordering of the symbols or their location in space (e.g., Straub et al., 1979; for general reviews, see Terrace, 1984b; Roitblat, 1986). Furthermore, it is clear that the pigeons learn the ordering rule rather than a simple linked chain of responses, since probes of subsets of two colors, such as the first and third or second and fourth, produce the properly ordered response sequence to the two. What is different about the sequence-controlled responses of the dolphins is that responses are not made to the symbols themselves but to their referents, that the response to a given referent can vary in kind depending on the nature of the other symbols in the sequence and their relationship within the sequence, and that the ordering rule is not specific to any particular set of symbols but to classes of symbols together with their particular meaning. The last property allows for the construction of new sequences that may be understood immediately without specific training.

A further, important distinction is that for many of the sentences given to the dolphins, both semantic and syntactic information processing were necessary for sentence understanding. Of all of the skills demonstrated, it is probably the ability to integrate the semantic with the syntactic component to reach an interpretation of a sentence that marks the performance of these animals as unusually adroit. California sea lions have an ability to process the semantic components of sentences and, in preliminary receptive tests, appear to be able to process some syntactical information as well. The time seems ripe for formal tests of similar receptive competencies in apes, animals that would be expected to show at least comparable capabilities to the marine mammals.

The syntax used in the studies of marine mammals was based on word-order rules. Word order is not a trivial type of syntactic rule. As discussed by Horgan (1980), citing work by Brown (1973) and others, word order is a central criterion for syntax. Horgan states: "Word order [in English] . . . is considered one of the best indications that the child possesses linguistic knowledge'' (1980, p. 129). For the marine mammals, the word-order rules were: Modifiers precede objects modified and direct object names precede action names, but these rules alone were not sufficient to cast a correct interpretation. A few examples will illustrate this point. For the sea lions, either one or two modifiers might occur before an object name, as in LARGE BALL FLIPPER-TOUCH versus LARGE WHITE BALL FLIPPER-TOUCH, so that a semantic interpretation had to be superimposed on the word-order rules to categorize the second symbol correctly as either attribute or object. For the dolphins, similar though at times more complex interactions of semantic- and syntactic-based interpretations were necessary, particularly for relational sentences. For the inverse grammar used with the dolphin Ake, a modifier might appear before a pair of object names or be sandwiched between the two, as in LEFT WATER PIPE FETCH versus WATER LEFT PIPE FETCH. Thus, as in this example, the location of a word in a sequence of words was not necessarily sufficient to interpret its grammatical function; a semantic evaluation had to be made as well. In Ake's grammar, the first word of a sentence might be a modifier, a direct object, or an indirect object. Additionally, the semantic value of the word might be insufficient to determine its grammatical function. For object words, a succeeding word(s) was necessary to determine whether the reference was to a direct or indirect object. Also, in Ake's grammar, the terminal word of the sentence determined the type of response to be taken toward an object, the type of relation expressed between two objects, or whether any action was to be taken to the object at all. In the latter case, the terminal word might be the interrogative requesting a report about an object, given by pressing one of two response paddles, or it might be the canceling term ERASE, requiring that the dolphin take no response at all other than remaining at her station to receive new instructions. Although Phoenix's linear grammar appears simpler than Ake's, word order was still a determinant of the grammatical function of a word as direct or indirect object. Reversals of the ordering of object names resulted in reversal of function, as was the case in Ake's language. Both dolphins were able to track a reversal of the ordering of object names by a reversal of the ordering of their responses. The processing of the semantic and syntactic features of the sentences was very general, as shown by the ability of the dolphins to understand sentences to which they had not been exposed previously.

Thus, in the receptive skills shown by the dolphins and, to a less complex degree, in those shown by the sea lions, syntactic and semantic processing go hand-in-hand to create a correct interpretation of a sentence, as is the case for human language. The work with apes has not yet convincingly shown whether these two fundamental attributes of language may be combined to enlarge the apes' communicative repertoire, either in production or comprehension. The emphasis on the semantic attribute in the current ape language studies is, however, in keeping with studies with children, showing the priority of semantics over syntax in early language development (e.g., C. Chomsky, 1969). It will be interesting to see, as the semantic work with apes progresses, whether Terrace's (1985) premise holds: that semantics, as evidenced by referential naming, is a precursor of syntax.

B. The Need for Teaching Receptive Skills

The work with marine mammals, as well as some work by Savage-Rumbaugh and by Premack with apes, shows that receptive competencies, like productive competencies, can be *taught* to animals. The work by Savage-Rumbaugh (but not Premack) suggests that there is unlikely to be direct or even easy transfer between the two poles of communication. Historically, there was seldom any concerted effort to teach receptive skills to apes, and where such teaching has occurred it has been constrained to rather limited experimental paradigms. Before the recent reports on the pygmy chimpanzee Kanzi (Savage-Rumbaugh *et al.*, 1985), it would have been easy to postulate that receptive skills *must* be expressly taught through formal pedagogical techniques. If further work with Kanzi demonstrates that observation alone, in the context of near-total immersion in the language being taught, is sufficient for attaining reasonable levels of receptive skill then the postulate, in its strong form, would have to be abandoned. Near-total immersion in a foreign language has proven effective for teaching second languages to children or adults (e.g., Lambert and Tucker, 1972) and has been used in most of the ape language signing projects. However, its previous use has always been in conjunction with rote drilling and other formal pedagogical techniques. Hence, Kanzi's progress and performance should be carefully monitored through objective assessments and his ability to make use of both semantic and syntactic components evaluated. If what is taught to animals in a language-learning paradigm is likened to second-language learning by humans, then it would be surprising if formal instruction based on pedagogical grammars (St. Clair, 1980) was not additionally facilitative for Kanzi.

C. Receptive versus Productive Competencies

Learning of languages by humans is generally characterized by a temporal gap in which comprehension precedes and exceeds production (Ingram, 1974), possibly because the cognitive processes involved in comprehension are less complex than those controlling production (although the processes controlling each may partially overlap) (Bloom, 1974; Schiefelbusch, 1974). The same may be true for the animals studied in languagelike tasks, judging by many of the results reviewed in this paper. As was noted, the work on comprehension in marine mammals has provided evidence for the abilities of these animals to use word order as information, a capability never fully realized within the language studies of apes emphasizing production.

This finding, in conjunction with other evidence for receptive skills of animals, as reviewed in this paper, suggests that there may be asymmetric developments in the productive and receptive competencies of animals, receptive competencies being greatly favored. Why should this be so? A major reason may lie in the need, common to all animals, to monitor and interpret the stream of diverse information constantly arriving at their senses from the physical and social worlds. There is far less need, it would seem, to produce information intentionally, and in any event, produced information would be limited in its value as communication to the social domain, a subset of the multiple domains with which the animal must deal. So we begin with asymmetric biological needs for receiving information versus producing information. To the extent that the social domain of the species grows in scope and complexity, productive skills can be expected to increase in usefulness to the individual animal. Indeed, social forces may be the prime mover for the evolution of productive skill (though not necessarily receptive skill), reaching a climax in the development of the extensive productive skills of humans.

Studying the receptive skills of animals is valuable from this theoretical perspective, and needs to be greatly expanded in future studies with animals. Ideally, one would want to examine both receptive and productive competencies in any species. Yet until there are clear demonstrations of receptive competencies, interpretations of the results of studies of productive skills remain equivocal. In part, this is because the many variables that potentially confound the interpretation of the results of language studies are better controlled in a comprehension design than in a production study.

Perhaps the closest approximation to the goal of exploring and documenting both production and comprehension successfully is the work by Savage-Rumbaugh and colleagues, showing competencies of the chimps Sherman and Austin for exchanging roles as sender and receiver in tool-using and food-sharing tasks (Savage-Rumbaugh and Rumbaugh, 1978; Savage-Rumbaugh et al., 1983). However, a limitation in that work (as well as in related work by Savage-Rumbaugh) is the emphasis on single symbols (words) rather than symbol strings (sentences). While the study of the word has illuminated the levels of semantic comprehension of the chimpanzees studied and their ability to use words to refer rather than simply to request, it would be important to know to what extent Sherman and Austin (or other apes) could understand versus produce sequences of words that transmitted both semantic and syntactic information.

D. THE RELATIONSHIP OF ANIMAL LANGUAGE STUDIES
   TO HUMAN LANGUAGE

The degree of overlap between animal language competencies and human language abilities is a continuing empirical question. It is far from a settled issue.

Although the development of language in the child may be governed and facilitated by specialized brain architecture or processing algorithms, studies of first- and second-language learning show that language is a set of sequentially developing skills mastered only over a protracted period of study or immersion (e.g., Bailey *et al.*, 1974; Brown, 1973; Dulay *et al.*, 1982). Consequently, it is unlikely that any short-term studies of languagelike skills of animals will reveal the extent of underlying competencies (or the extent of limitations).

Possibly, we can take for granted that at best what an animal learns through specific training in language paradigms is some subset, some fragment, of the language skills of the adult human; that it is not likely that even the fragmentary skills acquired will reflect the levels reached by young children; and that the sequence and mechanisms of learning may be different in animals and humans. Nevertheless, it is important and illuminating to identify the boundary conditions—the specific skills and their levels that can and cannot be learned by specific animals—in order to understand better some of the cognitive bases of language learning. If animals can learn to understand that the ordering or other structuring of symbol sequences is information, then that level of processing is not an exclusive property of human language. If the symbols manipulated by an animal come to be surrogates for their referents, then neither is "reference" an exclusive property of human language use. If animals comprehend more information than they can produce, then this is a correlate of human language characteristics. If animals cannot or do not use the acquired language systems to communicate beyond the boundaries of the materials or contexts taught, then this is a limitation in pragmatics that may fundamentally separate human developments in language from those attainable by animals. And, if animals cannot create symbols or sequences of symbols to expand their repertoire of reference, then this is a further stricture on their ability that may identify by default an exclusive human attribute of language use.

E.   SOME COMMENTS ON THE "ANIMAL
     LANGUAGE CONTROVERSY"

The attempts over the past two decades to study languagelike abilities in animals have been an exciting enterprise that has produced both information and dissension. As a result of this work, a better understanding of pertinent questions to ask about language has emerged, as well as a refinement of our conceptions of language itself. The work has expanded our knowledge of the cognitive characteristics of the animals studied in languagelike paradigms, including their cognitive abilities, specializations, and limitations. Also, the work has resulted in a better appreciation of the empirical tools, controls, and data generation and management techniques necessary for making valid inferences in this most difficult field. Of course, major questions remain unanswered or only partially answered, including those raised in the preceding sections.

Nevertheless, these positive outcomes have often been set within a contentious atmosphere that at times has gone well beyond the boundaries of objective and facilitative scientific criticism and rejoinder. Whole enterprises have been summarily dismissed as a result of these excesses, and some journals have ruled that they will no longer accept articles on teaching animals language. Clearly, some facts have been thrown out with the artifacts. On the other hand, some researchers have not sought to respond to valid criticism by rectifying their methods in new experiments or moderating their interpretations. Little of scientific value can come from such extreme stances. The better solution is to seek to build with new data and to integrate these data with the old, into refined concepts and theories of animal cognition and its relation to issues about language.

Despite Premack's (1986) view that "to get on with an understanding of our species, we shall have to relinquish our infatuation with language. . ." (p. 155), that infatuation is probably as fundamental a human attribute as is language itself. The language research with animals is likely to continue and to produce new evidence and new insights. It *is* valid to continue to ask questions about competencies of animals in languagelike tasks, because these are questions about behavior, cognitive structures and processes, communication, and the range of the animal and human mind, all issues of current scientific (and lay) interest that can be better attacked successfully through experiment and observation than through philosophy or fiat.

Acknowledgments

Preparation of this paper and the reported studies with dolphins were supported by grants or contracts from the National Science Foundation (BNS-8019653), the Office of Naval Research (Contract No. CA-9700-3-8028), and the Center for Field Research (Earthwatch). Release time from teaching provided through the Social Science Research Institute of the University of Hawaii facilitated the report preparation. I thank Paul Forestell, Carolyn Ristau, Herbert Roitblat, Amye Warren-Leubecker, and James Wolz for helpful comments on the manuscript.

References

Andrew, R. J. (1962). Evolution of intelligence and vocal mimicking. *Science* **137,** 585–589.
Bailey, N., Madden, C., and Krashen, S. D. (1974). Is there a "natural sequence" in adult second language learning? *Language Learning* **24,** 235–243.
Bates, E. (1976). "Language and Context: The Acquisition of Pragmatics." Academic Press, New York.
Bloom, L. (1974). Talking, understanding, and thinking: Developmental relationship between receptive and expressive language. *In* "Language Perspectives—Acquisition, Retardation, and Intervention" (R. L. Schiefelbusch and L. L. Lloyd, eds.), pp. 285–311. University Park Press, Baltimore.
Bronowski, J., and Bellugi, U. (1970). Language, name and concept. *Science* **168,** 669–673.

Brown, R. (1968). The development of wh questions in child speech. *J. Verb. Learn. Verb. Behav.* **7,** 277–290.

Brown, R. (1973). "A First Language." Harvard University Press, Cambridge, Massachusetts.

Bruner, J. (1983). "Child's Talk: Learning to Use Language." Norton, New York.

Caramazza, A., and Berndt, R. S. (1978). Semantic and syntactic processes in aphasia: A review of the literature. *Psychol. Bull.* **85,** 898–918.

Chapman, R. S. (1974). Discussion summary—Developmental relationship between receptive and expressive language. *In* "Language Perspectives—Acquisition, Retardation, and Intervention" (R. L. Schiefelbusch and L. L. Lloyd, eds.), pp. 335–344. University Park Press, Baltimore.

Chapman, R. S., and Miller, J. F. (1975). Word order in early two and three word utterances: Does production precede comprehension? *J. Speech Hear. Res.* **18,** 355–371.

Chomsky, C. (1969). "The Acquisition of Syntax in Children from 5 to 10." MIT Press, Cambridge, Massachusetts.

Chomsky, N. (1972) "Language and Mind" (enlarged edition). Harcourt Brace Jovanovich, New York.

Churchill, D. W. (1978). Language: The problem beyond conditioning. *In* "Autism" (M. Rutter and E. Schopler, eds.), pp. 71–84. Plenum, New York.

Curtiss, S. (1977). "Genie." Academic Press, New York.

D'Amato, M. R. (1973). Delayed matching and short-term memory in monkeys. *In* "The Psychology of Learning and Motivation: Advances in Research and Theory" (G. H. Bower, ed.), pp. 227–269. Academic Press, New York.

D'Amato, M. R., and Colombo, M. (1985). Auditory matching-to-sample in monkeys (*Cebus apella*). *Anim. Learn. Behav.* **13,** 375–382.

D'Amato, M. R., and Salmon, D. P. (1984). Processing and retention of complex auditory stimuli in monkeys (*Cebus apella*). *Can. J. Psychol.* **38,** 237–255.

de Villiers, J., and de Villiers, P. (1973). Development of the use of word order in comprehension. *J. Psycholing. Res.* **2,** 162–181.

Dulay, H., Burt, M., and Krashen, S. (1982). "Language Two." Oxford University Press, New York.

Essok, S., Gill, T., and Rumbaugh, D. M. (1977). Language relevant object- and color-naming by a chimpanzee. *In* "Language Learning by a Chimpanzee: The Lana Project" (D. M. Rumbaugh, ed.), pp. 193–206. Academic Press, New York.

Fodor, J. A., Bever, T. G., and Garrett, M. T. (1974). "The Psychology of Language." McGraw-Hill, New York.

Fouts, R. S. (1978). Sign language in chimpanzees: Implications of the visual mode and the comparative approach. *In* "Sign Language and Language Acquisition in Man and Ape: New Dimensions in Comparative Pedolinguistics" (F. C. Peng, ed.), pp. 121–136. Westview, Boulder, Colorado.

Fouts, R. S., Chown, B., and Goodin, L. (1976a). Transfer of signed responses in American Sign Language from vocal English stimuli to physical object stimuli by a chimpanzee (*Pan*). *Learning & Motivation* **7,** 458–475.

Fouts, R. S., Chown, W., Kimball, G., and Couch, J. (1976b). *Comprehension and production of American Sign Language by a chimpanzee (Pan).* Paper presented at the XXI International Congress of Psychology, Paris.

Fouts, R., Shapiro, G., and O'Neill, C. (1978). Studies of linguistic behavior in apes and children. *In* "Understanding Language through Sign Language Research" (P. Siple, ed.), pp. 163–183. Academic Press, New York.

Fraser, C., Bellugi, U., and Brown, R. W. (1963). Control of grammar in imitation, comprehension and production. *J. Verb. Learn. Verb. Behav.* **2,** 121–135.

Gardner, B. T., and Gardner, R. A. (1971). Two-way communication with an infant chimpanzee. *In*

"Behavior of Nonhuman Primates" (A. M. Schrier and F. Stollnitz, eds.), pp. 117–184. Academic Press, New York.

Gardner, B. T., and Gardner, R. A. (1975). Evidence for sentence constituents in the early utterances of child and chimpanzee. *J. Exp. Psychol.: Gen.* **104**, 244–267.

Gardner, B. T., and Gardner, R. A. (1979). Two comparative psychologists look at language acquisition. *In* "Children's Language," (K. E. Nelson, ed.), Vol. 2, pp. 309–369. Halsted, New York.

Gardner, R. A., and Gardner, B. T. (1969) Teaching sign language to a chimpanzee. *Science* **165**, 664–762.

Gardner, R. A., and Gardner, B. T. (1978). Comparative psychology and language acquisition. *Ann. N. Y. Acad. Sci.* **309**, 37–76.

Gardner, R. A., and Gardner, B. T. (1984). A vocabulary test for chimpanzees (*Pan troglodytes*). *J. Comp. Psychol.* **98**, 381–404.

Gould, J. L. (1976). The dance–language controversy. *Q. Rev. Biol.* **51**, 211–244.

Hearst, E. (1984). Absence as information: Some implications for learning, performance, and representational processes. *In* "Animal Cognition" (H. L. Roitblat, T. G. Bever, and H. S. Terrace, eds.), pp. 311–328. Erlbaum, Hillsdale, New Jersey.

Herman, L. M. (1980). Cognitive characteristics of dolphins. *In* "Cetacean Behavior: Mechanisms and Functions" (L. M. Herman, ed.), pp. 363–429. Wiley, New York.

Herman, L. M. (1986). Cognition and language competencies of bottlenosed dolphins. *In* "Dolphin Cognition and Behavior: A Comparative Approach" (R. Schusterman, J. Thomas, and F. Wood, eds.), pp. 221–252. Erlbaum, Hillsdale, New Jersey.

Herman, L. M., and Forestell, P. H. (1985). Reporting on the presence or absence of named objects by a language-trained dolphin. *Neurosci. Biobehav. Rev.* **9**, 667–681.

Herman, L. M., Wolz, J. P., and Richards, D. G. (1983). Processing of anomalous sentences by bottlenosed dolphins. Unpublished manuscript, University of Hawaii, Kewalo Basin Marine Mammal Laboratory, Honolulu.

Herman, L. M., Richards, D. G., and Wolz, J. P. (1984). Comprehension of sentences by bottlenosed dolphins. *Cognition* **16**, 129–219.

Hockett, C. F. (1960). Logical considerations in the study of animal communication. *In* "Animal Sounds and Communication" (W. E. Lanyon and W. N. Tavolga, eds.), pp. 392–430. American Institute of Biological Sciences, Pub. No. 7, Washington, DC.

Horgan, D. (1980). The importance of word order. *In* "New Approaches to Language Acquisition" (B. Kettemann and R. N. St. Clair, eds.), pp. 125–147. Narr, Tubingen.

Hovancik, J. R., Herman, L. M., Forestell, P. H., Gory, J. D., and Bradshaw, G. L. (1985). Processing of visual information by the bottlenosed dolphin. *In* Vision and learning. L. M. Herman, chair. Symposium conducted at the Sixth Biennial Conference on the Biology of Marine Mammals, Vancouver.

Ingram, D. (1974). The relationship between comprehension and production. *In* "Language Perspectives—Acquisition, Retardation, and Intervention" (R. L. Schiefelbusch and L. L. Lloyd, eds.), pp. 313–334. University Park Press, Baltimore.

Itard, J. M. G. (1932). "The Wild Boy of Aveyron" (translated by G. Humphrey and M. Humphrey). Century, New York.

Jerison, H. J. (1973). "Evolution of the Brain and Intelligence." Academic Press, New York.

Lambert, W. E., and Tucker, G. R. (1972). "Bilingual Education of Children: The St. Lambert Experiment." Newbury House, Rowley, Massachusetts.

Lieberman, P. (1985). "The Biology and Evolution of Language." Harvard Univ. Press, Cambridge, Massachusetts.

Miles, H. L. (1983). Apes and language: The search for communicative competence. *In* "Language in Primates" (J. deLuce and H. T. Wilder, eds.), pp. 43–61. Springer-Verlag, New York.

Muncer. S. J., and Ettlinger, G. (1981). Communication by a chimpanzee: First-trial mastery of word order that is critical for meaning, but failure to negate conjunctions. *Neuropsychologia* **19**, 73–78.

Murdock, B. B., Jr. (1962). The serial position effect of free recall. *J. Exp. Psychol.* **64**, 482–488.

Newman, J., Wolff, W. T., and Hearst, E. (1980). The feature-positive effect in adult human subjects. *J. Exp. Psychol.: Hum. Learn. Motiv.* **6**, 630–650.

Nottebohm, F. (1972). The origins of vocal learning. *Am. Nat.* **106**, 116–140.

Paivio, A., and Begg, I. (1981). "Psychology of Language." Prentice-Hall, Englewood Cliffs, New Jersey.

Patterson, F. G. (1978a). The gestures of a gorilla: Language acquisition in another pongid. *Brain Lang.* **5**, 72–97.

Patterson, F. G. (1978b). Linguistic capabilities of a young lowland gorilla. *In* "Sign Language and Language Acquisition in Man and Ape: New Dimensions in Comparative Pedolinguistics" (F. C. Peng, ed.), pp. 161–201. Westview, Boulder, Colorado.

Patterson, F., and Linden, E. (1981). "The Education of Koko." Holt, Rinehart and Winston, New York.

Pepperberg, I. M. (1981). Functional vocalizations by an African grey parrot (*Psittacus erithacus*). *Z. Tierpsychol.* **5**, 139–160.

Petitto, L. A., and Seidenberg, M. S. (1979). On the evidence for linguistic abilities in signing apes. *Brain Lang.* **8**, 162–183.

Premack, D. (1971). On the assessment of language competence in the chimpanzee. *In* "Behavior of Nonhuman Primates" (A. M. Schrier and F. Stollnitz, eds.), Vol. 4, pp. 186–228. Academic Press, New York.

Premack, D. (1976). "Intelligence in Ape and Man." Erlbaum, Hillsdale, New Jersey.

Premack, D. (1985). "Gavagai!" or the future history of the animal language controversy. *Cognition* **19**, 207–296.

Premack, D. (1986). " 'Gavagai!' or the Future History of the Animal Language Controversy." MIT Press, Cambridge, Massachusetts.

Premack, D., and Premack. A. J. (1983). "The Mind of an Ape." Norton, New York.

Rice, M. (1980). "Cognition to Language: Categories, Word Meanings, and Training." University Park Press, Baltimore.

Richards, D. G. (1986). Dolphin vocal mimicry and vocal object labeling. *In* "Dolphin Cognition and Behavior: A Comparative Approach" (R. Schusterman, J. Thomas, and F. Wood, eds.), pp. 273–288. Erlbaum, Hillsdale, New Jersey.

Richards, D. G., Wolz, J. P., and Herman, L. M. (1984). Mimicry of computer-generated sounds and vocal labeling of objects by a bottlenosed dolphin. *J. Comp. Psychol.* **98**, 10–28.

Ridgway, S. H., Carder, D. A., and Jeffries, M. M. (1985). Another "talking" male white whale. *In* "Proceedings of the Sixth Biennial Conference on the Biology of Marine Mammals." Vancouver (Abstract).

Ristau, C. A., and Robbins, D. (1982). Language in the great apes: A critical review. *In* "Advances in the Study of Behavior" (J. F. Rosenblatt, R. B. Hinde, C. Beer, and M-C. Busnel, eds.), Vol. 12, pp. 141–255. Academic Press, New York.

Roitblat, H. L. (1986). "Introduction to Comparative Cognition." Freeman, New York.

Rumbaugh, D. M. (ed.) (1977). "Language Learning by a Chimpanzee: The Lana Project." Academic Press, New York.

St. Clair, R. N. (1980). The parameters of second-language acquisition. *In* "New Approaches to Language Acquisition" (B. Ketteman and R. N. St. Clair, eds.), pp. 13–31. Narr, Tubingen.

Savage-Rumbaugh, E. S. (1981). Can apes use symbols to represent their world? *In* "The Clever Hans Phenomenon: Communication with Horses, Whales, Apes, and People" (Annals of the New York Academy of Sciences Vol. 364) (T. A. Sebeok and R. Rosenthal, eds.), pp. 35–59. New York Academy of Sciences, New York.

Savage-Rumbaugh, E. S. (1984a). Acquisition of functional symbol usage in apes and children. *In* "Animal Cognition" (H. L. Roitblat, T. G. Bever, and H. S. Terrace, eds.), pp. 291–310. Erlbaum, Hillsdale, New Jersey.

Savage-Rumbaugh, E. S. (1984b). *Pan paniscus* and *Pan troglodytes:* Contrasts in preverbal communicative competence. *In* "The Pygmy Chimpanzee" (R. L. Susman, ed.), pp. 395–413. Plenum, New York.

Savage-Rumbaugh, E. S., and Rumbaugh, D. M. (1978). Symbolization, language and chimpanzees: A theoretical reevaluation based on initial language acquisition processes in four young *Pan troglodytes. Brain Lang.* **6,** 265–300.

Savage-Rumbaugh, E. S., Rumbaugh, D. M., and Boysen, S. (1980a). Do apes use language? *Am. Sci.* **68,** 49–61.

Savage-Rumbaugh, E. S., Rumbaugh, D. M., Smith, S. T., and Lawson, J. (1980b). Reference— The linguistic essential. *Science* **210,** 922–925.

Savage-Rumbaugh, E. S., Pate, J. L., Lawson, J., Smith, S. T., and Rosenbaum, S. (1983). Can a chimpanzee make a statement? *J. Exp. Psychol.: Gen.* **112,** 457–492.

Savage-Rumbaugh, E. S., Rumbaugh, D. M., and McDonald, K. (1985). Language learning in two species of apes. *Neurosci. Biobehav. Rev.* **9,** 653–665.

Schiefelbusch, R. L. (1974). Summary. *In* "Language Perspectives—Acquisition, Retardation, and Intervention" (R. L. Schiefelbusch and L. L. Lloyd, eds.), pp. 647–660. University Park Press, Baltimore.

Schusterman, R. J. (1968). Experimental laboratory studies of pinniped behavior. *In* "The Behavior and Physiology of Pinnipeds" (R. J. Harrison, R. C. Hubbard, R. S. Peterson, C. E. Rice, and R. J. Schusterman, eds.), pp. 87–167. Appleton-Century-Crofts, New York.

Schusterman, R. J. (1981). Behavioral capabilities of seals and sea lions: A review of their hearing, visual, learning and diving skills. *Psychol. Rec.* **31,** 125–143.

Schusterman, R. J. (1984). *California sea lions comprehend novel symbol combinations.* Invited paper presented to a symposium on the "Cognitive behavior of marine animals" at the Second International Conference of the International Society for Comparative Psychology, Acapulco.

Schusterman, R., and Krieger, K. (1984). California sea lions are capable of semantic comprehension. *Psychol. Rec.* **34,** 3–23.

Seeley, T. (1977). Measurement of nest cavity volume by the honey bee (*Apis mellifera*). *Behav. Ecol. Sociobiol.* **2,** 201–227.

Seidenberg, M. S., and Petitto, L. A. (1979). Signing behavior in apes: A critical review. *Cognition* **7,** 177–215.

Seidenberg, M. S., and Petitto, L. A. (1981). Ape signing: Problems of method and interpretation. *In* "The Clever Hans Phenomenon: Communication with Horses, Whales, Apes, and People" (Annals of the New York Academy of Sciences Vol. 364) (T. A. Sebeok and R. Rosenthal, eds.), pp. 35–59. New York Academy of Sciences, New York.

Seyfarth, R. M., and Cheney, D. L. (1980). The ontogeny of vervet alarm calling behavior: A preliminary report. *Z. Tierpsychol.* **54,** 37–56.

Seyfarth, R. M., Cheney, D. L., and Marler, P. (1980). Vervet monkey alarm calls: Semantic communication in a free-ranging primate. *Anim. Behav.* **28,** 1070–1094.

Shipley, E. F., Smith, C. S., and Gleitman, L. R. (1969). A study in the acquisition of language: Free responses to commands. *Language* **45,** 322–342.

Straub, R. O., Seidenberg, M. S., Bever, T. G., and Terrace, H. S. (1979). Serial learning in the pigeon. *J. Exp. Anal. Behav.* **32,** 137–148.

Strohner, H., and Nelson, K. E. (1974). The young child's development of sentence comprehension: Influence of event probability, nonverbal context, syntactic form, and strategies. *Child Dev.* **45,** 567–576.

Terrace, H. S. (1979a). Is problem solving language? *J. Exp. Anal. Behav.* **31,** 161–175.

Terrace, H. S. (1979b). "Nim." Knopf, New York.

Terrace, H. S. (1984a). "Language" in apes. *In* "The Meaning of Primate Signals" (R. Harre and V. Reynolds, eds.), pp. 179–207. Cambridge University Press, Cambridge.

Terrace, H. S. (1984b). Animal cognition. *In* "Animal Cognition" (H. L. Roitblat, T. G. Bever, and H. S. Terrace, eds.), pp. 7–28. Erlbaum, Hillsdale, New Jersey.

Terrace, H. S. (1985). In the beginning was the "Name." *Am. Psychol.* **40,** 1011–1028.

Terrace, H. S., Petitto, L. A., Sanders, R. J., and Bever, T. G. (1979). Can an ape create a sentence? *Science* **200,** 891–902.

Terrace, H. S., Petitto, L. A., Sanders, R. J., and Bever, T. G. (1981). Ape language—Letter to *Science. Science* **211,** 87–88.

Terrace, H. S., Petitto, L. A., Sanders, R. J., and Bever, T. G. (1985). On the grammatical capacity of apes. *In* "Children's Language" (K. Nelson, ed.), Vol. 2, pp. 371–495. Gardner Press, New York.

Thompson, R. K. R., and Herman, L. M. (1977). Memory for lists of sounds by the bottlenosed dolphin: Convergence of memory processes with humans? *Science* **195,** 501–503.

Tyack, P. (1986). Whistle repertoires of two bottlenosed dolphins, *Tursiops truncatus:* Mimicry of signature whistles? *Behav. Ecol. Sociobiol.* **18,** 251–257.

von Frisch, K. (1967). "The Dance Language and Orientation of Bees." Harvard University Press, Cambridge, Massachusetts.

Wetstone, H. S., and Friedlander, B. Z. (1973). The effect of word order on young children's responses to simple questions and commands. *Child Devel.* **44,** 734–740.

Woodruff, G., and Premack, D. (1979). Intentional communication in the chimpanzee: The development of deception. *Cognition* **7,** 333–362.

Wright, A. A., Santiago, H. C., Sands, S. F., and Urcuioli, P. J. (1984). Pigeon and monkey serial probe recognition: Acquisition, strategies, and serial position effects. *In* "Animal Cognition" (H. L. Roitblat, T. G. Bever, and H. S. Terrace, eds.), pp. 353–388. Erlbaum, Hillsdale, New Jersey.

Self-Generated Experience and the Development of Lateralized Neurobehavioral Organization in Infants

George F. Michel

DEVELOPMENTAL PSYCHOBIOLOGY UNIT
DEPARTMENT OF PSYCHIATRIC RESEARCH
CHILDREN'S HOSPITAL MEDICAL CENTER
BOSTON, MASSACHUSETTS 02115

I. Introduction

The ability to use visual information to coordinate and regulate the adaptive movement patterns of the hands (eye–hand coordination) is a type of fine motor control which seems to undergo distinct changes of form during infancy (Bower, 1982). Because various aspects of this skill appear at different ages for different types of manual actions, eye–hand coordination plays an integral part in all measures of the sensorimotor development of the infant (Bruner, 1971; Uzgiris and Hunt, 1975). In general, eye–hand coordination seems to require a capacity of the nervous system to detect and process visual information, relate it to an internal body-centered spatial map, and translate that result into a well-executed motor pattern (Hein, 1980; Paillard, 1980). Therefore, identifying the mechanisms underlying the changes in eye–hand coordination during infancy involves the examination of a broad range of neural processes. However, despite the attention of many researchers, there is no unequivocal account either of the course of the development of eye–hand coordination or of the processes involved in its organization (Hay, 1984).

Although some of the neuromotor processes underlying eye–hand coordination may be present at birth (Mounoud, 1982; Trevarthen, 1982), it is generally believed that they are enhanced, refined, improved, and altered through visuomotor experience generated by the infant's use of the eyes and hands together in a variety of situations (Bullinger, 1983; Bushnell, 1985; Hein, 1974). Thus, visuomotor experience is one process involved in the development of eye–hand coordination. Unfortunately, few have identified which specific aspects of coordination are affected by visuomotor experience or which types of experience are effective (cf. White, 1970). So far, only rather extreme modes of deprivation (Bauer and Held, 1975) and rather gross forms of experiential enrichment

(White, 1970) have been shown to affect eye–hand coordination. Neither of these techniques can adequately assess the contribution of naturally occurring experience to the development of eye–hand coordination.

The preferred use of one hand for unimanual activities and the occurrence of consistent differences in performance between the hands during bimanual activities are common aspects of eye–hand coordination that may allow assessment of the effects of experience on the development of infant motor coordination. Infants show lateralized differences in motor coordination, but the lateralization is right biased in some individuals and left biased in others. Therefore, hypotheses about the role of experience in the development of one form of lateralization may be tested by specific predictions about the development of the other form of lateralization. For example, the hypothesis that neonatal head orientation preferences play a role in the development of infant right hand use preference was tested by specific predictions about infants with left hand use preferences (Michel, 1981, 1982, see below). Thus, systematic examination of the development of hand-use preferences in motor coordination, because of naturally occurring group differences in which hand is preferred, allows a form of hypothesis testing not generally available to the study of infant sensorimotor development.

In addition, skill differences between the hands are distinct and easily described during infancy and resemble the sort of improvement, enhancement, and alteration of neuromotor processes that might be expected to depend on visuomotor experience. Indeed, many have argued that preference in hand use results entirely from cultural proscription and training during childhood (Hildreth, 1949). However, an alternative argument may be proposed that it is not explicit training but the visuomotor experiences gained through using the eyes and hands together in a variety of situations that affects the development of infant eye–hand coordination. It is of interest to know, then, whether there are naturally occurring lateral biases in visuomotor experiences gained in the development of eye–hand coordination during infancy that could contribute to the development of skill differences between the hands (Michel, 1983). Cultural pressure and training during childhood may only accentuate a characteristic already present in the individual (Annett, 1978). Thus, one question that has guided my research program is whether self-generated experience during infancy contributes toward the development of lateralized neurobehavioral organization.

II. Some Biological Characteristics of Human Handedness

A. Handedness, Hemispheric Specialization, and the Right Bias

In adults, handedness does not merely indicate a lateralized asymmetry in eye–hand coordination. Rather, handedness contributes, as a major interactive variable, to the assessment of hemispheric specialization for speech (Annett, 1975) and to the prognosis for recovery of function after brain damage (Hecaen *et al.*, 1981). Indeed, handedness itself represents a form of hemispheric specialization of function (Beaumont, 1974; Kinsbourne and Hiscock, 1977). Patterns of handedness are related also to cognitive style (Mebert and Michel, 1980; Newland, 1984; Peterson, 1979), specific learning disabilities (Geschwind and Behan, 1982; Nichols and Chen, 1981), and certain developmental psychopathologies (Barry and James, 1978; Colby and Parkison, 1977). Therefore, if naturally occurring experience during infancy contributes to the development of the neuromotor process(es) underlying handedness, then an experiential factor will have been identified that is relevant for both theoretical accounts of brain–behavior relations and their clinical application.

Handedness, or limb use preference, is a general characteristic of mammals, especially those that use their forelimbs in ways other than in locomotion (Walker, 1980). However, humans are distinct in manifesting an uneven distribution of handedness in the population. Some 90% of adults in all cultures are righthanded (Hicks and Kinsbourne, 1978). In a survey of over 5000 years of art works representing unimanual tool use, Coren and Porac (1977) found that right-handedness predominated irrespective of century or geographic location. There is even evidence of right-handed tool manufacture and use for several fossil hominids (Spuhler, 1977; Steklis and Harnad, 1976; Toth, 1985). Therefore, the evolution of the predominance of right-handddness is an event of great antiquity but restricted to the hominid lineage. Any explanation of the development of handedness must account for the right bias in its distribution.

Although much speculation has centered on the question of why right-handedness prevails (Harris, 1980), the more fundamental question of why there is any bias at all in handedness distribution has been ignored. What is the advantage to the individual if his or her handedness is the same as that of the majority of people? Since the right bias in handedness distribution seems to be an ancient characteristic of the hominid lineage (Spennemann, 1984; Toth, 1985), it is likely that the bias in handedness arose from the same selection pressures by which humans evolved. Therefore, handedness should be associated with traits that are specifically human.

B.   ADAPTIVE VALUE OF CONCORDANCE IN HANDEDNESS

The manufacture and use of tools are traits strongly tied to the evolution of humans (Oakley, 1972). Tool working requires manual skill and, since handedness is a common feature of primates that affects manual skill, handedness may have been an important factor in the evolution of tool-working abilities (Falk, 1980; Frost, 1980; Toth, 1985). Toolmaking traditions are evident early in hominid evolution and imply the social transmission of manual skills. It is very likely that this early social transmission of skill traditions relied primarily on observational learning with little verbal mediation (Falk, 1980; Frost, 1980; Lieberman, 1975). Therefore, any characteristic that facilitated the nonverbal transmission of manual skills would be of some selective advantage to both observer and demonstrator. Since handedness affects manual skill, it is conceivable that concordance of handedness between observer and demonstrator, if it facilitated the learning of manual skills, could have been a selection pressure for the evolution of the bias in handedness distribution (Bradshaw and Nettleton, 1982).

In a study by Michel and Harkins (1985), left- and right-handed students were shown how to tie three different knots by either left- or right-handed teachers. Observational learning was significantly faster if student and teacher were both right-handed or both left-handed than if their handedness was discordant (Fig. 1). Therefore, the facilitation of manual-skill learning provided by concordance of handedness could have contributed to a selection pressure favoring a population bias in human handedness (see Bradshaw and Nettleton, 1982). A selection pressure against discordance of handedness would mean that any bias in the distribution of a lateral asymmetry during infancy could become the developmental precursor favoring the establishment of the bias in handedness distribu-

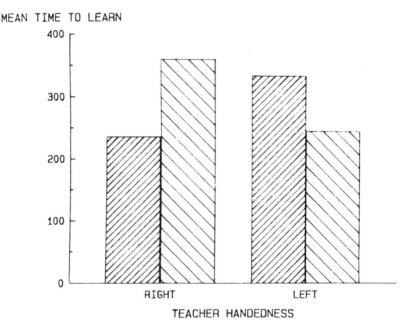

FIG. 1. The effect of the relation between handedness of demonstrator (teacher) and handedness of observer (student) on the mean amount of observation time (in seconds) required to learn how to tie one kind of knot. Narrow hatch, right-handed students; wide hatch, left-handed students. (Adapted with permission from Michel and Harkins, 1985.)

tion. If infant lateral asymmetries were biased toward the right side, then this might account for the right-handed bias in handedness distribution.

The advantage provided by the concordance in handedness raises the issue of why any individuals are discordant. Some have argued that all left-handedness results from pathological conditions (Bakan, 1971; Satz, 1972), but this is very unlikely for most left-handers (Hardyck and Petrinovich, 1977). Nevertheless, the maintenance in a population of different behavioral types (polyethism), like the maintenance of polymorphism, may mean that the minority type has associated characteristics that are relatively more advantageous than those associated with the majority type, but only for selected aspects of the population's ecology. Therefore, left-handedness may be maintained in the human population because certain characteristics associated with left-handedness provide the individuals with specific strengths and abilities that allow them to function somewhat better than right-handers for certain adaptively significant endeavors, such as a greater proficiency for employing spatial-orientation skills (Mebert and Michel, 1980). This would account for the nonrandom increase in proportion of left-handers among those who pursue careers requiring the use of visuospatial skills (e.g., architecture, painting, sculpture; cf. Peterson, 1979).

C. Genetic Analyses of Handedness

Although there is a genetic association between parental and offspring handedness (Annett, 1978), only about 40% of the offspring of two left-handed parents are left-handed (Annett, 1974). Therefore, left-handedness does not seem to require a specific genetic influence. To account for the geneological data, Annett (1978) proposed a model, based on a single allele which when present in an individual biases handedness to the right. In the absence of the allele (as in the offspring of two left-handed parents), handedness distributes randomly. The slight right bias observed in the distribution of handedness among the offspring of left-handed parents is thought to represent a relatively mild influence of cultural pressure. Of course, the allele proposed in Annett's model need not affect handedness directly: it might affect conditions, early in development, that induce a right bias in the development of eye–hand coordination.

McManus (1984) has criticized Annett's model for failing to distinguish between the "mode" or direction of lateralization in hand use (left versus right) and differences in degree of lateralization. According to Annett's model, as individuals exhibit less left-handedness (or right-handedness) in tasks, the more likely it is that they will be classified as right-handed (or left-handed). Rather than classifying individual handedness, Annett used measures of degree of lateralization to calculate heritability estimates and to examine the association of handedness among family members. By analyzing the familial association of handedness using distinct categories of left- and right-handedness, McManus

(1984) found a genetic influence in left-handedness. Therefore, McManus argued that any measure of handedness that represents the degree of lateralization "may represent either true individual differences or perhaps errors of measurement, and has no genetic component" whereas the mode of lateralization "is dichotomous, has a familial component, and hence is of genetic interest" (p. 128).

Of course, characters that exhibit continuous variation are often of genetic interest and can be examined by genetic analysis, but a dichotomous classification of handedness does make its family association more distinct. Therefore, there is some utility in classifying individual handedness rather than using some numerical representation of its degree. But by what criterion should a classification be made? Despite its obvious disadvantages, McManus (1984) chose writing hand (a criterion also sometimes chosen by Annett, 1972) as being the most valid criterion for classifying the handedness status of individuals. Unfortunately, this criterion is not useful for studying the handedness of infants. Therefore, most researchers have simply used the relative frequency of right and left hand use during the infant's play with objects to identify infant handedness status. In order to impose a distinct classification upon the continuum inherent in this mode of analysis, some researchers have used models of chance (usually Gaussian or binomial) to trichotomize the performance of the infants into right-handed, left-handed, and no-preference categories. By using a statistical model and conventional decision criteria for rejecting a null hypothesis, some infants would exhibit relative differences in hand use that would be considered random (no preference), whereas for other infants the differences between hands would be large enough that they would not be expected to occur by chance and would represent a preference in hand use (right or left).

III.   The Expression of Handedness during Infancy

A.   Reaching, Manipulation, and Complementary Bimanual Action

By whatever means handedness is classified, it is generally acknowledged that the initial establishment of the bias in handedness distribution must occur during infancy because even 2-year-old children show hand-use preferences with an adult-like right bias (Annett, 1972; Hildreth, 1949). However, it is generally believed that infant hand-use preferences are too variable and unstable to be related to, or predictive of, child or adult handedness status. This belief is based on studies of infant handedness that examined general differences between the use of the hands, irrespective of the demand characteristics of the tasks involved and the level of the infant's manual skill development (Michel, 1983). However, even adult handedness, when assessed by relative frequency of use across several tasks or by relative proficiency in performing a task, can appear to vary on repeated assessment depending on the individual's level of manual skill, the specific demands of the task(s), and the individual's previous experience with tasks having similar demand characteristics (Connolly and Elliott, 1972; Flowers, 1975; Provins and Cunliffe, 1972).

During infancy, specific manual skills appear at different ages and can exhibit different patterns of development. Therefore, in order to study hand-use preferences in infants, the preference must be assessed separately for each type of manual skill and then these separate assessments may be compared to provide a description of the infant's handedness status. These descriptions of infant handedness status may be presented within and across age groups to provide an account of the course of handedness development during infancy. Using this approach, we (Michel *et al.*, 1986) assessed the hand-use preferences of 96 infants (48 male), 6–13 months of age (12 in each month), in three different manual skills (reaching for objects, manipulating objects, and coordinating complementary bimanual actions).

Whether reaching for objects or manipulating them, the majority of infants showed a distinct preference for using one hand, and most preferred to use their right hand (Fig. 2). The infant's hand-use preference (right versus left) exhibited during reaching was significantly and strongly associated ($\chi^2 = 32.9$, $N = 96$, $p < 0.01$, contingency coefficient $= 0.6$) with the preference exhibited during manipulation. Fewer than 10% of the infants had opposite hand-use preferences

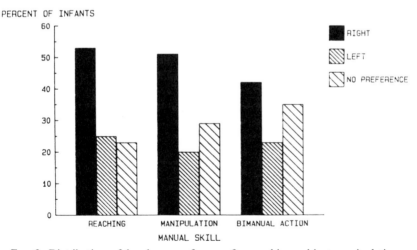

FIG. 2. Distribution of hand-use preference for reaching, object manipulation, and bimanual action of 96 infants, 6–13 months of age. (Reproduced with permission from Michel *et al.*, 1986.)

across these two measures. Infants with a right hand use preference for reaching predominated over those with a left preference at every age except 13 months (Fig. 3). For measures of object manipulation, every age had more right- than left-handed infants.

It is possible that at any age both hands may occasionally manipulate the same object. However, complementary bimanual manipulation (one hand supports the object as the other hand manipulates it) is not exhibited by all infants until 12 months, although it appears, infrequently, in a few infants 9 to 11 months of age. When this bimanual manipulation appears, most infants show a right hand use preference (Fig. 2). These observations confirm those of Ramsay *et al.* (1979).

Comparing the hand-use preference that the infants showed during reaching with that shown during bimanual manipulation demonstrates the importance of taking account of the level of the infant's sensorimotor skill relative to the task demands for assigning handedness status. In our sample, 75% of the 12-month infants were right-handed and 17% left-handed on measures of bimanual manipulation. No 12-month-old infant showed a reaching hand-use preference that was opposite to the preference showed during bimanual action. However, 56% of the 13-month infants showed preferences during reaching that were opposite to those they showed during bimanual manipulation. Such data could be used to support the notion that infant hand-use preferences for reaching are unstable across ages and tasks or that infant hand-use preferences fluctuate during development, as

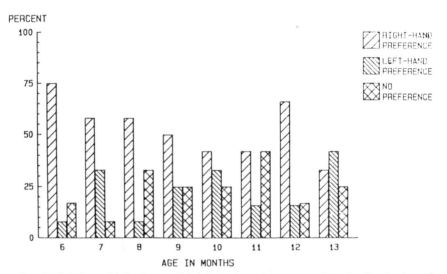

FIG. 3. Relation of infant's age (12 infants in each age group) to the distribution of hand-use preference for reaching. Note apparent left bias at 13 months. (Adapted with permission from data presented in Michel *et al.*, 1986.)

argued by Gesell and Ames (1950). There is, however, another way of interpreting these data.

Complementary bimanual manipulation of objects only becomes a common skill in the infant's repertoire during the infant's twelfth month. Once a sensorimotor skill is mastered, it can be incorporated into the network of other skills. A theoretical feature of such incorporation is that previously independent skills may influence one another's expression (Bruner, 1971; Piaget, 1952). Thus, reaching can be deployed for the purpose of bimanual manipulation. It is conceivable, then, that many of the reaches by 13-month infants involved the nonpreferred hand so that complementary bimanual manipulation could begin immediately without violating the infant's handedness status. If this account of infant handedness is correct. and it deserves further experimental examination, then it may be concluded that infants at all ages during the second half of the first year show a dextral bias in the distribution of handedness not unlike that present in children and adults.

In a separate study (Michel and Harkins, 1986), the consistency or stability of hand-use preferences during infancy was determined by assessing the reaching preferences of 20 infants at eight different times from 3 to 18 months postpartum. Of these infants, 90% maintained quite consistent hand-use preferences during this age span; 45% never changed their preference across the eight assessment visits and 45% had only one visit in which their hand-use preference appeared to be different from that of the other seven assessment visits. These results demonstrate that infant hand-use preferences are stable and, when combined with the results of the previous study, we can conclude that infants show the right bias in handedness distribution similar to that found in children and adults. Therefore, if experiential factors affect the initial development of infant hand-use preferences, they must operate early in infancy and they must be capable of inducing a right bias in the distribution of those preferences.

B. SELF-GENERATED EXPERIENCE AND INFANT HANDEDNESS DEVELOPMENT

Neonates adopt a limited number of different postures when supine, prone, seated, or carried (Casaer, 1979) which reflect, in part, a continuation of patterns of behavioral organization relevant to intrauterine conditions (Casaer, 1979; Michel and Goodwin, 1979; de Vries et al., 1982). These postures affect the neonate's interactions with objects (Bullinger, 1983; Michel, 1982) and caregivers (Ginsburg et al., 1979). One prevalent characteristic of neonatal postures is a preference to orient the head to one side (Fig. 4), usually the right (Gesell and Ames, 1950; Michel, 1981; Turkewitz et al., 1965). This neonatal head-orientation preference is expressed for about 8–10 weeks after birth and is associated with asymmetries of hand regard and movement of the arms (Coryell

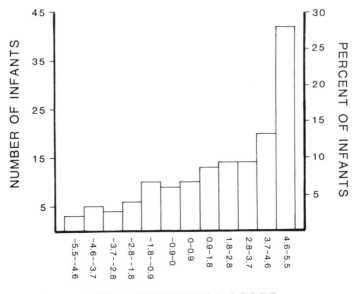

MEAN PREFERENCE SCORE

FIG. 4. Distribution of head orientation preference scores (mean of two assessments obtained between 16 and 48 hr after birth) of 150 neonates (see Michel, 1981 for details of the assessment procedure and scoring technique). Scores of 1.8 or larger and −1.8 or smaller represent significant rightward and leftward head orientation preferences, respectively. (Adapted with permission from Michel, 1981.)

and Michel, 1978; Michel and Harkins, 1986). It is conceivable, then, that differences in movement, proprioception, and visual experience of the hands, as induced by the neonate's asymmetrical postural preference, could contribute to the development of a lateral bias in eye–hand coordination. If so, then the rightward bias in the distribution of neonatal postural asymmetries could be the source of the right bias in the distribution of infant hand-use preferences.

The question of the relation between neonatal postural asymmetries and the development of hand-use preference was examined in a longitudinal study of 20 infants from birth to 18 months of age. Ten infants had a leftward neonatal head-orientation preference, and 10 had a rightward neonatal head-orientation preference. If neonatal head-orientation preference is a precursor of infant hand-use preference, then the lateral asymmetries of motor coordination and visuomotor experience should be quite different for these two groups of infants. Indeed, the difference between the groups in neonatal head-orientation preference was maintained through the first 2 months (Michel, 1981; Michel and Harkins, 1986; Fig. 5). During this 2-month period, those infants with a rightward head-orientation preference saw their right hand more than their left hand, and those infants with a

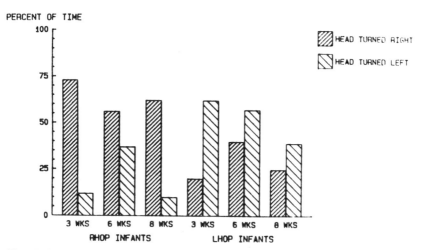

FIG. 5. Supine head orientation (mean percentage of time for 4-minute observation period) for three assessments conducted during the 2-month period after birth for infants with an initial neonatal preference to turn their heads rightward (RHOP, $n = 10$) or leftward (LHOP, $n = 10$). The total time that the head is oriented right is significantly longer than the time that the head is oriented left for the RHOP infants whereas the reverse is true for the LHOP infants. (Adapted with permission from data in Michel and Harkins, 1986.)

leftward head-orientation preference saw their left hand more [$F (1,16) = 71.2$, $p < 0.001$, Fig. 6]. Also, the face-side hand was the more frequently active hand for both groups [$F(1,16) = 71.2, p < 0.01$, Fig. 7]. The infant exhibits a head-orientation preference not only when supine but also when seated in an infant chair. When sitting, the infant's head orientation continues to affect arm and hand movements, especially if the infant's head orients to a visual object. Perhaps this is one source of the "proto-" or "prereaching" movements so often reported for neonates.

Infants with a leftward head-orientation preference during their first 2 months preferred to reach for objects with their left hand during the subsequent 12 to 74-week period (Fig. 8). Infants with a rightward head-orientation preference preferred to reach with their right hand. Therefore, the neonate's head-orientation preference predicts the infant's hand-use preference when reaching for objects [$F(1,16) = 13.8, p < 0.005$].

Since little bimanual manipulation or intermanual object transfer occurs for several months after reaching preferences first appear (Michel et al., 1986; Provine and Westerman, 1979; Ramsay et al., 1979), the preferred hand can obtain more objects and engage in more manipulation and oral and visual inspection of them than the nonpreferred hand. This difference in experience, in turn,

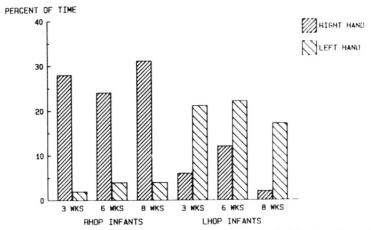

FIG. 6. Mean percentage time of 4-minute assessment period for visual regard of right and left hand while supine for RHOP and LHOP infants during the 2-month postnatal period. (Adapted with permission from data presented in Michel and Harkins, 1986.)

could promote skill differences in unimanual object manipulation and subsequently the adoption of different strategies of right- and left-hand performance during bimanual manipulation.

An allele that promotes conditions encouraging a rightward bias in infant head-orientation preferences could result in a dextral bias in handedness through a process of self-generated experience. That is, head orientation preference induces an asymmetry of limb movements and visual regard of the hands that

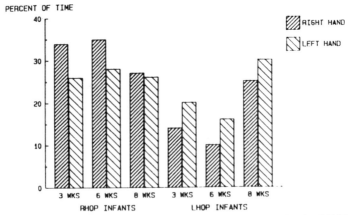

FIG. 7. Mean percentage time that right and left hands are active for RHOP and LHOP infants during the 2-month postnatal period. (Adapted with permission from data in Michel and Harkins, 1986.)

PREFERENCE SCORE

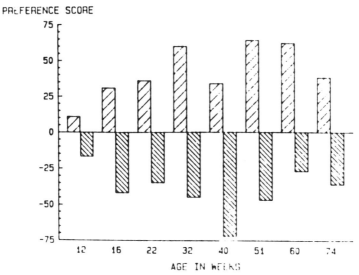

FIG. 8. Median hand-use preference scores for reaching during the 3- to 18-month postnatal period for infants who showed consistent preferences to turn their heads rightward (n = 8) or leftward (n = 7) when supine during the 2-month postnatal period. Positive score indicates right-hand preference; negative score indicates left-hand preference. ▨, Supine head right preference; ▧, supine head left preference. (Adapted with permission from Michel and Harkins, 1986.)

results in an asymmetry of eye–hand coordination skill between the hands. The lateral bias in skill leads to a hand-use preference in reaching which, in turn, expands, as a consequence of differential experience with objects, into additional lateral differences in eye–hand coordination and manual skill. A right bias in the distribution of neonatal head-orientation preferences would then be a conceivable source for the right bias in the distribution of hand-use preferences among infants. Although no step in this sequence is obligatory, it does show how the self-generated experiences created by normal spontaneous neonatal postures and movements can contribute to the formation of new patterns of neuromotor organization, with potentially long-term consequences for the neurological character of the individual.

Of course, it could be argued that the head-orientation preference and lateral asymmetry of hand movements are independent representations of the same underlying asymmetry of brain function (Kinsbourne and Hiscock, 1983). However, when the infant's head is centered in a midline position, there are no lateral differences in hand activity (Michel and Harkins, 1986). If lateral differences in hand activity, head orientation, and hand-use preference were independent representations of the same underlying asymmetry of neural functioning, then the midline orientation of the head should not have eliminated the lateral asymmetry of hand activity. The data suggest that the differential activity of the hands is induced by the infant's head-orientation preference. The evidence is consistent with the hypothesis that early head-orientation preference contributes to the development of infant handedness by inducing laterally asymmetric sensorimotor experiences which, in a majority of infants, will produce a right preference in hand use. An early leftward head-orientation preference in a minority of infants is associated with a left-hand bias in sensorimotor experience and a later left preference in hand use. Therefore, it is conceivable that self-generated sensorimotor experiences provided by the infant's head-orientation preference contribute to the development of handedness.

C. Infant Handedness and Development of Hemispheric Specialization

Infant hand-use preferences may have more subtle and extensive consequences for neural organization than simply as preparation for adult handedness. Evidence from callosectomized monkeys and humans shows that the corpus callosum is essential for interhemispheric (intermanual) transfer of certain types of tactile learning and haptic (manual) experience (Ebner and Myers, 1962; Geffen et al., 1985; Sperry et al., 1969). Measurement of cortical-evoked potentials to stimulation of a hand shows that an ipsilateral response (presumably dependent on a functional corpus callosum) does not appear before 7 months of age (Cernacek and Podivinsky, 1971), and it seems to take several years before the ipsilateral response has the characteristics of the adult (Salamy, 1978). If callosally mediated interhemispheric transfer was absent during infancy, certain forms of haptic experience would then be confined to one hemisphere.

Using a head-turn conditioning procedure, 35 infants (7–14 months) were tested to assess intermanual (interhemispheric) transfer of tactile discrimination learning (Michel et al., 1984). A pair of textured stimuli (rough vs smooth) was used. One texture (e.g., smooth), when placed in the infant's right hand, signaled that 5 sec later someone would appear to the infant's right side and play "peek-a-boo" for 5 sec. The other texture, when placed in the infant's right hand, would signal that 5 sec later someone would appear to the infant's left side and play peek-a-boo. The direction of the infant's initial "anticipatory" head turn during the pre-peek-a-boo interval was recorded to assess discrimination learning. When the infant learned the discrimination, intermanual transfer of the learning was assessed by presenting the stimuli to the untrained hand. Failure of intermanual transfer could indicate immature callosal functioning.

A criterion of directionally appropriate anticipatory head turning for four consecutive presentations of the stimuli signified that the infant had learned the discrimination. Only seven infants learned (ages 7, 9, 9, 11, 11, 12, 14 months). For these seven infants, an extinction phase immediately followed with four presentations of the stimuli to the infant's right hand without the occurrence of a peek-a-boo. If the infant's initial head turns were directionally appropriate for all four of these presentations (i.e., the infants showed no extinction), then intermanual transfer was assessed by presenting the stimuli, without peek-a-boos, four times to the untrained left hand. If head turning was directionally appropriate for these presentations (i.e., no extinction), then interhemispheric transfer was presumed to have occurred. If head turning was not directionally appropriate during these presentations, then the stimuli were presented without peek-a-boos twice to the right (trained) hand. If directionally appropriate head turning occurred during these last two presentations to the trained hand, then the previous inappropriate responding during testing of the untrained hand could be assumed to have resulted from a lack of intermanual (interhemispheric) transfer of the learning rather than from extinction of the response.

No infant showed intermanual transfer of the discrimination (Fig. 9). Indeed, they seemed completely ignorant about the task, showing neither directionally appropriate nor inappropriate head turning when the stimuli were placed in their untrained hand. Although preliminary, these results are consistent with the notion that infants do not transfer tactile–haptic experiences between their hemispheres during their first year.

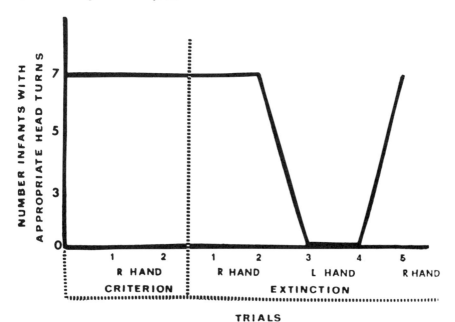

FIG. 9. Number of infants showing appropriate haptic–tactile discrimination learning (criterion trials 1, 2 and extinction trials 1, 2, 5) and intermanual transfer (extinction trials 3, 4) of the learned discrimination.

Since infants manifest hand-use preferences when playing with objects during this time, it is likely that one hemisphere receives tactile experience that is quite different from, and not shared with, the other. Under these conditions, it is quite possible for each hemisphere to establish separate manual sensorimotor skills, even when each hemisphere has access to visual information about the use of both hands (Trevarthen, 1978). Thus, the developmental elaboration of hemispheric specialization of function may depend, in part, on an early form of neural organization which restricts interhemispheric transfer of certain haptic and manual experience. This restriction combines with the infant's hand-use preference to insure that the infant's spontaneous, self-generated play with objects will provide each hemisphere with somewhat different capacities for programming and controlling sensorimotor skills.

D. INFANT HANDEDNESS AS
AN ONTOGENETIC ADAPTATION

Early phases in development are often not fully understood unless they are considered as adaptations to current situations as well as preparations for adult characteristics (Oppenheim, 1981, 1982; Prechtl, 1981). Therefore, the neuromotor organization represented in the infant's hand-use preference likely serves some immediate requirements of infancy. For adults, handedness not only improves efficiency in the performance of manual skills (Flowers, 1975; Tudor and Doane, 1977), but also reduces decision time for the initiation and execution of manual actions by removing the "choice-of-hand" step from the information processing (Flowers, 1975). For young infants, a preferred hand will be more skillful and successful in reaching for objects, obtaining them, and investigating their properties. Therefore, hand-use preference could play an important role in the organization of sensorimotor skills and problem solving strategies during infancy. Eight-month-old infants with distinct hand-use preferences are more advanced on tests of sensorimotor intelligence than infants without clear preferences (Cohen, 1966). However, this association could reflect maturation of neural functioning common to both sensorimotor intelligence and handedness.

During the second half of their first year, infants show bimanual coordination of arm movements in a number of activities from crawling to manipulating objects. In adults, coordinated use of the arms often involves the temporal and spatial linkage of their movement (Kelso et al., 1983). For example, when reaching bimanually to two targets, each at different distances, both hands contact the targets simultaneously because the timing of the movements of each hand is adjusted to match the other. If the task requires one hand to change the trajectory of its movement, the trajectory of the other hand changes, as well. Such linkage of movement is thought to allow the nervous system to more easily control the actions of several joints during complex movement patterns (Bernstein, 1967).

In a recent study, we (Goldfield and Michel, 1986b) showed that spatial and temporal linkage of the movements of the arms is present also in infants. By using a large, transparent, toy-filled box, bimanual reaching can be reliably elicited by 7 months of age, and it occurs with equal frequency throughout the remainder of the infant's first year. However, although both 7- and 11-month-old infants exhibit bimanual reaching, the spatial and temporal linkages of their arm movements are not the same.

The timing of the movements of one arm is more tightly linked to that of the other for 7- than for 11-month infants. Also, at 7 months, the hands tend to move together in isomorphic directions (i.e., if one hand moves to the left, the other also moves to the left). At 11 months, the hands tend to move in complementary directions (i.e., if one hand moves left, the other moves right). Thus, during bimanual reaching at 11 months, the hands seem to converge on the target, with greater independence in the timing of their movement. At 7 months, however, the hands seem to ''home'' on the target with little independence in the timing or direction of their movement. Thus, although both 7- and 11-month-old infants can reach bimanually, the spatio-temporal coordination of the movement of the hands is quite different at these two ages. Whether one hand is controlling the linkage of the hands at 7 months is not yet known.

The infant's handedness status does affect some aspects of coordination during bimanual reaching (Goldfield and Michel, 1986a), both when there is a low barrier (8 cm high) in the path of either hand and when there is no barrier. Without a barrier, one hand (the preferred hand) tends to lead during bimanual reaching only for those infants with a hand-use preference. The presence of the low barrier disrupted this pattern of bimanual reaching coordination in 7- and 8-month-old infants but not in 11-month infants. Also, the younger infants were more likely to hit the barrier when it was in the path of their nonpreferred hand than when it was in the path of their preferred hand. Thus, the specific character of the disruption of bimanual coordination produced by the barrier depended on the infant's age and handedness status. In younger infants (7–9 months), the barrier was more of a disturbance to coordination for infants with a hand-use preference than for infants with no hand-use preference. In older infants (10–12 months), the barrier disturbed coordination more for infants with no hand-use preference than for those with a preference. These results demonstrate that the formation of temporary linkages of joints in the coordination of bimanual reaching changes as a function of the infant's age and handedness status.

Thus, infant handedness, particularly in its different sensorimotor manifestations, can contribute to, as well as reflect, the organization of the neuromotor processes governing the coordination of movements. It is likely that further research will reveal many more instances in which the infant's handedness contributes to the adaptive organization of motor performance. Infant handedness not only serves as preparation for subsequent phases of development but also has behavioral consequences that are of immediate functional significance.

IV. Summary Remarks

Skill differences between the hands likely played an important role in the evolution of human tool-working abilities. Handedness would have affected performance during complementary bimanual manipulation of raw materials (required for manufacturing tools) and consistency of the use of the hands during practice (required for skillful tool use). As the social transmission of the manual skills employed in tool working took on greater significance in human evolution, so too would the influence of handedness on such transmission. If discordance of handedness between the teacher of the skill and the student disrupted the progress of learning and concordance facilitated learning, then the observational learning of manual skill could have been a selection pressure responsible for the evolution of the bias in the distribution of human handedness. Thus, both handedness and a right bias in handedness are significant parts of our human evolutionary heritage. The motor processes involved in their development are of substantial theoretical interest for this reason as well as because of the presumed relation of motor development with neurological and cognitive development. It is conceivable that evolutionary changes in the motor processes selected to support tool use and the social transmission of tool-working skills contributed to specifically human cognitive, intellectual, and social capacities.

The developmental sequence of lateralized motor processes in infancy reveals how handedness and the right bias in handedness may have developed. The rightward head-orientation bias in the posture of most neonates is the likely developmental precursor affecting the ''choice'' of the right hand for the bias in handedness. As the infant's head orientation induces lateral asymmetries of visuomotor experience of the hands, hand-use preferences will become apparent first during reaching and later during object manipulation. When infant hand-use preferences combine with relatively inefficient interhemispheric transmission of manual experience, the subsequent course of the development of hemispheric specialization of function can be affected. This is one means whereby handedness could come to affect the development of differences between the hemispheres in efficiency of motor programming and control (Freeman, 1984) as well as to reflect these differences.

The developmental sequence underlying handedness illustrates how particular patterns of motor coordination can emerge through self-generated processes and suggests how motor processes may contribute to other aspects of neuropsychological functioning. The motor aspects of hand use are particularly valuable in this regard because of individual differences in handedness and lateralized neural functioning. These individual differences allow different predictions to be made for left- and right-biased individuals and thus permit stronger tests of hypotheses about the development of hemispheric specialization of function than are usually possible with humans (Michel, 1983).

Infant hand-use preferences are not just expressions of current patterns of lateralization in the organization of the infant's neuromotor processes. Although more research is needed on the role of handedness in the development of the infant's ability to program and control motor performance, it is encouraging to find that handedness affects the infant's ability to coordinate common bimanual actions. Handedness also affects the infant's ability to develop subsequent manifestations of lateralized neurobehavioral organization. Although modern research is far from a full description of the specific neuromotor processes that regulate the developmental changes in the infant's ability to organize and coordinate motor performance, it is certain that such a description will refer to processes involved in the development of eye–hand coordination and hence, hand-use preferences. Thus, studies of the processes involved in the development of hand-use preferences will continue to be important in efforts to relate neuromotor processes to the development of other psychological capacities.

Because self-generated experience contributes to the development of infant hand-use preferences, any account of the processes governing the development of neuromotor organization, especially as it involves the upper limbs, must examine the role of experience. In the study of the development of new patterns of psychological organization in humans, too little attention has been given to the possibility that these new patterns arise from the experiences generated as a consequence of the behavior associated with earlier patterns. The study of the early development of handedness during infancy demonstrates that attending to the effects of self-generated experience on the development of the infant's motor repertoire may reveal more about the character of the infant's neuromotor processes and their relation to the development of other psychological characteristics than traditional approaches which focus on assessing reflexes and the age of achievement of certain motor "milestones."

Acknowledgments

The collection of some of the data presented in this article was supported by grants from the National Institute of Mental Health (1R03 MH35528 and 1R03 MH37749), the National Institute of Child Health and Human Development (5F 32 HD 05667), and the CLM/JLM Foundation.

References

Annett, M. (1972). The distribution of manual asymmetry. *Br. J. Psychol.* **63**, 343–358.
Annett, M. (1974). Handedness in children of two left-handed parents. *Br. J. Psychol.* **65**, 129–131.
Annett, M. (1975). Hand preference and laterality of cerebral speech. *Cortex* **11**, 305–328.
Annett, M. (1978). Genetic and nongenetic influences on handedness. *Behav. Genet.* **8**, 227–249.
Bakan, P. (1971). Birth order in handedness. *Nature (London)* **229**, 195.

Barry, R., and James, A. (1978). Handedness in autistics, retardates, and normals of a wide age range. *J. Autism Child. Schizophr.* **8,** 315–323.

Bauer, J. A., and Held, R. (1975). Comparison of visually-guided reaching in normal and deprived infant monkeys. *J. Exp. Psychol.: Animal Behavior Processes* **1,** 298–308.

Beaumont, J. (1974). Handedness and hemisphere function. *In* "Hemisphere Function in the Human Brain" (S. Dimond and J. Beaumont, eds.), pp. 89–120. Wiley, New York.

Bernstein, N. (1967). "The Coordination and Regulation of Movement." Pergamon Press, New York.

Bower, T. G. R. (1982). "Development in Infancy," 2nd Ed. Freeman, San Francisco.

Bradshaw, J. L., and Nettleton, N. C. (1982). Language lateralization to the dominant hemisphere: Tool use, gesture and language in hominid evolution. *Current Psychol. Rev.* **2,** 171–192.

Bruner, J. S. (1971). The growth and structure of skill. *In* "Motor Skills in Infancy" (K. J. Connolly, ed.), pp. 245–269. Academic Press, New York.

Bullinger, A. (1983). Space, the organism and objects, their cognitive elaboration in the infant. *In* "Spatially Oriented Behavior" (A. Hein and M. Jeannerod, eds.), pp. 215–222. Springer-Verlag, New York.

Bushnell, E. W. (1985). The decline of visually-guided reaching. *Infant Behav. Dev.* **8,** 139–155.

Casaer, P. (1979). "Postural Behavior in Newborn Infants." Clinics in Developmental Medicine (No. 72). Lippincott, Philadelphia.

Cernacek, J., and Podivinsky, F. (1971). Ontogenesis of handedness and somatosensory cortical response. *Neuropsychologia* **9,** 219–232.

Cohen, A. (1966). Hand preference and developmental status of infants. *J. Genet. Psychol.* **108,** 337–345.

Colby, K., and Parkison, C. (1977). Handedness in autistic children. *J. Autism Child. Schizophr.* **7,** 3–9.

Connolly, K., and Elliott, J. (1972). The evolution and ontogeny of hand function. *In* "Ethological Studies of Child Behaviour" (N. B. Jones, ed.), pp. 329–383. Cambridge University Press, Cambridge.

Coren, S., and Porac, C. (1977). Fifty centuries of right-handedness: The historical record. *Science* **198,** 631–632.

Coryell, J. F., and Michel, G. F. (1978). How supine postural preferences of infants can contribute toward the development of handedness. *Infant Behav. Dev.* **1,** 245–257.

de Vries, J. I. P., Visser, G. H. A., and Prechtl, H. F. R. (1982). The emergence of fetal behaviour. I. Qualitative aspects. *Early Hum. Dev.* **7,** 301–322.

Ebner, F. F., and Myers, R. E. (1962). Corpus callosum and the interhemispheric transmission of tactual learning. *J. Neurophysiol.* **25,** 380–391.

Falk, D. (1980). Language, handedness and primate brains: Did the Australopithecines sign? *Am. Anthropol.* **82,** 72–79.

Flowers, K. (1975). Handedness and controlled movement. *Br. J. Psychol.* **66,** 39–52.

Freeman, R. B., Jr. (1984). The apraxias, purposeful motor behavior, and left-hemisphere function. *In* "Cognitive and Motor Processes" (W. Prinz and A. F. Sanders, eds.), pp. 29–50. Springer-Verlag, New York.

Frost, G. T. (1980). Tool behavior and the origins of laterality. *J. Hum. Evol.* **9,** 447–459.

Geffen, G., Nilsson, J., Quinn, K., and Teng, E. L. (1985). The effect of lesions of the corpus callosum on finger localization. *Neuropsychologia* **23,** 497–514.

Geschwind, N., and Behan, P. (1982). Left-handedness: Association with immune disease, migraine, and developmental learning disorder. *Proc. Nat. Acad. Sci. U.S.A.* **79,** 5097–5100.

Gesell, A., and Ames, L. B. (1950). Tonic neck reflex and symmetrotonic behavior. *J. Genet. Psychol.* **70,** 155–175.

Ginsburg, H. J., Fling, S., Hope, M. L., Musgrove, D., and Andrews, C. (1979). Maternal holding preferences: A consequence of newborn head-turning response. *Child Dev.* **50,** 280–281.

Goldfield, E. C., and Michel, G. F. (1986a). Ontogeny of infant bimanual reaching during the first year. *Infant Behav. Dev.* **9,** 81–89.

Goldfield, E. C., and Michel, G. F. (1986b). Spatiotemporal linkage in infant interlimb coordination. *Dev. Psychobiol.* **18,** 97–102.

Hardyck, C., and Petrinovich, L. F. (1977). Left-handedness. *Psychol. Bull.* **84,** 385–404.

Harris, L. J. (1980). Left-handedness: Early theories, facts, and fancies. *In* "Neuropsychology of Left-Handedness" (J. Herron, ed.), pp. 3–78. Academic Press, New York.

Hay, L. (1984). Discontinuity in the development of motor control in children. *In* "Cognitive and Motor Processes" (W. Prinz and A. F. Sanders, eds.), pp. 351–360. Springer-Verlag, New York.

Hecaen, H., De Agostini, M., and Monzon-Montes, A. (1981). Cerebral organization in left-handers. *Brain Lang.* **12,** 261–284.

Hein, A. (1974). Prerequisite for development of visually guided reaching in the kitten. *Brain Res.* **71,** 259–263.

Hein, A. (1980). The development of visually guided behavior. *In* "Visual Coding and Adaptability" (C. S. Harris, ed.), pp. 51–68. Erlbaum, Hillsdale, NJ.

Hicks, R. E., and Kinsbourne, M. (1978). Human handedness. *In* "Asymmetrical Function of the Brain" (M. Kinsbourne, ed.), pp. 151–187. Cambridge University Press, Cambridge.

Hildreth, G. (1949). The development and training of hand dominance: I, II, III. *J. Genet. Psychol.* **75,** 197–275.

Kelso, J. A. S., Putnam, C. A., and Goodman, D. (1983). On the space–time structure of human interlimb coordination. *Quart. J. Exp. Psychol.* **35A,** 347–375.

Kinsbourne, M., and Hiscock, M. (1977). Does cerebral dominance develop? *In* "Language Development and Neurological Theory" (S. Segalowitz and F. Gruber, eds.), pp. 171–191. Academic Press, New York.

Kinsbourne, M., and Hiscock, M. (1983). The normal and deviant development of functional lateralization of the brain. *In* "Infancy and Developmental Psychobiology", Handbook of Child Psychology, vol. II (M. M. Haith and J. J. Campos, eds.), pp. 157–280. Wiley, New York.

Lieberman, P. (1975). "On the Origins of Language: An Introduction to the Evolution of Human Speech." Macmillan, New York.

McManus, I. C. (1984). Genetics of handedness in relation to language disorder. *In* "Advances in Neurology," Vol. 42, "Progress in Aphasiology" (F. C. Rose, ed.), pp. 125–138. Raven Press, New York.

Mebert, C. J., and Michel, G. F. (1980). Handedness in artists. *In* "Neuropsychology of Left-Handedness" (J. Herron, ed.), pp. 273–280. Academic Press, New York.

Michel, G. F. (1981). Right-handedness: A consequence of infant supine head-orientation preferences? *Science* **212** 685–687.

Michel, G. F. (1982). Ontogenetic precursors of infant handedness. *Infant Behav. Dev.* **5,** 156.

Michel, G. F. (1983). Development of hand-use preference during infancy. *In* "Manual Specialization and the Developing Brain" (G. Young, S. Segalowitz, C. Corter, and S. Trehub, eds.), pp. 33–70. Academic Press, New York.

Michel, G. F., and Goodwin, R. (1979). Intrauterine birth position predicts newborn supine head position preferences. *Infant Behav. Dev.* **2,** 29–38.

Michel, G. F., and Harkins, D. A. (1985). Concordance of handedness between teacher and student facilitates learning manual skills. *J. Human Evol.* **14,** 30–34.

Michel, G. F., and Harkins, D. A. (1986). Postural and lateral asymmetries in the ontogeny of handedness during infancy. *Dev. Psychobiol.* **18,** 85–96.

Michel, G. F., Ovrut, M. R., and Harkins, D. A. (1984). Intermanual transfer of tactile discrimination. *Infant Behav. Dev.* **7**, 247.

Michel, G. F., Ovrut, M. R., and Harkins, D. A. (1986). Hand-use preferences for reaching and object manipulation in 6–13 month-old infants. *Genetic, Social and General Psychology Monographs* 409–427.

Mounoud, P. (1982). Revolutionary periods in early development. *In* "Regressions in Mental Development" (T. B. Bever, ed.), pp. 119–132. Erlbaum, Hillsdale, New Jersey.

Newland, G. A. (1984). Left-handedness and field-independence. *Neuropsychologica* **22**, 617–619.

Nichols, P., and Chen, T. (1981). "Minimal Brain Dysfunction: A Prospective Study." Erlbaum, Hillsdale, New Jersey.

Oakley, K. P. (1972). Skill as a human possession. *In* "Perspectives on Human Evolution," Vol. 2 (S. L. Washburn and P. Dolhinow, eds.), pp. 14–50. Holt, Rinehart and Winston, New York.

Oppenheim, R. W. (1981). Ontogenetic adaptations and retrogressive processes in the development of the nervous system and behavior: A neuroembryological perspective. *In* "Maturation and Development: Biological and Psychological Perspectives" (K. J. Connolly and H. F. R. Prechtl, eds.), pp. 73–109. Lippincott, Philadelphia, Pennsylvania.

Oppenheim, R. W. (1982). The neuroembryological study of behavior: Progress, problems, perspectives. *In* "Current Topics in Developmental Biology, Vol. 17, Neural Development, Part III" (R. K. Hurt, ed.), pp. 257–309. Academic Press, New York.

Paillard, J. (1980). The multichanneling of visual cues and the organization of a visually guided response. *In* "Tutorials in Motor Behavior" (G. E. Stelmach and J. Requin, eds.), pp. 259–280. North-Holland, New York.

Peterson, J. M. (1979). Left-handedness: Differences between student artists and scientists. *Percept. Motor Skills* **48**, 961.

Piaget, J. (1952). "The Origins of Intelligence in Children." International Universities Press, New York.

Prechtl, H. F. R. (1981). The study of neural development as a perspective of clinical problems. *In* "Maturation and Development: Biological and Psychological Processes" (K. J. Connolly and H. F. R. Prechtl, eds.), pp. 198–215. Lippincott, Philadelphia, Pennsylvania.

Provine, R., and Westerman, J. (1979). Crossing the midline: Limits of early eye–hand behavior. *Child Dev.* **50**, 437–441.

Provins, K. A., and Cunliffe, P. (1972). The reliability of some motor performance tests of handedness. *Neuropsychologia* **10**, 199–206.

Ramsay, D. S., Campos, J. J., and Fenson, L. (1979). Onset of bimanual handedness in infants. *Infant Behav. Dev.* **2**, 69–76.

Salamy, A. (1978). Commissural transmission: Maturational changes in humans. *Science* **200**, 1409–1411.

Satz, P. (1972). Pathological left-handedness: An explanatory model. *Cortex* **8**, 121–135.

Spennemann, D. R. (1984). Handedness data on the European neolithic. *Neuropsychologica* **22**, 613–615.

Sperry, R. W., Gazzaniga, M. S., and Bogen, J. E. (1969). Interhemispheric relationships: The neocortical commissures; syndromes of hemisphere disconnection. *In* "Handbook of Clinical Neurology," Vol. 4 (P. J. Vinken and G. W. Bruyn, eds.), pp. 273–290. North Holland, New York.

Spuhler, J. N. (1977). Biology, speech, and language. *Annu. Rev. Anthropol.* **6**, 509–561.

Steklis, H. D., and Harnad, S. R. (1976). From hand to mouth: Some critical stages in the evolution of language. *Ann. N. Y. Acad. Sci.* **280**, 445–455.

Todor, J. L., and Doane, T. (1977). Handedness classification: Preference versus proficiency. *Percept. Motor Skills* **45**, 1041–1042.

Toth, N. (1985). Archeological evidence for preferential right-handedness in the lower and middle Pleistocene, and its possible implications. *J. Human Evol.* **14**, 35–40.

Trevarthen, C. (1978). Manipulative strategies of baboons and origins of cerebral asymmetry. *In* "Asymmetrical Function of the Brain" (M. Kinsbourne, ed.). Cambridge University Press, Cambridge.

Trevarthen, C. (1982). Basic patterns of psychogenetic change in infancy. *In* "Regressions in Mental Development" (T. G. Bever. ed.), pp. 7–46. Erlbaum, Hillsdale, New Jersey.

Turkewitz, G., Gordon, E. W., and Birch, H. G. (1965). Head turning in the human neonate: Spontaneous patterns. *J Genet. Psychol.* **107**, 143–158.

Uzgiris, I. C., and Hunt, J. McV. (1975). "Assessment in Infancy." University of Illinois Press, Chicago.

Walker, S. F. (1980). Lateralization of function in the vertebrate brain: A review. *Br. J. Psychol.* **71**, 329–367.

White, B. L. (1970). Experience and the development of motor mechanisms in infancy. *In* "Mechanisms of Motor Skill Development" (K. Connolly, ed.). Academic Press, New York.

Behavioral Ecology: Theory into Practice

Neil B. Metcalfe and Pat Monaghan

DEPARTMENT OF ZOOLOGY
UNIVERSITY OF GLASGOW
GLASGOW G12 8QQ, SCOTLAND

I. Introduction

The contributions of the science of animal behavior to the fields of animal welfare and husbandry are comparatively clear and well recognized, for example in the assessment of stress in captive animals and the design of housing systems (Monaghan, 1984). While the benefits of ethological studies to agriculture are becoming increasingly apparent (e.g., Broom, 1981; Wood-Gush, 1983) the application of ethological methods and principles in other fields of both practical and commercial value is not widely appreciated. It needs to be emphasized that applied ethology is not only concerned with farm animals. Moreover, there is now a considerable body of knowledge which could be put to practical use, but which remains relatively untapped at present. This is because advances and theoretical developments in the behavioral sciences since the mid 1970s, particularly in behavioral ecology, have not been wholly matched by an increase in the scope of applied ethology. For example, we now have a far greater understanding of the economics of decision making in animals in a wide variety of contexts, and the potential exists for the costs and benefits of particular acts to be altered in order to change the way in which an animal behaves; such manipulation of animal decision making, rather than force, could be used more extensively in managing the behavior of pests or commercially valuable species.

The aim of this article is to review the ways in which theoretical developments in behavioral ecology, such as optimization in foraging and reproductive strategies, are being, or could be, put to practical use. We have taken three aspects of behavior (foraging, spacing, and breeding) which often require control by man. Each has been broken down into its components (e.g., what animals eat, where they feed), and the factors which influence these are discussed with reference to current theories and their practical value. It is not our intention to provide a comprehensive review of the applications of these theories. Rather, we have chosen pertinent examples to illustrate how the theories and methods of behavioral ecology can help solve some of the problems we face in relation to animals in our service, those with which we compete for resources, and those whose populations we strive to conserve. Where we have not found relevant examples, we have tried to suggest ways in which current theories might be applied. In doing so, we hope to demonstrate that working in an applied context can be exciting and challenging, as well as useful.

II. CONTROL OF FORAGING

Much of behavioral ecology rests on the assumption that animals have been shaped by natural selection to maximize the net benefits resulting from particular behaviors, while recognizing the possibility that different individuals may achieve this end by different means. Optimization models provide a method of testing our understanding of the selection pressures involved. Such models have been widely used to predict how animals choose where and what to eat. The profitabilities of potential food types are calculated, taking into account parameters such as encounter rates, handling times, and calorific values; prey choice and movement between patches are then modeled on the basis of maximizing net intake rates. Such models are tested and refined using field and laboratory observations of foraging animals. Foraging models have been further developed to encompass situations where animals need to sample their environments in order to assess the quality of different food patches and prey types, and when animals will risk feeding in situations where returns are highly variable (Krebs *et al.* 1983). The ways in which animals allocate their time between foraging and other potentially conflicting activities (such as looking out for predators) can also be predicted on the basis of theoretical models (e.g., Caraco, 1979).

Competition with other animals for food or other resources is the basis of many of our conflicts with wild animal populations. Population reduction as a means of controlling species which have become pests is often tried, but rarely effective. In most cases, even if the necessary scale of culling could be condoned and is feasible, such measures are often too drastic and too expensive. An alternative is to try to control where and on what the animals feed. Such an approach can also be used where it is necessary to control food intake in order to maximize productivity in animal husbandry. In identifying the key parameters involved in these foraging decisions, optimal foraging models highlight potential factors which could be manipulated in order to change the ways in which animals behave.

A. WHAT ANIMALS EAT

Preventing animals from eating particular foods, either because these items are required for human consumption or because we wish to conserve them for other reasons, is one of the most common pest-control problems. It may be possible to make the foodstuff undesirable by altering its palatability or inducing an aversive conditioning through a poison avoidance response (Bourne, 1982; Burns, 1983; Horn, 1983). Such chemical treatments, particularly of crops, often tend to be of limited duration and effectiveness and may also have adverse effects on the product involved. Studies of the factors influencing prey choice in animals in the field, including both palatability and profitability, may increase our understanding of why they avoid particular foods and thereby lead to the development of more efficient and harmless treatments. An understanding of the factors which control diet choice is also essential to animal husbandry, since feed design and presentation can then be manipulated to fit requirements.

1. Palatability and Profitability

An approach to pest control based on the determinants of prey choice is being successfully developed by P. W. Greig-Smith and colleagues at the Ministry of Agriculture, Fisheries and Food in the United Kingdom in a broad program of research into the behavioral ecology of foraging in the bullfinch *Pyrrhula pyrrhula*. The aim of these studies is to develop methods of diverting these birds from eating the buds of fruit trees in commercial orchards, a habit which can result in serious economic losses to fruit growers. Identification of plant compounds which act as deterrents to herbivores is sometimes undertaken in an attempt to improve the efficacy of chemical spraying (Harborne, 1982). Greig-Smith has combined such work with studies on how the birds select food items and the factors which influence foraging rates, both in the field and in the laboratory.

It has been demonstrated that bullfinches prefer the buds of the pear cultivar Conference to the Comice variety and that this relates to differences in the flavor of the two as well as differences in their nutritional content. This preferential selection of Conference buds results in Comice trees suffering a uniform low level of damage irrespective of the level of bud loss suffered by neighboring Conference trees (Greig-Smith, 1985). These results suggest that the birds must sample both cultivars in order to establish their preference and thereafter avoid the Comice trees. If the birds were selecting buds only on the basis of nutritional content, changing the relative abundance of the two tree varieties in an orchard might be expected to even out the damage and thereby reduce fruit loss (see Section II,B,3). For this to work, the abundance of the preferred type would have to be lower than the level at which, according to optimal foraging theory, the birds should ignore the less-preferred type regardless of its abundance (MacArthur and Pianka, 1966). However, since palatability is also involved in seed selection, management based only on nutritional content is likely to have limited, if any, success.

Further work with bullfinches has demonstrated that, in addition to a study of food preferences, an analysis of the economics of foraging is also necessary in understanding the basis of diet choice. In a study of bullfinches foraging on ash trees, an investigation of the relationship between feeding preferences and the phenolic content of seeds was coupled with a study of how diet choice related to the nutritional value of the seed, seed size, and the behavioral costs of foraging (Greig-Smith and Wilson, 1985). Phenolic compounds in plants affect both the taste of the food and its digestability, and apparently act as deterrents (Rosenthal and Janzen, 1979). Behavioral parameters contributing to the attack rate on seeds were measured, including the time taken to find and handle seeds, the probabilities of failure to pluck seeds from the trees, and rejection and dropping rates, in relation to seed phenolic content. Seed-handling times did not increase with seed size, while seed preference was positively related to the fat content of seeds. It therefore paid the bullfinches to select bigger seeds, which contain more fat. Since bigger seeds also contain more phenols, the finches also appeared to have a preference for seeds with more phenol. However, for seeds of a constant fat content, the bullfinches' seed preference had in fact a negative relationship with phenolic content. Thus the bullfinches' tendency to feed in individual ash trees was increased by a high fat content in the seed and reduced by a high phenol content. These effects only became clear when the rates at which the bullfinches ingested these components were calculated. In this case the bullfinches appear to arrive at a trade off between nutrient content, the presence of aversive chemicals, and the behavioral costs of foraging. They prefer bigger seeds, which have more fat and more phenols than smaller seeds, but try to select big, fatty seeds with comparatively low phenol content. This work demonstrates that it is not sufficient simply to seek broad correlations between a measure of food preference and the concentration of a chemical, without taking into account other components which influence the profitability of feeding.

Problems with what animals eat are, of course, not always concerned with prevention. It may be necessary to monitor or control diet choice in order to maximize growth rates or productivity of commercial species, while keeping the financial costs of the feed within certain economic constraints. Special problems of this kind arise in the feeding of farmed fish, where the farmer aims to feed the fish in such a way that they will grow at the maximum rate, without undue waste of expensive fish food. This requires tailoring the size of the food particles to the body size of the fish. The use of optimal foraging theory can enable this to be done very precisely, as illustrated by a consideration of juvenile Atlantic salmon (*Salmo salar*) feeding behavior.

In their juvenile freshwater phase, salmon are essentially "sit and wait" predators, intercepting food particles as they are carried past in the drift of the stream. There are thus three stages in the foraging process—particle detection, travel to intercept the particle, and particle handling time. Visual acuity is important in the ability of salmon to locate food, and larger particles are detected at greater distances (Fig. 1A; Wankowski, 1979, 1981). Salmon parr eat prey items

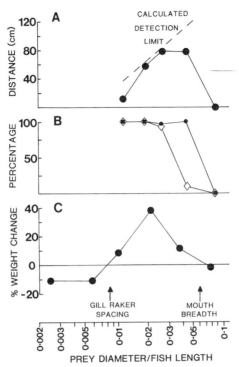

FIG. 1. Foraging behavior and growth of juvenile salmon in relation to food particle diameter (expressed as a proportion of fish length). (A) The maximum distance at which fish could detect particles (calculated from their visual activity), and the maximum distance (●) over which they were observed to move when striking at prey. (B) The percentages of passing prey that were captured (●) and ingested (◇). (C) The growth of fish reared for 20 days on diets of various particle sizes. Also indicated is the distance between the gill-rakers and the mean mouth breadth. (After Wankowski, 1979, 1981).

whole, and the range of particles which they could potentially eat is determined by the mouth breadth, which sets the upper limit, and the distance between the gill rakers, which sets the lower limit, since particles smaller than this are not retained in the mouth (Wankowski, 1979). Within this range of potential food sizes, optimal foraging theory predicts that salmon will only eat those particles for which the costs of obtaining the food do not outweigh the benefits of so doing. Thus fish tend to ignore particles which are unprofitable. Furthermore, since some particles are more profitable than others, the problem for the fish farmer is to ensure that the particle sizes made available to the fish are the most profitable; thus food intake rate, and thereby fish growth rate, will be maximized.

Work with other fish species (Werner, 1974) has shown that prey handling time increases exponentially as prey size nears the fish's mouth breadth. Handling time therefore remains low until prey size approaches that of the mouth breadth, whereupon it rises steeply (Fig. 2). To forage optimally, fish should reject the larger particles because of their high handling costs and ignore more distant small particles because of the disproportionate costs in travel time. The extent to which these less-profitable sizes should be included in the diet will vary with the abundance of different prey sizes.

Studies of feeding salmon have confirmed these predictions. They rarely intercept particles too large or too small to eat, and they will not travel long distances for small but detectable particles (Fig. 1A); particles close to, but less than, the mouth breadth are often rejected after interception (Fig. 1B), presumably on the basis of their potentially long handling time (Wankowski and Thorpe, 1979). While the travel time to these rejected particles represents a cost for which there is no compensatory benefit (since they are not eaten), this may occur because, at a distance, the salmon cannot discriminate finely within the small range of particle sizes over which handling time increases very rapidly (Fig. 2). It may also be a consequence of the "apparent size" problem, which can potentially cause misselection of prey due to near, small objects resembling farther, larger ones (O'Brien et al., 1976). The most profitable particle size for a given size class of fish (i.e., that which optimizes the trade off of detection distance and energetic content with handling time) can be accurately predicted to be in the region of 42% of the mouth breadth (Wankowski, 1979). Experimental work has demonstrated that fish fed on this size category of particle do indeed grow faster

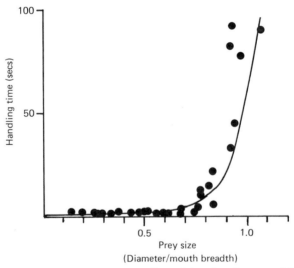

FIG. 2. Time (in seconds) taken by bluegill sunfish to handle prey of different diameters (expressed as proportions of mouth breadth). (After Werner, 1974.)

than those fed on slightly larger or smaller particles (Fig. 1C; Wankowski and Thorpe, 1979). Since mouth breadth increases allometrically with fish length, optimal particle size can thus be expressed as a constant percentage of fish length and thereby tailored to maximize growth rates. Furthermore, since the range of profitable prey is proportional to body size, in absolute terms large-size fish have a wider range of prey sizes close to the optimum than do small fish (Werner, 1974). This means that the fish farmer must be more rigorous in controlling the particle size fed to small fish, since slight variations in particle size will deviate farther from the optimum for small fish than for large.

2. Learning Effects

An alternative approach to manipulating what animals eat, often tried with species which are themselves protected but causing a local nuisance, is to try to lure the animals to feed on the same foods provided in special refuges and thereby reduce their competition with agriculture. Such refuges have been extensively developed for grazing geese and other wildfowl in North America and are increasing in Europe. However, apart from the problems encountered in getting the animals to concentrate in the refuge, such practices may hasten the trend for geese to switch from traditional food sources to agricultural crops (Owen, 1980). In other words, they learn that foraging on these crops is profitable and selectively search for abundant patches of them in other locations when the supply in the refuge becomes somewhat depleted or while on migration. Such an approach could have serious consequences with the brent goose (*Branta bernicla*) in Britain, for example, since the majority of these birds still feed on traditional mudflats where, although threatened by loss of habitat in some areas, they do not cause any problems.

3. The Costs of Finding the Food

Optimal foraging models have clearly identified search time as an important component of diet choice. Time spent in searching for a particular food has to be weighed against its nutritional value in comparison with other available foods, and studies which examine only the profitability of foods, without taking into account their availability, can be misleading. Search time (and therefore rates of consumption) will be influenced by the spacing of potential foods as well as their vulnerability. For example, feral dogs (*Canis familiaris*) are becoming increasingly serious predators of marine iguanas (*Amblyrhyncus cristatus*) on the Galapagos Islands. These dogs prey preferentially on large adult males. However, studies by Kruuk and Snell (1981) demonstrated that this is not in fact a preference by the dogs for larger and more profitable prey. Rather, it comes about because these adult males, in defending their territories, have shorter reaction distances and sleep in more exposed places than does the rest of the iguana population. The dogs are simply taking the most vulnerable prey. Similarly, selective predation by blue tits (*Parus caeruleus*) on female rather than male codling moth larvae (*Cydia pomonella*) was found not to be related to larval size, but to the increased vulnerability of female larvae to predation. Having a larger head capsule than males, the females have more difficulty in becoming completely concealed in crevices in trees (Glen *et al.*, 1981). Such selective predation is important in the control of codling moths which are significant pests of fruit trees in commercial orchards in Britain. Where tits are present, only 35% of larvae which survive the overwinter tit predation are female, whereas in the absence of tits the sex ratio of surviving moths is equal. The decision on whether to apply insecticide to an orchard is taken on the basis of the number of male moths caught in pheromone traps, which is presumed to be representative of the number of females present and therefore the likely larval production. However, where overwinter predation by tits has occurred, a higher catch of males can be tolerated before spraying need be undertaken, since the sex ratio is biased in favor of males (Glen *et al.*, 1981).

Controlling diet choice in species kept in natural or seminatural conditions, where a range of prey species is available, is potentially more difficult, since food availability is less easily manipulated. This is generally the case with fish stocks kept in ponds and lakes, where the fish feed on naturally occurring prey. In this situation, consideration needs to be given to the structural complexity of the habitat, since the presence of refuges for the prey reduces their vulnerability, thus increasing the predator's search time. Though prey abundance may be high, availability is low. Optimality models of diet breadth predict that when search time for the preferred prey increases, the predator should widen its diet breadth (Stein, 1977; Cooper and Crowder, 1979), which will result in growth rates falling below the previous optimal level. On the other hand, if the habitat has no structural complexity, prey vulnerability will be so high that populations of the optimal prey will quickly become depleted, which will also give rise to a broadening of the predator's diet breadth (Werner, 1977). Thus habitat complexity needs to be managed in order to ensure that the predator concentrates on the optimal prey type. Crowder and Cooper (1982) tested these predictions by manipulating the macrophyte density, and thereby the amount of prey refuge, in a pond in which bluegill sunfish (*Lepornis macrochirus*) were being reared. While variation in prey abundance presented difficulties in the analysis of prey selectivity, the growth rates of the bluegills were found to be highest at intermediate macrophyte densities as predicted (Table I).

The above theories could also be used to overcome the problem of stunting in commercial fish species in ponds. Stunting can result from high intraspecific competition. For example, when bluegill sunfish reach 50 mm in length, they compete with the larger adults in the pond for the same size classes of prey. The younger, smaller fish, being more maneuverable, are more successful than the adults, and the growth rate of the latter decreases. Small fish then grow to a point

TABLE I
MEAN GROWTH RATES OF BLUEGILL SUNFISH
KEPT IN PONDS WITH DIFFERENT
AVAILABILITY OF PREY REFUGES[a]

Refuge availability[b]	Mean fish growth[c]
Low	0.490
Intermediate	0.775
High	0.440

[a] After Crowder and Cooper (1982).

[b] Measured in terms of macrophyte density.

[c] Growth expressed as percentage increase in body weight per day; differences between the fish groups were significant (ANOVA, $p < 0.01$).

where they themselves lose out in competition to smaller fish. This creates a size bottleneck where few fish grow above the intermediate size. One solution to this would be to net a proportion of the young fish to decrease the amount of competition. However, this is time-consuming and costly. An alternative is to introduce a predator on small bluegills, such as bass (*Micropterus salmoides*), and to manage the structural complexity of the pond to maintain the degree of predation on these small fish at the desired level. (This is discussed further in Section I,B.1.)

In addition to vulnerability to predation, spacing of potential foods may influence search time and thereby how much is consumed. Foraging theories predict that manipulation of this spacing should influence diet choice, depending on the availability of alternative foods. [As demonstrated with the bullfinches and the pear cultivars (Section II,A,1), palatability may also need to be taken into account.] Detailed studies of how diet choice relates to the spacing patterns of potential foods could be used, for example, in controlling damage to vegetation where this is giving cause for concern. Such is the case with the "elephant problems" experienced in many African national parks. In Ruaha Park, Tanzania, special concern is being expressed for two species of tree, *Acacia albida* and *Comiphora ugogensis*, which are heavily damaged and killed by browsing elephants (*Loxodonta africana*). Counts of the number of damaged trees in relation to tree density have shown that while the proportion of *A. albida* killed is positively correlated with tree density, this is not the case for *C. ugogensis*. In addition to affecting tree abundance, elephant browsing is altering the dispersion of the former but not the latter. Simulation models have suggested that massive culls of elephants would be necessary to control this problem, involving the shooting of more than 12,000 animals (Barnes, 1983). Elephants eat a wide range of vegetation types, and detailed studies of their actual foraging behavior and food preferences may, by increasing our understanding of how they select their foods, suggest ways in which tree damage could be minimized by adjusting the spacing of the trees such that it becomes unprofitable for the elephants to concentrate on a particular type.

Captive animals, which are provided with a highly profitable food supply, requiring little search or travel time, often pose a different problem. Rather than operating under time constraints, these animals may be inactive for long periods of time, which can lead to the development of undesirable, stereotypic behaviors. For example, feral horses in the Camargue spend 56% of their time eating, while stabled horses spend only 25% of their time eating; the latter may therefore have 14 hr of the day in which to do nothing (Duncan, 1980; M. Kiley-Worthington, personal communication). Many zoo animals also suffer similar "boredom" syndromes, and zoo visitors are distressed to see animals engaging in stereotypic movements, aberrant sexual behavior, and so on. Such problems can be overcome by making it necessary for the animals to search for their food, rather than providing it on a plate, so to speak. Hancocks (1980) prevented the development of stereotypies among primates in the Seattle zoo by piling hay thickly on the floors of their cages and scattering sunflower seeds and raisins among it. The animals now spend several hours each day in an activity similar to natural foraging.

A further use of optimal foraging models in controlling the diet choice of pests is in predicting the probability that a particular species is likely to become a pest when a locally abundant, potential food source is created. as in the growing of a new crop or the siting of a fish farm. For example, central-place foraging theory (based on animals carrying food to a central location such as a nest site) predicts that predators carrying more than one prey item back to the central place should remain in a foraging patch for longer the farther that patch is from the central location (Orians and Pearson, 1979). Predators carrying a single item should become more selective with increasing distance from the nest, thus taking only the most profitable prey when travel time is long (Lessells and Stephens, 1983). Such theories could be used to predict whether breeding birds such as ospreys (*Pandion haliaetus*) or cormorants (*Phalacrocorax carbo*) are likely to become important pests at fish farms if location of the nests and preferred size classes of prey are known. Those size classes of prey likely to prove profitable to the birds when carrying food back to the nest could either not be kept in large numbers or be given special protection. Further uses of central-place foraging in predicting where animals feed are discussed in Section II,B,3.

B.   Where Animals Feed

In addition, or in some cases as an alternative, to manipulating what foods animals eat, it may be necessary to control where they feed. Such action may be needed to prevent localized damage to crops or livestock, to conserve a vulnerable population, or to maximize growth rates in commercial species. To do this we need to understand the social and environmental factors which influence an animal's decision on where to forage and the factors which determine how long it will remain in a particular patch before moving elsewhere. The foraging and time-budget studies of behavioral ecology have identified, and enable us to quantify, many of these parameters.

Animals tend to feed in areas where the costs of obtaining food are outweighed by the benefits which result; the marginal value theorem predicts that they will leave particular food patches when their average intake rate falls below the average food intake per unit time for the habitat as a whole (Charnov, 1976). Thus the availability and the distances between food patches within the animal's habitat, the abundance and distribution of food within these patches, and the risks of predation are key parameters which need to be taken into account in predicting where animals will feed. They are also parameters which can be manipulated in order to alter the animals' behavior.

1. The Effects of Predation Risk

Increasing the perceived risk of predation in a particular food patch may cause the animal to move elsewhere, provided, of course, it has an alternative feeding site. In some cases, the presence of a predator may alter the social behavior of the animals, for example, causing them to group more tightly or become more vigilant, rather than leave the area (Bertram, 1978). Animals may tolerate high predation risks if the alternative is starving to death, and there is likely to be a trade off between risk of predation and the value of the food resource. Such a trade off has been demonstrated in bluegill sunfish. Studies of the optimum diet of bluegills of different sizes feeding in different food patches in a pond lead to the prediction that, in order to maximize food intake, all sizes of fish should switch from the vegetated areas to open water partway through the summer period, as the profitabilities of these different food patches change (Mittelbach, 1981; Werner et al., 1983a). In the absence of bass, a predator of small bluegills, all fish move as predicted (Werner et al., 1983a). However, when bass are present, the more vulnerable small bluegills remain in the vegetation despite the poorer feeding conditions (Werner et al., 1983b). A consequence of this reduced foraging efficiency is that the growth rate of the small fish is reduced by 27%, while the large fish grow faster due to the reduced competition (Table II). The period of vulnerability of small fish to predation is therefore extended, since they take longer to reach a size too large for bass to handle. The introduction of the predator prevents the development of stunted populations of fish, as mentioned in section I,A,3, since the growth rate of the larger bluegills is not held in check by the effect of competition from smaller fish.

However, while direct use of a predator can be successful, there are often

TABLE II

GROWTH RATES OF THREE DIFFERENT SIZE CLASSES OF BLUEGILL SUNFISH KEPT IN PONDS
WITH OR WITHOUT A PREDATOR[a]

	Sunfish size					
	Small		Medium		Large	
	P[b]	NP[b]	P	NP	P	NP
Mean weight increment						
per fish during	0.62	0.85	3.10	3.00	5.53	5.00
experiment (g)	($p < 0.01$)		(N.S.)		($p < 0.01$)	
Total weight increment						
of population (g)	191.0	265.5	768.8	750.0	392.6	320.0
Difference in						
population		−78.5		+18.8		−72.6
increment (g)						

[a] After Werner et al. (1983b).
[b] P, Predator; NP, no predator.

problems in the number of manhours involved and in controlling the predator's behavior. Considerable effort has gone into designing appropriate predator mimics which, when deployed in sensitive areas, increase the apparent predation risk and thereby make these areas unattractive to foraging animals. In general, abiotic deterrents such as loud noises or flashing lights are of limited success, since the animals cease responding after repeated presentation of the stimulus. The problem of habituation is less marked with biotic signals, which may mimic the predator's presence. For example, broadcasting the call of the killer whale (*Orcinus orca*) is used to prevent beluga whales (*Delphinapterus leucas*) from feeding on concentrations of Pacific salmon smolts (*Oncorhynchus* spp.) at estuary mouths (Meacham and Clark, 1979); the same call, however, did not deter another killer whale prey species, the fur seal (*Arctocephalus pusillus*), from feeding around fishing nets (Shaughnessy et al., 1981); more detailed studies of seal foraging may explain why this is so.

Alternatively, the deterrent can mimic the predator's effects. The presence of a model of a dead pigeon, with wings outstretched to display the white wing bars, is aversive to wood pigeons (*Columba palumbus*), presumably because it signals the presence of a predator (or poison), and increasing the area of the wing marks enhances this effect (Inglis and Isaacson, 1984). Many birds emit distress calls when caught by a predator (Inglis et al., 1982), and these can be used as deterrents. The response of conspecifics to these signals is often to approach the source of the call and give alarm calls (thereby presumably gaining information on the nature of the predator), and then leave the area. The producer of the distress call may benefit from calling by being released by a predator which has been startled or confused either by the call itself or by its effects on conspecifics; it might also gain kin-selection benefits through enhancing the survival of close relatives (Gochfeld, 1981). Distress calls can be induced in birds by chemically treating foodstuffs but, since this is presumably a consequence of the affected individuals being in considerable pain, this inhumane approach is banned in many countries (Wright, 1980), and taped distress calls are broadcast instead. Both distress and alarm calls may in fact be more complex than has been appreciated, since they may give information on the level of distress and, for some species such as the vervet monkey (*Cercopithecus aethiops*), the nature of the threat is also encoded in the alarm call (Bremond, 1980; Seyfarth *et al.*, 1980). The context in which the call is given also affects the response (Bremond, 1980; Monaghan, 1984). Work is in progress to produce supernormal calls, which would ideally work interspecifically and when broadcast would not attenuate or degrade with distance from the source to the same extent as normal calls. Such calls have been produced but have yet to be fully tested in the field (Bremond, personal communication). The broadcast of species-specific taped distress calls has been successful in a variety of situations, for example, in deterring roosting birds (Benton *et al.*, 1983), but in this situation, and with foraging birds, the predation risk tolerated will vary with the nature of the resource and with the cost of moving elsewhere. For example, while distress calls have been shown to decrease the number of night herons (*Nycticorax nycticorax*) found at fish ponds (Spanier, 1980), such calls tend to be more effective during the day than at dusk when feeding motivation is high (Behlert, 1977). Moreover, simply reducing the numbers of birds present may not in fact be reducing the amount of damage. Draulens and van Vessen (1985) studied feeding rates and activity budgets of grey herons (*Ardea cinerea*) at fish ponds and observed their response to different levels of disturbance. They found that herons took the maximum number of fish within the first half hour of their arrival, thereafter feeding at a much reduced rate. Therefore, the most likely birds to leave after a disturbance would be those which have already fed, while those which remain or are first to return will inflict maximal damage. Kenward (1978) also found that the shorter the time wood pigeons had spent feeding before an interruption, the sooner they returned after it. The risks foragers will take are thus influenced by their feeding motivation and by the other options open to them; the delay before herons returned to feed after a disturbance at the fish farm decreased as the winter progressed and was inversely proportional to weather severity, reflecting both their relative food demands and the availability of alternative feeding sites (Fig. 3; Draulens and van Vessen, 1985).

    In selecting a place to feed, many animals are influenced by the presence of conspecifics which may indicate that the feeding patch is a good one (Krebs, 1974; Murton *et al.*, 1974). Such findings have encouraged people to try to lure animals to feed in particular places using conspecific models. Time budget

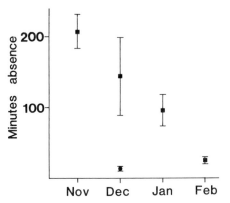

FIG. 3. Time (expressed as means ± SE) for the first herons to return to a fish farm after having been disturbed by the fish farmer. Data presented for the winter of 1982–83 (squares), when the weather was mild in December, and December 1983 (circle), when it was severe. (After Draulens and van Vessem, 1985.)

studies in relation to group size have shown that, for many species, the amount of time individuals spend scanning for predators decreases as group size increases; the overall vigilance of the group increases, but at a reduced time cost to the individual who can thus devote more time to foraging (e.g., Lazarus, 1978; Barnard, 1980; Sullivan, 1984; Monaghan and Metcalfe, 1985). These studies predict that the ratio of vigilant to nonvigilant animals in a bird flock may influence the decision of birds on whether or not to join the flock. Too many vigilant individuals may suggest an increased predation risk; furthermore, since for some species a proportion of scanning may involve searching for food (Inglis and Isaacson, 1978), this may also indicate a poor feeding site. (On the other hand, too few individuals scanning may suggest that the corporate vigilance of the group is poor and thereby deter arriving individuals from joining the flock!) Field studies are clearly necessary to determine optimum head-down/head-up ratios under different conditions. Drent and Swierstra (1977) carried out a series of field experiments on this effect using models of barnacle geese (*Branta leucopis*) in grazing and alert postures. They expected bigger flocks to attract more geese, but found that a flock of 36 models was not noticeably more effective in attracting geese than a flock of 9. They had, however, kept the ratio of grazers to alert individuals constant, whereas in natural flocks, the proportion alert would have decreased with flock size. The experiment was repeated with two flocks of 30 model geese, with different proportions of alert individuals (Table III). Flocks with a low proportion of alert models attracted comparatively more arriving geese which formed larger groups and remained for longer periods. Inglis and Isaacson (1978) obtained similar results with model brent geese and also showed that a high proportion of alert models in the flock deters birds from landing. Such

TABLE III

ATTRACTIVENESS OF MODEL FLOCKS OF BARNACLE GEESE
TO ARRIVING GEESE IN RELATION TO THE PROPORTION OF
MODELS IN THE ALERT POSTURE[a]

Number of models in flock	30	30
Percentage alert	17%	50%
Proportion of arriving birds landing	74%	14%
Initial flock size (range)	1–299	1–69
Goose-minutes spent grazing in vicinity of models during test	38,219	2,048

[a] After Drent and Swierstra (1977).

effects thus need to be taken into account when attempting to influence the distribution of foragers using models.

Since visibility also affects the amount of time birds spend vigilant (Metcalfe, 1984), changing the extent to which they can view the surrounding area when feeding may serve as a deterrent. Milsom *et al.* (1985), in a study of lapwing (*Vanellus vanellus*) foraging on airfields, demonstrated that these birds prefer short grass for feeding and do not use long grass even for roosting. In addition to reducing the visibility of approaching predators, long grass areas probably contain lower earthworm densities than regularly mown short grass areas. Furthermore, since lapwing feed by scanning the ground in front of them for prey items (Metcalfe, 1985), long grass also reduces foraging efficiency. Growing grass longer on airfields is thus an important management strategy in deterring birds from feeding (Brough and Bridgeman, 1980; Milson *et al.*, 1985). Distances from places where predators may be concealed also affects where birds feed (Thompson and Barnard, 1983). Pink-footed geese (*Anser brachyrhynchus*), for example, do not forage in fields less than 500 m in diameter and avoid windbreaks and areas near roads. Thus fields in refuges for these birds must have widths of 1 km or more and have areas more than 500 m from roadways (Madsen, 1985).

2. Food Quality and Quantity

Animals generally move between food patches in response to depletion, as observed in wintering geese, which use several areas in succession and move when a certain level of usage has accumulated. Drent and Swierstra (1977) estimated bite size of foraging geese by calculating intake rates and counting the number of bites; barnacle geese were found to compensate for decreased vegetation height by increasing both their peck rates and the time spent foraging. However, when sward height is reduced to around 2 cm, bite size decreases markedly. Wild geese spend approximately 50 min/hr of daylight foraging, and, since peck rates are already high, have little capacity to compensate for decreasing bite size. Thus, when sward height is 2 cm or less, they cannot maintain a profitable intake rate and move to other areas. Reserves must contain adequate areas for the foraging geese; otherwise, since there is strong selection pressure to reduce travel time between patches, they will move onto adjacent farmland and thus come into conflict with agriculture.

The quality of the forage is also an important parameter affecting patch use and can vary both spatially and temporally, as do the animals' needs. For example, in spring, geese must build up nutrient reserves upon which their subsequent breeding success depends, and they may move from pastureland to other areas at this time. The level of protein in their food is particularly important, and grazing increases protein levels by stimulating plant regrowth. It may therefore pay geese to utilize the same areas in rotation and adjust their grazing intensity to the regrowth potential of the plant. In brent geese, a combination of the bite size and a 4-day revisit interval maximizes the harvest of young plant tissue, and thereby protein intake rate (Prins *et al.*, 1980; Ydenberg and Prins, 1981). Goose refuges must therefore contain enough grazing areas to permit this successive grazing pattern. This effect may operate in many herbivores, and it is important for the maintenance of range and pasture lands to know how grazing animals make use of their forage. In addition, animal productivity can be more efficiently maintained if the relationship between the condition of the forage and the animals' behavior can be quantified and used in management (Low *et al.*, 1981).

An alternative for the animals is to migrate when food supplies in a habitat become limiting. Anadromous fish, for example, migrate because the food supply in rivers only allows growth to a certain size, as demonstrated in salmon (Bachmann, 1982). Salmon must choose the optimum velocity of water in which to sit and wait for prey in streams. However, while there is a linear increase in intake with current velocity, the energy required for maintenance increases exponentially with current velocity due to the cost of swimming. Maintenance costs are also higher for large fish, and a size is eventually reached where the available energy is no greater than that expended (Bachmann, 1982). Thus if the fish is to continue growing, it must move to a more profitable site which, in the case of salmon, involves becoming a seagoing active predator.

A form of risk other than predation which foraging animals face in their choice of feeding site relates to temporal variability in food abundance. Caraco *et al.* (1981) have pointed out that, while two potential feeding patches may have the same mean density of food, one patch may offer a very predictable reward while the returns from the other may fluctuate wildly in an unpredictable manner. Caraco *et al.* have suggested that foragers faced with a choice between such patches should normally favor the more predictable situation (i.e., be "risk averse"), since opting for the unpredictable patch carries the risk of going hungry. However, should the mean reward rate of both patches fall below the animal's intake requirement, it should adopt the opposite policy (i.e., be "risk prone"), since it then has some chance of achieving its required intake (Caraco *et al.*, 1981). The idea that foragers should normally choose the less variable of two food sources might in some cases explain their preferences for man-created food supplies, since on the whole these tend to be more predictable in space and time than natural foods. A deliberate reduction in this predictability would be a novel approach to tackling opportunistic pests; the sporadic use of deterrents where their full-time deployment is not practicable (for example, at refuse dumps to deter feeding gulls) may help to reduce the abundance of pests at all times, since the pests may opt for food patches with a more predictable access to food.

3. The Importance of Travel Time

Since foraging animals are designed to minimize the costs of obtaining food, they tend to concentrate on areas of abundant food which involve the lowest travel costs. Thus, if the animal is moving from a roost or nest site to a foraging area, patches nearest to this route will be depleted most. This can result in severe localized damage to a crop, which would be less costly to the farmer if feeding were more spread out.

For example, bullfinches tend to make excursions from surrounding hedges or woods into orchards to feed, returning to the refuge again when satiated or disturbed. This foraging pattern results in high levels of bud damage at the edge of the orchard, with comparatively little damage to central trees. Fruit trees can compensate for some bud loss, the fruit yield being reduced only when bud damage exceeds 50–60% (Summers and Pollock, 1978; Greig-Smith and Wilson, 1984). Thus, if the foraging effort of the bullfinches were more evenly spread over the orchard, rather than concentrated on the edge, economic losses to the fruit grower would be considerably reduced.

Greig-Smith has examined this problem in detail and applied mathematical models of foraging, coupled with laboratory simulations and field observations, in order to identify parameters which might be modified to manipulate the bullfinches' foraging pattern. In Greig-Smith (1986), he has adapted the model of central-place foraging (see Section II,A,3) developed by Andersson (1978) to encompass the comparatively long and unidirectional foraging trips typical of bullfinches traveling from their refuge (the central place) into orchards to feed. Both in the field and in the laboratory, the feeding effort of bullfinches was shown to decline linearly with distance from the refuge as predicted by the model. Theoretical considerations of the costs and benefits of foraging suggested four potential methods which might be employed to influence the bullfinches' behavior: (1) providing alternative food in the refuge, (2) creating a gap between the refuge and the food source, (3) providing alternative food in the created gap, and (4) concealing the foods to increase searching effort. Greig-Smith's laboratory simulations suggest that creation of a gap between the refuge and the orchard is likely to be the most feasible control method, since this consistently causes more widespread foraging. This work therefore suggests that a simple and practical way of spreading out bullfinch bud damage would be to net the outermost trees in an orchard. Further work is in progress to test this method in the field and predict the optimal gap width.

III. Control of Spacing and Social Behavior

Animals very rarely space themselves randomly. The observed variation in spacing, which ranges from strict individual territoriality through overlapping home ranges and loose aggregations to obligate group living, can be interpreted as a consequence of variation both in the distribution and predictability of key resources and in the nature of interactions between individuals. Thus territoriality should only be favored when a resource is economically defendable and the benefits of exclusive use of that resource outweigh the costs of defending it; the optimum territory size is that which maximizes the net benefits (Brown, 1964; Davies and Houston, 1984). Similar cost–benefit analyses can be used to predict whether animals should live in groups or not. Being a member of a group will often reduce the risk of being predated; the effect on food intake depends on the nature of the food and the foraging method employed (Bertram, 1978). By quantifying the importance of these various parameters, it is possible both to understand the function of the spacing patterns observed and to predict the consequences of any changes in parameter values.

A. Density and Dispersion

1. The Problem of Territoriality

Individual spacing patterns can cause great problems when animals are reared commercially in wild or captive conditions, where the aim is usually to maintain as high a rearing density as possible. For example, while it has been known for some time that juvenile stream-living salmonids are often territorial (e.g., Kalleberg, 1958), experimental manipulations have demonstrated that the size of territories is dependent on food supply, rather than on population size. Slaney and Northcote (1974) showed that decreasing the food abundance led to the more dominant rainbow trout (*Salmo gairdneri*) in a population increasing the size of their territories within hours, forcing previously resident subordinates to migrate downstream (Fig. 4). This is of obvious importance when it comes to restocking streams: the numbers of residents cannot be increased beyond the level determined by territoriality, unless the food supply is also increased. A benefit of this spacing behavior is that the growth rates of those fish that obtain territories is density independent and so will not be reduced by overstocking. This contrasts

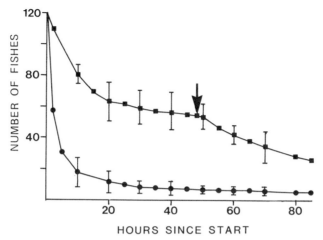

FIG. 4. Number of juvenile rainbow trout (means with 95% confidence limits) remaining in sections of two experimental streams with time since initial stocking. The decrease in numbers present was due to emigration downstream by fish unable to obtain a territory. One stream (the upper line) received supplementary food until the point indicated by the arrow; territory sizes of the remaining fish more than doubled within four hours of the reduction in food supply. (After Slaney and Northcote, 1974.)

with salmonid fish living in lakes, where they are nonterritorial, adopting an active searching rather than a sit-and-wait foraging strategy due to the reduced spatial and temporal predictability of the food supply; they therefore experience density-dependent growth, which can lead to the problem of a stunted population if the initial stocking density is too high (Johnston, 1965).

One way to circumvent the limitations on density normally produced by territoriality would be to increase the density artificially to a point where the costs of territorial defense are so high, due to the rate of intrusions into the territory, that it no longer becomes economically viable to defend a territory. The cessation of territorial defense may then result in a reduction of aggression and reduced variability between individuals in the feeding conditions they experience (Kawanabe, 1968). However, the success of this approach will depend on whether all animals can obtain enough food and whether other aspects of their behavior are also seriously disrupted by the potentially stressful conditions of crowding.

2. Resource Distribution and Competitive Ability

All animals are not equal, and since they are all attempting to maximize their own inclusive fitness, it would obviously be naive to assume that resources will necessarily be shared so that all individuals will receive an equal amount. Yet, in many cases, commercial animal-rearing systems do little to overcome the inequalities in resource acquisition that often result when animals are forced to compete. For instance, the common agricultural practice of locally supplementing the food supply of livestock rarely takes into consideration the effects it may have on competition and the use of space by the animals concerned. When feed blocks are used to supplement the available forage, they are usually left in a very small number of patches. Creation of an extremely patchy food resource encourages intense competition at the feed blocks. This results in levels of aggression that are abnormally high for a grazing animal, a situation which could cause chronic stress in subordinates. In addition, the animals may reduce the extent of their ranging to the neighborhood of the blocks, which leads to overgrazing of these areas and undergrazing of the rest, so exacerbating the original problem (as found in hill sheep, A. Lawrence, personal communication). There is great potential here for the use of theoretical models of dispersion such as the Ideal Free Distribution (Fretwell and Lucas, 1970) in predicting the distribution of the population in the habitat in relation to the distribution of resources, and the effect on this distribution of differences in competitive ability among individuals (Regelmann, 1984; Sutherland and Parker, 1985). One solution to the problem with feed blocks would be to reduce the spatial variability in food supply by decreasing the size and increasing the number of food depots, so reducing both the intensity of competition at depots and the overlap of individual home ranges.

A similar lack of attention to the consequences of competition on the natural spacing and feeding behavior of juvenile salmonids has led to growth problems in fish reared in the high-density rearing tanks increasingly employed on fish farms. The conventional tank design for fish such as Atlantic salmon is either round or square, approximately 2 m in diameter, with a water inlet pipe arranged to produce a tangential water flow around the tank. Food is dropped into this flow, and the water, uneaten food, and feces pass out through a drain in the center of the tank floor. The problem with this design is that the water flow is far from even, and eddies and countercurrents create localized areas of high velocity. For sit and wait predators intercepting food carried by the water current, the profitability of a waiting position is directly related to the velocity of the neighboring current (Fausch, 1984); thus there is a great variation in food availability according to the position of the fish in the tank. This results in the fish becoming very unevenly distributed (Thorpe and Wankowski, 1979). Dominant fish tend to be able to monopolize the most profitable conditions (Fausch, 1984), while subordinates may be forced either to take up unsheltered positions in fast currents (which ensures a high intake but is energetically expensive) or to opt for energy conservation by remaining in calmer water (so obtaining a very low food-intake rate); either way, their energetic efficiency and growth rate will be inferior to that of dominants (Metcalfe, 1986). The consequence of this is that growth rates vary according to dominance status, a phenomenon described in various species and known as growth depensation (e.g., Magnusson, 1962; Jobling, 1985).

The major problem to be countered in conventional tanks is the uneven spatial distribution of food, since the extent to which dominant individuals can monopolize a resource is dependent on its dispersion (see Davies and Houston, 1984; and empirical studies by Yamagishi, 1962; Monaghan and Metcalfe, 1985). By taking greater account of this and of the behavioral response of the fish, John Thorpe and his colleagues at the Department of Agriculture and Fisheries for Scotland Freshwater Fisheries Laboratory, Pitlochry, were able to design a salmon tank that considerably reduced the variability in growth rates. By using a circular tank with a downward-pointing water inlet pipe positioned in the center of the tank, they created a radial water flow across the floor of the tank out from the center to a ring of drains around the outer edge. Therefore, if the fish could be persuaded to form a ring around the middle of the tank, each fish pointing inwards, they would all experience an identical water velocity; by adding the food to the water as it entered the tank, they should also receive the same amount of food. Fish can be made to align in this way by exploiting another aspect of their natural behavior: given a choice, salmon will sit underneath overhead cover rather than remain in the open, presumably to gain greater concealment from overhead predators. By providing a ring of cover just under the water surface, it is possible to manipulate the fish so that they adopt the required spacing pattern.

The performance of this radial-flow tank design was compared to the conventional tangential-flow tanks in a series of salmon growth trials (Thorpe and Wankowski, 1979). It was found that this design did indeed reduce the variability in growth within the fish population, but that the mean growth rate of the fish in radial tanks was in fact slightly lower than that in the conventional design. Rather ironically, the reason for this poorer average growth was the reduced variance in growth rates. Since the optimal food pellet size for growth is very precisely correlated with fish size (see Section II,A,5), and since commercial foods, although size graded, contain a spectrum of pellet sizes, the majority of the fish in radial tanks were feeding on the same restricted band of optimal pellet sizes at any one time. This led to greater competition for certain sizes of pellet and inefficient utilization of the food provided. In contrast, the variation in growth rates of fish in tangential tanks resulted in less competition for certain pellet sizes, since the smallest fish could feed profitably on the smaller pellets ignored by larger fish, resulting in more efficient use of the food from the point of view of the fish farmer. Therefore, the only way of obtaining the full benefit of the radial-flow design would be to reduce further the variability in size of pellets presented at any one time, so achieving a more precise matching of pellet size to fish size.

Differential access to resources due to aggressive defense by dominants is often easy to detect; rather harder, although no less serious, is the interference in the foraging of subordinates that is caused by threat and intimidation. Koebele (1985) showed that the same phenomenon of growth depensation can occur in the absence of any physical aggression or monopolization of resources: the mere sight of a dominant, seen through a glass partition, is enough to reduce the food intake of subordinate cichlids (*Tilapia zillii*). These problems are not restricted to fish; domestic pigs kept in groups soon form hierarchies (James, 1967), and the common procedure of feeding them from troughs presents the dominant individuals with a defendable food resource which they are able to monopolize. Stolba (1985, personal communication) carried out a series of behavioral experiments in which he varied the way in which food was presented to pigs, and by monitoring the feeding behavior of different individuals was able to pinpoint those conditions which minimized the differential effects of dominance status. Increasing the length of troughs decreased their defendability and allowed subordinates to feed without being in close contact with dominants; however, dominant pigs were still able to deter other pigs by facial threat displays. This could easily be countered by dividing the trough into individual sections using small screens placed along its length. By thus preventing each pig at the trough from seeing the head of its neighbor, Stolba was able to reduce both the incidence and effect of threat posturing by dominants. This demonstrates the tremendous potential of the ethological approach, in that a simple and practicable solution to a complex problem has been produced by careful experimental study of the behavioral causes.

An alternative approach to the problems of dominance and resource access is to enlarge the group size, so increasing the complexity and hence reducing the stability and polarity of the dominance hierarchy. Yamagishi (1962) found that the extent of growth depensation in rainbow trout decreased as he increased population size from 6 to 120 fish, controlling for density by increasing tank size; in addition, survival rates and mean growth rates were much higher in the larger populations. He suggested that the reduction in the effects of dominance were due to dominant fish being less able to intimidate all fish simultaneously in a larger group. In some situations the problem can also be tackled by lengthening the period over which animals can feed, so increasing the temporal rather than spatial availability of the resource. If the daily frequency of feeds is greater than that required by any one individual, subordinates can alter their time of feeding so as to avoid conflict with dominants; the interindividual variation in food intake should therefore increase with decreasing number of feeds per day. Experimental work with Arctic charr (*Salvelinus alpinus*) has shown that this result may be obtained even when the fish are presented with food ad lib at each feeding time, indicating the extent to which the presence of feeding dominants can suppress the feeding behavior of subordinates even when food is plentiful (Jobling, 1983).

Intraspecific variation in competitive ability and dominance in affecting the feeding distribution of animals, may also have consequences for their potential to become pests. For example, a high proportion of the "nuisance" bears in American national parks are males which have not managed to secure a territory; these bears range widely in search of food and come into more contact with humans as a result (McArthur, 1981). Differences in the feeding localities used by dominant and subordinate animals may also influence their capacity to carry disease, as is the case with the herring gull (*Larus argentatus*). In feeding interactions, female herring gulls tend to be subordinate to their larger male counterparts and, as a consequence, are more likely to occupy the less-preferred feeding areas (Greig *et al.,* 1985; Monaghan *et al.,* 1985). In Scotland, female herring gulls predominate at garbage dumps, where they are often concentrated on the older, more putrid feeding areas. As a result, more than double the proportion of females compared with males carry the *Salmonellae,* causative agents of food poisoning in man and domestic animals (Monaghan *et al.,* 1985).

B.   GROUP SIZE AND PREDATION RISK

While the optimal solution for a sheep farmer is to have the sheep dispersed, the opposite may be true for anyone raising animals that suffer a high predation rate. Numerous studies (both theoretical and empirical) have suggested that the risk of predation tends to be much higher for solitary individuals than for members of a group, although the causes of this effect vary (reviewed in Bertram, 1978; Pulliam and Caraco, 1984). For instance, Neill and Cullen (1974) found that a variety of predators were much less successful when faced with fish schools than when attacking solitary fish, probably due to the ''confusion effect'' of being unable to concentrate on one particular fish when in the presence of a throng of rapidly moving potential victims. Knowledge of the interaction between group size and predation risk can be used to reduce losses due to predation. When Lake Kinnert in Israel was stocked with silver carp (*Hypophthalmichthys molitrix*) by simply pouring them into the lake, the majority were quickly consumed by resident cichlids (*Tilapia zillii*). This problem was largely solved by holding the fry in the lake behind a protective net for an hour prior to release. This allowed the fish to recover from the initial stresses of being transported to the lake and enabled them to form schools again. When the net was removed, the schools of fish were far less vulnerable to attack, resulting in a much lower initial mortality (Henderson, 1980).

However, this tendency to group can be exploited by man as a predator: while schooling is an effective antipredatory strategy against natural predators, it offers no protection against fishing nets, which, if skillfully managed, catch the entire school. Commercially important species that are obligate schoolers, such as the herring *Clupea harengus,* sardine *Sardina pilchardus,* and tuna *Thunnus* spp., present a distribution of extremely profitable patches to the human predator. Furthermore, the advent of school-finding fishing technology such as sonars makes it increasingly easy to locate the position of these patches. Since search time for fishing boats tends to be small once the fishing grounds are reached, and since the elimination of the school once it is located makes it a nonrenewable patch, patches will disappear at an almost constant rate regardless of their abundance. There is also evidence that school sizes of obligate schooling fish may be independent of population size above a certain threshold; this will result in the "intake rate" of fishing boats remaining steady even if the fish population is in serious decline. The implication for fisheries management is that there may be very little warning of any decline in the abundance of obligate schooling fish until the population has almost disappeared (Murphy, 1980); a depressing example of this is the Atlanto-Scandian herring fishery, which crashed from a catch of 1.7 million tons in 1966 to 21,000 tons within 4 years, due to the virtual elimination of the fish.

IV. CONTROL OF BREEDING

Behavioral ecology should have an important part to play in our attempts to control the reproduction of animals. Manipulation of breeding behavior is desirable in a wide variety of contexts, including the improved productivity of commercial species, the conservation of endangered species by captive breeding, and the control of pests by reducing their reproductive rate. Theories such as those of mate choice, kin recognition and incest avoidance, parent–parent and parent–offspring conflict, parental investment, resource allocation, and life-history strategies may all potentially contribute; they have led to a far greater understanding of how and why animals select mates and breeding sites, what determines their maturation rate and investment in reproduction, and ultimately, what influences their reproductive output. Many of these theories have not penetrated the applied field, but those examples that do exist, together with empirical studies on noncommercial species, indicate the scope for further applications.

A. MATE CHOICE

1. Courtship

It is a common assumption of many captive breeding programs that sexually mature animals will be equally willing to breed with any mature conspecific of the opposite sex. Thus animals are often denied the opportunity to choose mates. Does this have any effect on reproductive output? Theoretical considerations (see Partridge and Halliday, 1984) suggest that, unless the time and resource costs of breeding are minimal, it is advantageous for individuals to discriminate between potential mates on the basis of factors that will affect inclusive fitness. While as yet there have been few direct tests of this, those that have been carried out suggest that giving animals the opportunity to chose their mates increases mean reproductive rates (e.g., Partridge, 1980). Thus an animal husbandry system that arbitrarily creates pairs may produce suboptimal results, as might any which interferes with those aspects of courtship and breeding behavior involved in the assessment of mate quality. It has been shown that courtship may be important even when using artificial insemination: in pigs, the conception rate in sows that are courted by a boar prior to artificial insemination is 86.7%, compared to 62.1% for females denied courtship (Hemsworth *et al.,* 1978).

A study by Bluhm (in press) of breeding canvasback ducks (*Aythya valisineria*) in captivity aptly illustrates the importance of natural courtship and mate selection in reproduction. Canvasbacks, like many waterfowl, normally pair on their wintering grounds after a prolonged period of courtship. Courting by males occurs within winter flocks; eventually a female will perform the "inciting" display to one or more males, until one of them is able to maintain position beside her. The pair then remain close together, with the male defending the female's feeding territory and the female chasing off other males. Bluhm found that canvasbacks taken from a flock of displaying birds and randomly assigned as male and female pairs to breeding cubicles did not produce eggs. Birds that had been displaying when in the flock, but unpaired, stopped displaying when forced into pairs. More dramatically, those female canvasbacks that had previously been paired when in the flock behaved so aggressively to their new mates that the majority of these males actually died. In contrast, birds that were transferred as natural pairs to breeding cubicles continued courtship, with the result that almost all bred successfully (Table IV). Clearly, both the breakup of existing pairs and the lack of mate choice can result in reproductive failure in canvasbacks. These effects may vary between species, and further research will allow us to predict the conditions under which they occur. Moreover, attempts to

TABLE IV
BREEDING SUCCESS OF CANVASBACK DUCKS IN CAPTIVITY,
IN RELATION TO MATE CHOICE[a]

Pair type[b]	Aggressive females[c] (%)	Females laying eggs (%)	Mean number eggs/pair
Natural (*n* = 19)	5	89	18.8
Forced type I (*n* = 12)	17	0	0.0
Forced type II (*n* = 7)	86	0	0.0

[a] After Bluhm (in press).

[b] Type of pair: Natural, naturally formed pairs; forced type I, previously displaying but unpaired birds formed into random pairs; forced type II, birds separated from their naturally formed mate and given a new mate.

[c] Percentage of females aggressive to their assigned mates.

improve captive breeding programs will, in addition to their applied benefits, contribute to our understanding of mate choice in animals.

2. Optimal Inbreeding

A further problem in breeding captive animals is the avoidance of inbreeding. There is now substantial evidence of the deleterious effects which can result from mating between closely related individuals, the most obvious of these being high juvenile mortality (Ballou and Ralls, 1982; O'Brien et al., 1985). It has been suggested (Bateson, 1978) that there is an optimal level of inbreeding which balances the costs of both inbreeding (the unmasking of deleterious recessive genes through increased homozygosity), and distant outbreeding (the breakup of favorable gene complexes). There are several behavioral mechanisms that potentially allow animals in the wild to optimize their degree of inbreeding. First, natal dispersal: In the majority of species for which there are adequate data, one sex disperses farther from the natal area than does the other, thus reducing the likelihood of sibling matings (Greenwood, 1980). Second, kin recognition: There is increasing evidence that animals ranging from arthropods to mammals may be able to recognize their close kin, even without prior contact (e.g., Kareem and Barnard, 1982). By thus being able to crudely estimate the degree of relatedness to potential mates through phenotypic traits, it is possible for animals to select mates of approximately the optimal degree of relatedness. Laboratory Japanese quails (Coturnix coturnix japonica) prefer first cousins, apparently on the basis of plumage pattern (Bateson, 1982), while female great tits (Parus major) tend to mate with males singing song types similar to (but not the same as) their father's (McGregor and Krebs, 1982). Although little studied, there is evidence that the relatedness of potential mates may also alter reproductive behavior in some species. For instance, female mice (Mus musculus) frequently abort if pregnant, or accelerate estrus if not, when exposed to the pheromones of unfamiliar and unrelated males; these effects (which increase the chances of mating with the new male) do not occur if the male is closely related, even if unfamiliar (Lendrem, 1985, personal communication).

Such mechanisms for the avoidance of inbreeding are usually of little use in small captive populations. They may even backfire, since it is likely that in many species individuals estimate close kinship partly on the basis of early experience and so will preferentially avoid mating with any individual with which they have been raised, regardless of actual genetic relatedness. Thus zoos may have to exchange animals in order to overcome these barriers to breeding imposed by raising even unrelated individuals together, and attempts to conserve highly endangered species by captive breeding must take great care to stop the over-familiarization of young animals that could reduce the likelihood of their breeding together when older.

B. Life-History Strategies

1. Time of First Breeding

The study of life-history strategies, which combines aspects of behavioral, evolutionary, and physiological ecology, has immense potential value in the understanding, and ultimately control, of reproductive rates and population demography. For example, the age of sexual maturation in Atlantic salmon is extremely plastic, and there is great variation among river systems in the mean age at which fish return from the sea to breed. Schaffer and Elson (1975) were able to interpret this variability by utilizing the concept of life-history strategies. They found that, for undisturbed Canadian salmon populations, age of return could largely be explained in terms of the difficulty of upstream migration: fish that spawned in long rivers (and thus had to accomplish a long upriver migration) delayed their return until they were older (and hence larger and stronger) than those ascending short rivers. However, in rivers that had long been subjected to fishing, the mean age at return was negatively correlated with fishing intensity, so the higher the adult mortality, the lower the age of first breeding, as would be predicted by life-history theories (e.g, Gadgil and Bossert, 1970; Schaffer, 1974).

A similar result was obtained by Boyce (1981) for the demography of different populations of the beaver (*Caster canadensis*). In an unexploited population, beavers were usually forced to disperse before being able to breed, and the costs of dispersal favored delayed maturation. In contrast, the reduced life expectancy of adult beavers in areas exploited by fur trappers led to more vacancies in the breeding population, and hence removed the need for dispersal. It also created a selection pressure for early maturation, leading to females ceasing growth and maturing at 3 years of age instead of 4. The outcome of this was different age structures of the two populations but almost identical densities, indicating that the beavers were well capable of responding to and withstanding the level of exploitation.

The same result can occur when man is actually trying to reduce the abundance of a pest species. A well-documented example is the response of the herring gull (*Larus argentatus*) population on the Isle of May to annual culling of breeding adults. The colony, which is on a Scottish nature reserve, had been expanding at the rale of 13%/yr throughout much of this century. In 1972, when the colony had reached over 14,000 pairs, it was decided that it should be reduced and regulated by culling, in an attempt to protect the vegetation of the island. The colony has now been reduced to around 3000 pairs, but at a cost of killing over 40,000 birds. This management policy has removed several of the constraints on the reproductive rate of the remaining birds and changed the social structure of the colony. The preferred breeding sites for young herring gulls recruiting into the breeding population are the areas at the center of a colony (Chabrzyk and Coulson, 1976); competition for these sites is generally fierce, since the low natural mortality of adult gulls results in few vacant breeding sites arising each year. In an undisturbed colony, young birds unable to obtain a central site may either defer breeding or breed on the colony periphery, an area in which there is a higher predation risk and lower reproductive success. The culling procedure adopted on the Isle of May reduces the colony density overall rather than completely clearing areas, thereby allowing a greater proportion of young birds to recruit into the preferred areas at an early age. Thus the mean age of first breeding has decreased by over a year, dropping from 5.6 to 4.3 years (Coulson *et al.*, 1982). Furthermore, those young birds returning to the colony to breed have attained a larger body size and lay larger eggs, presumably due to the reduced competition. The reduction in the breeding population of the herring gulls appears to have increased the reproductive success in the colony through these density-dependent effects and has also reduced social constraints on reproduction. The present need for an annual commitment to slaughtering hundreds of gulls could be avoided by completely clearing areas of the colony of nesting gulls, making these areas unattractive to recruiting birds and increasing the competition for socially acceptable nest sites (Monaghan, 1984).

2. The Costs of Breeding

Animals that have a life expectancy of more than one breeding season may differentially allocate their reproductive investment between breeding attempts, balancing the costs and likely success of any one breeding attempt against their residual reproductive value (Schaffer, 1974). Thus an individual with an expectancy of several breeding attempts in the future may maximize its fitness by abandoning the current breeding attempt altogether if conditions appear unfavorable, since the decision on whether to continue should be dependent on the trade off between the likely outcome of this attempt and its effect on future reproduction, rather than on the effort already invested (Dawkins and Carlisle, 1976).

Decisions on whether to breed or not are apparently made annually on the basis of those physiological, environmental, and social conditions which affect the cost of a breeding attempt; a greater understanding of these parameters should lead to our being able to modify the costs of breeding and so manipulate the decision. It may therefore prove possible to reduce the reproductive rate of pests by increasing the costs of breeding attempts, causing a greater proportion of the population to defer breeding for another year.

It has been pointed out by Owen (1980) that, in attempting to reduce the damage to drops caused by wintering geese, man may have actually increased the proportion of the geese that subsequently breed, making the problem worse! There is wide year-to-year variation in the reproductive rates of geese populations, which is largely due to variation in the body condition of birds as they arrive on the breeding grounds: the better the female's body condition, the more likely she is to breed and the more eggs she will lay (Ankney and MacInnes, 1978). Breeding body condition is dependent on the quality of spring forage, and so the creation of good quality goose forage on refuges (in an attempt to lure geese from the adjacent agricultural land) may increase the reproductive rate through lowering one of the main costs of breeding (Owen, 1980). One solution might be to move geese onto refuges by making valuable crops less attractive (by deterrents, see Section I,B,1), rather than by making the refuge more profitable.

3.   Sexual Maturation versus Growth

While many animals continue to grow through life, the rate of growth is not constant; sexual maturation tends to put a brake on their growth, since resources are diverted into gonadal rather than somatic tissue (Calow, 1981). When such animals are commercially harvested, this reduction in growth rate with maturity represents a loss in potential yield; when sexual maturation occurs precociously, with the animal only one hundredth of the normal adult size, it can be a commercial disaster. Thus, while the existence of tiny precociously mature salmon presents an intriguing challenge for the life-history theoretician, it is also a problem of considerable economic importance.

The presence of precocious male salmon (usually approximately 10–15 cm in length, and only a few grams in weight) was initially viewed as a curious anomaly (Jones and King, 1952). The development of theories of alternative reproductive strategies has led to a reexamination of the phenomenon in terms of its adaptive significance. Gross (1984) has shown that, while the largest coho salmon (*Oncorhynchus kisutch*) are able to gain access to spawning females by fighting, the smallest (precocious) males can achieve the same end by "sneaking" close, escaping detection by being able to hide behind stones on the stream bed. After taking into account the probabilities of the two forms of male (i.e., precocious and "normal") acquiring access to spawning females, and their relative survival rates, Gross considered the situation in the river he studied to be one of a mixed Evolutionary Stable Strategy, with both forms being maintained in the population due to their approximately equal fitness. If this is the case, then manipulations of the parameters which determine the relative fitness of the two options for male salmon could tip the balance away from the equilibrium, favoring one form of male over the other.

Commercial hatcheries of salmonids run the risk of upsetting this balance, since in increasing the growth rate of juvenile fish they may create an environment which favors the development of precocious maturation. It has now been established in a wide variety of fish species that faster growth is correlated with a reduced age at maturity (reviewed by Thorpe, in press); the fastest growing salmon within a cohort are those most likely to mature precociously (e.g., Hager and Noble, 1976; Dalley *et al.*, 1983). Paradoxically, the conditions that therefore maximize the final yield of a fish farm are poorer than those that maximize growth rate, since the latter situation will cause a much higher proportion of fish to become sexually mature at a small size (Bailey *et al.*, 1980; Thorpe, 1986).

This problem is not restricted to captive populations, since some wild stocks experience conditions for growth so favorable that the majority of male salmon and even some females mature precociously. In some cases this has apparently been created by a decrease in competition among juveniles when overfishing of adult fish has reduced the reproductive output of the population. The high postbreeding mortality of fish that have precociously matured (Dalley *et al.*, 1983) further reduces the stocks of adult fish, creating a positive feedback in the decline of the fishing industry (Thorpe, 1986). One solution, which at first sight seems to run counter to all theories of animal production, is to raise juvenile fish in captivity in conditions that are *worse* than those in the wild, in an attempt to reduce growth rates and hence the proportion of fish which opt for precocious maturation. This procedure is currently being tried in Japan with stocks of Hime salmon (*Oncorhynchus nerka*), which in the wild have fast growth rates due to the streams being warmed by volcanic activity; their growth rate can be reduced by using colder water in fish farms (J. E. Thorpe, personal communication).

V.   CONCLUSIONS

For the most part, the rise of behavioral ecology represents a progression of ideas rather than techniques (Krebs and Davies, 1984). What it offers applied ethology is a new theoretical framework for understanding, and thereby predicting, how animals behave. Being essentially functional in approach, behavioral ecology complements the causal approach to behavior on which much of applied ethology has hitherto been based. Many of the theories discussed in this paper in relation to particular problems could well be applied in other, related contexts. For example, theories developed to predict where animals will feed are relevant to animals whose use of other resources, such as roost sites, needs to be controlled. Furthermore, attempting to solve practical problems, such as why animals do not breed under certain conditions, can highlight weaknesses in theories and suggest new avenues of research. As in many other branches of science, the most rigorous test of the adequacy of the theoretical basis of behavioral ecology lies in its practical application.

Acknowledgments

We would like to thank Cynthia Bluhm, Peter Greig-Smith, Denis Lendrem, and John Thorpe for access to unpublished manuscripts and John Thorpe, Malcolm Beveridge, and David Wood-Gush for helpful discussions. Peter Greig-Smith, Sarah Lenington, and the editors made many useful comments. We would also like to thank Colin Beer for his "which" hunt, which greatly improved the manuscript.

References

Andersson, M. (1978). Optimal foraging area: Size and allocation of search effort. *Theor. Popul. Biol.* **13**, 397–409.

Ankney, C. D., and MacInnes, C. D. (1978). Nutrient reserves and reproductive performance of female lesser snow geese. *Auk* **95**, 459–471.

Bachman, R. A. (1982). A growth model for drift-feeding salmonids: A selective pressure for migration. *In* "Proceedings of Salmon and Trout Migratory Behavior Symposium" (E. L. Brannan and E. O. Salo, eds.), pp. 128–135. University of Washington, Seattle.

Bailey, J. K., Saunders, R. L., and Buzeta, M. I. (1980). Influence of parental smolt age and sea age on growth and smolting of hatchery-reared Atlantic salmon (*Salmo salar*). *Can. J. Fish. Aqua. Sci.* **37**, 1379–1386.

Ballou, J., and Ralls, K. (1982). Inbreeding and juvenile mortality in small populations of ungulates: A detailed analysis. *Biol. Conserv.* **24**, 239–272.

Barnard, C. J. (1980). Flock feeding and time budgets in the house sparrow (*Passer domesticus* L.). *Anim. Behav.* **28**, 295–309.

Barnes, R. F. W. (1983). Effects of elephant browsing on woodlands in a Tanzanian national park: Measurements, models and management. *J. Appl. Ecol.* **20**, 521–539.

Bateson, P. P. G. (1978). Sexual imprinting and optimal outbreeding. *Nature (London)* **273**, 659–660.

Bateson, P. P. G. (1982). Preferences for cousins in Japanese quail. *Nature London* **295**, 236–237.

Behlert, V. R. (1977). (Acoustic method for scaring herons from fish hatcheries). In German. *Z. Jagdwiss* **23**, 144–152.

Benton, C., Khan, F., Monaghan, P., Richards, W. N., and Shedden, C. B. (1983). The contamination of major water supply by gulls (*Larus* sp.). *Water Res.* **17**, 789–798.

Bertram, B. C. R. (1978). Living in groups: Predators and prey. *In* "Behavioral Ecology: An Evolutionary Approach" (J. R. Krebs and N. B. Davies, eds.), pp. 64–96. Blackwell Scientific Publications, Oxford.

Bluhm, C. (in press). Male preferences and mating patterns of canvasback ducks (*Athya valisineria*). *In* "Avian Monogamy" (P. A. Gowaty and D. Mock, eds.). American Ornithologists Union Monographs.

Bourne, J. (1982). A field test of lithium chloride aversion to reduce coyote predation on domestic sheep. *J. Wildl. Manage.* **46**, 235–239.

Boyce, M. S. (1981). Beaver life-history responses to exploitation. *J. Appl. Ecol.* **18**, 749–753.

Bremond, J-C. (1980). Prospects for making acoustic super-stimuli. *In* "Bird Problems in Agriculture" (E. N. Wright, I. R. Inglis, and C. J. Feare, eds.), pp. 115–120. British Crop Protection Council, Croydon.

Broom, D. (1981). "Biology of Behaviour." Cambridge Univ. Press, Cambridge.

Brough, T., and Bridgman, C. J. (1980). An evaluation of long grass as a bird deterrent on British airfields. *J. Appl. Ecol.* **17**, 243–253.

Brown, J. L. (1964). The evolution of diversity in avian territorial systems. *Wilson Bull.* **76**, 160–169.

Burns, R. J. (1983). Microencapsulated lithium chloride bait aversion did not stop coyote predation on sheep. *J. Wildl. Manage.* **47**, 1010–1017.

Calow, P. (1981). Resource utilization and reproduction. *In* "Physiological Ecology: An Evolutionary Approach to Resource Use" (C. R. Townsend and P. Calow, eds.), pp. 245–273. Blackwell Scientific Publications, Oxford.

Caraco, T. (1979). Time budgeting and group size: A theory. *Ecology* **60**, 611–617.

Caraco, T., Martindale, S., and Whitham, T. S. (1980). An empirical demonstration of risk-sensitive foraging preferences. *Anim. Behav.* **28**, 820–830.

Chabrzyk, G., and Coulson, J. C. (1976). Survival and recruitment in the herring gull *Larus argentatus*. *J. Anim. Ecol.* **45**, 187–203.

Charnov, E. L. (1976). Optimal foraging: The marginal value theorem. *Theor. Popul. Biol.* **9**, 129–136.

Cooper, W. E., and Crowder, L. B. (1979). Patterns of predation in simple and complex environments. *In* "Predator-Prey Systems in Fisheries Management" (R. H. Strand and H. Clepper, eds.), pp. 257–267. Sport Fishing Institute, Washington, DC.

Coulson, J. C., Duncan, N., and Thomas, C. S. (1982). Changes in the breeding biology of the herring gull (*Larus argentatus*) induced by reduction in the size and density of the colony. *J. Anim. Ecol.* **51**, 739–756.

Crowder, L. B.. and Cooper, W. E. (1982). Habitat structural complexity and the interaction between bluegills and their prey. *Ecology* **63**, 1802–1813.

Dalley, E. L., Andrews, L. W., and Green, J. M. (1983). Precocious male Atlantic salmon parr (*Salmo salar*) in insular Newfoundland. *Can. J. Fish. Aqua. Sci.* **40**, 647–652.

Davies, N. B., and Houston, A. I. (1984). Territory economics. *In* "Behavioural Ecology: An Evolutionary Approach" (J. R. Krebs amd N. B. Davies, eds.), 2nd ed., pp. 148–169. Blackwell Scientific Publications, Oxford.

Dawkins, R., and Carlisle, T. R. (1976). Parental investment, mate desertion and a fallacy. *Nature (London)* **262**, 131–133.

Draulens, D., and van Vessen J. (1985). The effect of disturbance on nocturnal abundance and behaviour of grey herons (*Ardea cinerae*) at a fish-farm in winter. *J. Appl. Ecol.* **22**, 19–27.

Drent, R., and Swierstra, P. (1977). Goose flocks and food finding: Field experiments with barnacle geese in winter. *Wildfowl* **28**, 15–20.

Duncan, P., (1980). Time budgets of Camargue horses. II. Time budgets of adults and sub-adults. *Behavior* **72**, 26–49.

Fausch, K. D. (1984). Profitable stream positions for salmonids: Relating specific growth rate to net energy gain. *Can. J. Zool.* **62**, 441–451.

Fretwell, S. D., and Lucas, H. L. (1970). On territorial behaviour and other factors influencing habitat distribution in birds. *Acta Biotheor.* **19**, 16–36.

Gadgil, M., and Bossert, W. (1970). Life historical consequences of natural selection. *Am. Nat.* **104**, 1–24.

Glen, D. M., Milson, N. F., and Wiltshire, C. W. (1981). The effect of predation by blue tits (*Parus caeruleus*) on the sex ratio of codling moths (*Cydia pamonella*). *J. Appl. Ecol.* **18**, 133–140.

Gochfeld, M. (1981). Responses of young black skimmers to high intensity distress notes. *Anim. Behav.* **29**, 1137–1145.

Greenwood, P. J. (1980). Mating systems, philopatry and dispersal in birds and mammals. *Anim. Behav.* **28**, 1140–1162.

Greig, S. A., Coulson, J. C., and Monaghan, P. (1985). Feeding strategies of male and female herring gulls (*Larus argentatus*). *Behaviour* **94**, 41–59.

Greig-Smith, P. W. (1985). The importance of flavour in determining the feeding preferences of bullfinches (*Pyrrhula pyrrhula*) for the buds of two pear cultivars. *J. Appl. Ecol.* **22**, 29–37.

Greig-Smith, P. W. (1986). Bud-feeding by bullfinches: Methods for spreading damage evenly within orchards. *J. Appl. Ecol.* In Press.

Greig-Smith, P. W., and Wilson, G. (1984). Patterns of activity and habitat use by a population of bullfinches (*Pyrrhula pyrrhula*) in relation to bud feeding in orchards. *J. Appl. Ecol.* **21**, 401–422.

Greig-Smith, P. W., and Wilson, M. F. (1985). Influences of seed size, nutrient composition and phenolic content on the preferences of bullfinches feeding in ash trees. *Oikos* **44**, 47–54.

Gross, M. R. (1985). Disruptive selection for alternative life histories in salmon. *Nature (London)* **313**, 47–48.

Hager, R. C., and Hoble, R. E. (1976). Relation of size at release of hatchery-reared coho salmon to age, size and sex composition of returning adults. *Prog. Fish-Cult.* **38**, 144–147.

Hancocks, D. (1980). Bringing nature into the zoo! Inexpensive solutions for zoo environments. *Int. J. Stud. Anim. Prob.* **13**, 170–177.

Harborne, J. (1982). "Introduction to Ecological Biochemistry," 2nd ed. Academic Press, New York.

Hemsworth, P. H., Beilharz, R. G., and Brown, W. J. (1978). The importance of the courting behaviour of the boar on the success of natural and artificial mating. *Appl. Anim. Ethol.* **4**, 341–347.

Henderson, H. F. (1980). Behavioral adjustment of fishes to release into a new habitat. *In* "Fish Behavior and Its Use in the Capture and Culture of Fishes" (J. E. Bardach, J. J. Magnusson, R. C. May, and J. M. Reinhart, eds.), pp. 331–344. ICLARM Conference Proceedings Vol. 5. ICLARM, Manila, Philippines.

Horn, S. W. (1983). An evaluation of predatory suppression in coyotes using lithium chloride induced illness. *J. Wildl. Manage.* **47**, 999–1009.

Inglis, I. R., and Isaacson, A. J. (1978). The responses of dark-bellied brent geese to models of geese in various postures. *Anim. Behav.* **26**, 953–958.

Inglis, I. E., and Isaacson, A. J. (1984). The responses of wood pigeons (*Columba palumbus*) to pigeon decoys in various postures: A quest for a super-normal alarm stimulus. *Behaviour* **90**, 224–240.

Inglis, I. R., Fletcher, M. R., Feare, C. J., Greig-Smith, P. W., and Land, S. (1982). The incidence of distress calling among British birds. *Ibis* **124**, 351–355.

James, J. W. (1967). The value of social status to cattle and pigs. *Proc. Ecol. Soc. Aust.* **2**, 171–181.

Jobling, M. (1983). Effect of feeding frequency on food intake and growth of Arctic charr. *Salvelinus alpinus* (L). *J. Fish Biol.* **23**, 177–185.

Jobling, M. (1985). Physiological and social constraints on growth of fish with special reference to Arctic charr, *Salvelinus alpinus* L. *Aquaculture* **44**, 83–90.

Johnston, W. E. (1965). On mechanisms of self-regulation of population abundance in *Oncorhynchus nerka. Mitt. Int. Ver. Theor. Ange. Limnol.* **13**, 66–87.

Jones, J. W., and King, G. M. (1952). Spawning of the male salmon parr (*Salmo salar* Linn. juv.). *Nature (London)* **169**, 882.

Kalleberg, H. (1958). Observations in a stream tank of territoriality and competition in juvenile salmon and trout (*Salmo salar* L. and *S. trutta* L.). *Inst. Freshwater Res., Drottningholm* **39**, 55–98.

Kareem, A. M., and Barnard, C. J. (1982). The importance of kinship and familiarity in social interactions between mice. *Anim. Behav.* **30**, 594–601.

Kawanabe, H. (1968). The significance of social structure in production of the "Ayu," *Plecoglossus attivelis. In* "Symposium on Salmon and Trout in Streams" (T. H. Northcote, ed.), pp. 243–252. A. R. MacMillan Lectures in Fisheries, University of British Columbia.

Kenward, R. E. (1978). The influence of human and goshawk *Accipiter gentilis* activity on wood-pigeons *Columba palambus* at brassica feeding sites. *Ann. Appl. Biol.* **89**, 277–286.

Koebele, B. P. (1985). Growth and the size hierarchy effect: An experimental assessment of three proposed mechanisms; activity differences, disproportional food acquisition, physiological stress. *Environ. Biol. Fishes* **12**, 181–188.

Krebs, J. R. (1974). Colonial nesting and social feeding as strategies for exploiting food resources in the great blue heron (*Ardea herodias*). *Behaviour*, **51**, 99–134.

Krebs, J. R., and Davies, N. B. (eds.) (1984). "Behavioural Ecology," 2nd Ed. Blackwell Scientific Publications, London.

Krebs, J. R., Stephens, D. W., and Sutherland, W. J. (1983). Perspectives in optimal foraging. *In* "Perspectives in Ornithology" (G. A. Clark and A. H. Brush, eds.), pp. 165–216. Cambridge Univ. Press, New York.

Kruuk, H., and Snell, H. (1981). Prey selection by feral dogs from a population of marine iguanas (*Amblyrhyncus cristatus*). *J. Appl. Ecol.* **18**, 197–204.

Lazarus, J. (1978). Vigilance, flock size and the domain of danger in the white-fronted goose. *Wildfowl* **29**, 139–145.

Lendrem, D. W. (1985). Kinship affects puberty acceleration in mice (*Mus musculus*). *Behav. Ecol. Sociobiol.* **17**, 397–399.

Lessells, C. M.,and Stephens, D. W. (1983). Central place foraging: Single-prey loaders again. *Anim. Behav.* **31**, 238–243.

Low, W. A., Dudzinski, M. L., and Muller, W. J. (1981). The influence of forage and climatic conditions on range community preference of shorthorn cattle in Central America. *J. Appl. Ecol.* **18**, 11–26.

McArthur, K. L. (1981). Factors contributing to the effectiveness of black bear transplants. *J. Wildl. Manage.* **45**, 102–110.

MacArthur, R. H., and Pianka, E. R. (1966). On the optimal use of a patchy environment. *Amer. Nat.* **100**, 603–609.

MacGregor, P. K., and Krebs, J. R. (1982). Mating and song types in the great tit. *Nature (London)* **297**, 60–61.

Madsen, J. (1985). Impact of disturbance on field utilization of pink-footed geese in West Jutland, Denmark. *Biol. Conserv.* **33**, 53–63.

Magnuson, J. J. (1962). An analysis of aggressive behavior, growth, and competition for food and space in Medaka (*Oryzias latipes* (Pisces: Cyprinodontidae)). *Can. J. Zool.* **40**, 313–363.

Meacham, C. P., and Clark, J. H. (1979). Management to increase anadromous salmon production. *In* "Predator-Prey Systems in Fisheries Management" (R. H. Stroud and H. Clepper, eds.), pp. 377–386. Sport Fishing Institute, Washington, DC.

Metcalfe, N. B. (1984). The effects of habitat on the vigilance of shore birds: Is visibility important? *Anim. Behav.* **32**, 981–985.

Metcalfe, N. B. (1985). Prey detection by intertidally feeding lapwings. *Z. Tierpsychol.* **67**, 45–57.

Metcalfe, N. B. (1986). Intraspecific variation in competitive ability and food intake in salmonids: Consequence for energy budgets and growth rates. *J. Fish Biol.* **28**, 525–531.

Milsom, T. P., Holditch, R. S., and Rochard, J. B. A. (1985). Diurnal use of an airfield and adjacent agricultural habitats by lapwings *Vanellus vanellus*. *J. Appl. Ecol.* **22**, 313–327.

Mittelbach, G. G. (1981). Foraging efficiency and body size: A study of optimal diet and habitat use by bluegills. *Ecology* **62**, 1370–1386.

Monaghan, P. (1984). Applied ethology. *Anim. Behav.* **32**, 908–915.

Monaghan, P., and Metcalfe, N. B. (1985). Group foraging in brown hares: Effects of resource distribution and social status. *Anim. Behav.* **33**, 993–999.

Monaghan, P., Shedden, C. B., Ensor, K., Fricker, C. R., and Gridwood, R. W. A. (1985). Salmonella carriage by herring gulls in the Clyde area of Scotland in relation to their feeding ecology. *J. Appl. Ecol.* **22**, 669–680.

Murphy, G. I. (1980). Schooling and the ecology and management of marine fish. *In* "Fish Behaviour and Its Use in the Capture and Culture of Fishes" (J. E. Bardach, J. J. Magnusson, R. C. May, and J. M. Reinhart, eds.), pp. 400–414. ICLARM Conference Proceedings Vol. 5, ICLARM, Manila, Philippines.

Murton, R. K., Westwood, N. J., and Isaacson, A. J. (1974). A study of woodpigeon shooting: The exploitation of a natural animal population. *J. Appl. Ecol.* **11,** 61–81.

Neill, S. R. St. J., and Cullen, J. M. (1974). Experiments on whether schooling by their prey affects the hunting behaviour of cephalopods and fish predators. *J. Zool.* **172,** 549–569.

O'Brien, S. J., Roelke, M. E., Marker, L., Newman, A., Winkler, C. A., Meltzer, D., Colly, L., Evermann, J. F., Bush, M., and Wildt, D. E. (1985). Genetic basis for species vulnerability in the cheetah. *Science* **227,** 1428–1434.

O'Brien, W. J., Slade, N. A., and Vinyard, G. L. (1976). Apparent size as the determinant of prey selection by bluegill sunfish (*Lepomis macrochirus*). *Ecology* **57,** 1304–1310.

Orians, G. H., and Pearson, N. E. (1979). On the theory of central place foraging. *In* "Analysis of Biological Systems" (D. J. Horn, G. R. Stairs, and R. Mitchell, eds.), pp. 154–177. Ohio State Univ. Press, Columbus.

Owen, M. (1980). The role of refuges in wildlife management. *In* "Bird Problems in Agriculture" (E. N. Wright, I. R. Inglis, and C. J. Feare, eds.), pp. 144–156. British Crop Protection Council, Croydon.

Partridge, L. (1980). Mate choice increases a component of offspring fitness in fruit flies. *Nature (London)* **283,** 290–291.

Partridge, L., and Halliday, T. M. (1984). Mating patterns and mate choice. *In* "Behavioural Ecology: An Evolutionary Approach" (J. R. Krebs and N. B. Davies, eds.), 2nd ed., pp. 222–250. Blackwell Scientific Publications, Oxford.

Prins, H. H. Th., Ydenberg, R. C., and Drent, R. H. (1980). The interaction of brent geese *Branta bernicla* and sea plantain *Plantago maritima* during spring sowing: Field observations and experiments. *Acta Bot. Neerl.* **29,** 585–596.

Pulliam, H. R., and Caraco, T. (1984). Living in groups: Is there an optimal group size? *In* "Behavioural Ecology: An Evolutionary Approach" (J. R. Krebs and N. B. Davies, eds.), 2nd ed., pp. 122–147. Blackwell Scientific Publications, Oxford.

Regelmann, K. (1984). Competitive resource sharing: A simulation model. *Anim. Behav.* **32,** 226–232.

Rosenthal, G. A., and Janzen, D. H. (1979). "Herbivores: Their Interaction with Secondary Plant Metabolites." Academic Press, London.

Schaffer, W. M. (1974). Selection for optimal life histories: The effects of age structure. *Ecology* **55,** 291–303.

Schaffer, W. M., and Elson, P. F. (1975). The adaptive significance of variations in life history among local populations of Atlantic salmon in North America. *Ecology* **56,** 577–590.

Seyfarth, R. M., Cheney, D. L., and Marler, P. (1980). Monkey responses to three different alarm calls: Evidence of predator classification and semantic communication. *Science* **210,** 801–803.

Shaughnessy, P. D., Semmelink, A., Cooper, J., and Frost, P. G. H. (1981). Attempts to develop accoustic methods of keeping cape fur seals *Arctocephalus pusillus* from fishing nets. *Biol. Conserv.* **21,** 141–158.

Slaney, P. A., and Northcote, T. G. (1974). Effects of prey abundance on density and territorial behavior of young rainbow trout. (*Salmo gairdneri*) in laboratory stream channels. *J. Fish. Res. Board Can.* **31,** 1201–1209.

Spanier, E. (1980). The use of distress calls to repel night herons (*Nycticorax nycticorax*) from fish ponds. *J. Appl. Ecol.* **17,** 287–294.

Stein, R. A. (1977). Selective predation, optimal foraging, and the predator–prey interaction between fish and crayfish. *Ecology* **58,** 1237–1253.

Stolba, A. (1985). Minimizing social interference during feeding in pig groups. *In* "Abstracts of the 19th International Ethological Conference, Vol. 2," p. 460. Toulouse, France.

Sullivan, K. A. (1984). The advantages of social foraging in downy woodpeckers. *Anim. Behav.* **32,** 16–22.

Summers, D. D. B., and Pollock, M. R. (1978). The effects of bullfinch damage on the yield of pear trees. *Ann. Appl. Biol.* **88,** 342–345.

Sutherland, W. J., and Parker, G. A. (1985). Distribution of unequal competitors. *In* "Behavioural Ecology: Ecological Consequences of Adaptive Behaviour" (R. M. Sibly and R. H. Smith, eds.), pp. 255–273. Blackwell Scientific Publications, Oxford.

Thompson, D. B. A., and Barnard, C. J. (1983). Anti-predator responses in mixed-species associations of lapwings, golden plovers and black-headed gulls. *Anim. Behav.* **31,** 585–593.

Thorpe, J. E. (1986). Age at first maturity in Atlantic salmon, *Salmo salar* L: Freshwater period influences and conflicts with smolting. *In* "Salmonid Age of Maturity" (D. J. Meerburg, ed.). *Can. Spec. Publ. Aquat. Sci.* **89,** 7–14.

Thorpe, J. E., and Wankowski, J. W. J. (1979). Feed presentation and food particle size for juvenile Atlantic salmon, *Salmo salar* L. *In* "Finfish Nutrition and Fishfeed Technology" (J. E. Halver and K. Tiews, eds.), pp. 501–513. Heenemann, Berlin.

Wankowski, J. W. J. (1979). Morphological limitations, prey size selectivity, and growth response of juvenile Atlantic salmon, *Salmo salar. J. Fish Biol.* **14,** 89–100.

Wankowski, J. W. J. (1981). Behavioural aspects of predation by juvenile salmon (*Salmo salar* L.) on particulate prey. *Anim. Behav.* **29,** 557–571.

Wankowski, J. W. J., and Thorpe, J. E. (1979). The role of food particle size in the growth of juvenile Atlantic salmon (*Salmo salar* L.) *J. Fish Biol.* **14,** 351–370.

Werner, E. E. (1974). The fish size, prey size, handling time relation in several sunfishes and some implications. *J. Fish Res. Board Can.* **31,** 1531–1536.

Werner, E. E. (1977). Species packing and niche complementarity in three sunfishes. *Am. Nat.* **111,** 553–578.

Werner, E. E., Mittelbach, G. G., Hall, D. J., and Gilliam, J. F. (1983a). Experimental tests of optimal habitat use in fish: The role of relative habitat profitability. *Ecology* **64,** 1525–1539.

Werner, E. E., Gilliam, J. F., Hall, D. J., and Mittelbach, G. G. (1983b). An experimental test of the effects of predation risk on habitat use in fish. *Ecology* **64,** 1540–1548.

Wood-Gush, D. G. M. (1983). "Elements of Ethology: A Textbook for Agricultural and Veterinary Students." Chapman and Hall, London.

Wright, E. N. (1980). Chemical repellents—A review. *In* "Bird Problems in Agriculture" (E. N. Wright, I. R. Inglis, and C. J. Feare, eds.), pp. 164–172. British Crop Protection Council, Croydon.

Yamagishi, H. (1962). Growth relation in some small experimental populations of rainbow trout fry, *Salmo gairdneri* Richardson, with special reference to social relations among individuals. *Jpn. J. Ecol.* **12,** 43–53.

Ydenberg, R. C., and Prins, H. H. Th. (1981). Spring grazing and the manipulation of food quality by barnacle geese. *J. Appl. Ecol.* **18,** 443–453.

The Dwarf Mongoose: A Study of Behavior and Social Structure in Relation to Ecology in a Small, Social Carnivore

O. Anne E. Rasa

LEHRSTUHL FÜR TIERPHYSIOLOGIE
UNIVERSITÄT BAYREUTH
BAYREUTH, FEDERAL REPUBLIC OF GERMANY

I. Introduction

In most ethological studies, one of the key questions asked is what a particular behavior pattern is "good" for. In the Darwinian sense, this presupposes that behavior patterns now extant have been selected for during evolution because they enhance fitness in the species concerned. In this context, fitness refers to the number of surviving offspring an individual produces. Such behavior patterns are predominantly phylogenetically fixed traits with only a minor learning component, if any, in their makeup. However, although a behavior pattern may be adaptive in one context, this should not be taken to mean that it is adaptive per se, that is, in all contexts. Behavior patterns can also be considered, in certain cases, as maladaptive since their presence imposes constraints on the species. These constraints can exert their effects in the realms of behavior, sociology, or ecology. Either the species is restricted in one or more of these realms by the presence of such a behavior pattern or mechanisms are necessary to compensate for it, mechanisms which would not have been needed had the constraining behavior pattern been more flexible. From this point of view, such behavior patterns can be considered analogous to morphological adaptations which can also have far-reaching effects, imposing constraints in one direction while enhancing fitness in another. An attempt is made in this article to examine two phylogenetically fixed traits in the behavioral repertoire of the dwarf mongoose, indicate the constraints they place on the species from behavioral, sociological, or ecological standpoints, and show how these constraints have been circumvented through the evolution of behavior patterns or social systems which compensate for their presence.

In general, the adaptiveness of a particular behavior pattern is considered as its positive effect on survival and reproductive success. Such considerations, however, are often confined to the proximate advantages—those that can be seen directly at the level of the individual. Some behavior patterns have, however, important ultimate effects in addition, these only being evident at the level of the social group or even the population. To determine such ultimate effects, long-term field studies of populations of known individuals of the species concerned are necessary. Immediate consequences, however, are best studied in detail under controlled laboratory conditions which allow for the experimental manipulation of the behavior pattern in question. To obtain an accurate picture of the adaptive significance of particular traits at all levels of the social structure of a species, both approaches are necessary. The presence of phylogenetically fixed behavior patterns has been shown to have far-reaching effects on the ecology and sociology of the dwarf mongoose, these effects exerting themselves at both the proximate and ultimate levels of behavioral and social organization.

Studies of mammalian social systems have mainly been restricted to the primates (Abegglen, 1976; Kummer, 1968; Lawick-Goodall, 1968; Itani *et al.*, 1963; Schaller, 1963), large herbivores (Gosling, 1974; Jarman, 1974; Klingel, 1969; Sinclair, 1977) and large carnivores (Bertram, 1975; Kruuk, 1972; Mech, 1966; Moehlman, 1983; Schaller, 1972; Reich, 1981), to name only a few (see Crook *et al.*, 1976, for a review). The majority of these studies have had their focus on the demography, general behavior, and sociology of the species in the field. There are far fewer long-term studies of known individuals within mammal societies (Clutton-Brock *et al.*, 1982; Drickamer and Vessey, 1973; Lawick-Goodall, 1973; Sade, 1972; Vogel, 1976; Winkler *et al.*, 1984) and, of these, fewer still have concerned themselves with an integration of both detailed laboratory studies of particular behavioral aspects and long-term field observations or experiments (Kummer, 1968, 1971; Kummer *et al.*, 1974).

It is through such an integration of detailed laboratory studies at the level of a particular behavior pattern or group of patterns, their relationship to social structure, and the correlation of this with long-term population studies on individually known groups in the field that it is possible for the adaptiveness of a particular behavior pattern to be determined for the individual and for its effects on the society or even the species to be understood. The proximate and ultimate effects of such behavior patterns and the means by which the individuals of a species have adapted to the constraints imposed by them can then be determined. Examples of two such behavior patterns are given to illustrate the far-reaching effects they have had on the sociology and ecology of the dwarf mongoose.

II. METHODS

Laboratory studies were conducted on three captive groups of 18, 11, and 8 individuals, which consisted in all cases of a pair of animals and their offspring over several years. Observations were made on these groups during a 16-year period for a total of 30 group years. Groups were housed in large inside enclosures with access to outside pens. The average enclosure size (including inside and outside pens) was approximately 80 m²/group. Rasa (1977a) gives details of food, feeding regime, temperature, lighting, enclosure furnishings, and so on. One-hour observations were made three times daily at 10 A.M., 1 P.M., and 4 P.M., and the data were entered on check sheets. Individuals were marked by clipping hair from various parts of the body. Rank orders were determined by using the methods described by Rasa (1972).

The field observations were conducted in a 15 km² area of the Taru Desert, Kenya, from January to May yearly between 1979 and 1985. Groups present in the area were monitored on a monthly basis and four target groups with adjacent territories selected for detailed study. Observations were made from a stationary car using 12 × 50 binoculars, and the data were entered on check sheets. Maps of foraging routes were made daily. The car was positioned 20–30 m away from the termite mound in which the group was sleeping before daybreak and only moved, if necessary, during the heat of the day when the animals had retired to sleep in another mound. The car remained in position until after dark. This observation method resulted in minimal disturbance, not only to the mongoose group under observation, but also to predators in the area. Target groups were followed continually for about 3 to 4 weeks until they had completed a circuit of their territory. Focus was then placed on another target group. Individuals were identified using natural cues (i.e., sex, age, facial configuration, color variation, scars), these characteristics being entered on cards together with a sketch of the animal showing the key characteristics. A high level of accuracy in identification was achieved with this method, and individuals remained recognizable from one year to the next. Behavior patterns performed by group members, intergroup interactions, and group/predator interactions were compiled daily for the target group under observation. Data on mortality, group-member loss, fate of splinter groups, and individuals lost to natal groups were collected not only for the target groups but, when possible, for the entire population in the 15 km² area ($n = 19$ groups), at least on a yearly basis.

III. Social Structure and Territory

The dwarf mongoose, *Helogale,* lives in family groups throughout the semi-desert, savannah bush regions of Africa wherever sufficient hiding places (termite mounds, rocks, hollow trees) are available. Dwarf mongooses are the smallest African carnivores, their total body length averaging 47 cm and adult individuals weighing approximately 400 g. The group is a matriarchy led by an alpha pair with a lifelong bond (Rasa, 1972, 1977a), the remainder of the group consisting predominantly of their offspring from several successive breeding cycles with females ranking higher than males in each age group and young animals higher than their older siblings. Within these groups, the level of division of labor and altruism is the highest that has been recorded for a mammal. Analyses of age and sex roles in the division of labor (e.g., guarding, babysitting, attacking predators, attacking conspecific intruders), the various rank orders within the group (e.g., priorities, social attractiveness, social activity, and 'popularity'), and interindividual relationships between group members have been published in detail elsewhere (Rasa, 1972, 1977a, 1977b, 1979, 1986a).

In the Taru Desert, groups inhabit territories containing up to 200 or more termite mounds with a network of ventilation shafts in which the mongooses sleep and which are used as refuges from predators. The territories measured varied in size from 0.65 to 0.96 km^2 (mean $= 0.78$ km^2, $n = 4$), and groups themselves ranged in size between 2 and 32 individuals with a mean of 12.3 ($n = 22$). One of the main factors influencing territory size appears to be the effective duration of the anal marking secretion.

Dwarf mongooses mark upright or horizontal objects in their territory with both their cheek glands and their anal glands. Such objects are almost always close to or on the termite mounds the group sleeps in, and 82% of these marking posts are situated in the northern quadrant of the mound. The prevalent winds (trades) blow from the north-northeast for nearly the entire year, thus the odor from these marking posts blows almost directly over the mounds adjacent to them. Ewer (1973, p. 245) states: "The familiar smell of the animal's own mark has the effect of making him more self-assured and less anxious." The positioning of these marking posts may therefore be associated with the impregnation of a group's resting places with their own odor, this having a calming effect.

All members of the group mark at marking posts. Marking frequency and order in which marks are deposited by individuals are correlated with the priorities rank order rather than other measures of social rank (Rasa, 1972, 1977a). The anal-marking secretion has been found to remain detectable for 20–25 days in the laboratory (Rasa 1973b), and dwarf mongoose groups were found to take an average of 21.8 days (range 18–26, $n = 7$) to make a complete circuit of their territory. These data were collected by following groups continually from dawn to dusk every day until they had returned to the mound on which they were first sighted. To determine the extent of variation in territory utilization, one group of nine animals was followed continuously for over 2 consecutive months. Although a different pattern of sleeping-mound utilization was recorded and daily foraging paths used varied between the three circuits, the boundaries of the territory were the same, as was the approximate time taken to make a complete circuit of the area (21, 23, and 25 days, respectively).

These findings strongly suggest that a circuit of the territory is timed to coincide with the viability of the anal-marking secretion on marking posts within it. Since the anal secretion is individually identifiable (Rasa, 1973a), the deposition of this by all group members on the marking post would result in a "group smell" (Ewer, 1973) which may be of importance in identifying the group which has deposited it.

There is little overlap between territories. Data indicate no correlation between territory size and group size ($r = 0.35$, $p > 0.05$, $n = 4$). There is evidence that territories may be traditional. In one case, loss of 60% of a group's members to disease resulted in a decrease of only 31.5% in the area used, this reduction being restricted to the fringes. After the extinction of this group in the following year, the area remained untenanted for over 2 years. Two of the four groups under detailed observation have shown no change in the size of their territories over the 6-year observation period despite fluctuations in group size. One group ranged from -12.5 to $+32.0\%$ of its original size, the other from -28.0 to $+18.6\%$. These findings are similar to those described for the European badger (*Meles meles*) (Cheeseman *et al.*, 1981). In this respect, dwarf mongooses can be considered contractors rather than expansionists, maintaining the smallest economically defensible area which will encompass sufficient resources for the group and for reproduction (Kruuk and McDonald, 1985).

IV. Constraining Behavior Patterns and Compensatory Mechanisms

Two behavior patterns in the repertoire of the dwarf mongoose are considered here to illustrate their intrinsic involvement with the ecology and sociology of the species from the point of view of adaptation and imposed constraints and their proximate and ultimate effects on survival. Their association with territoriality and their relationship with predation avoidance is considered in the Discussion, as are the advantages and disadvantages of group territoriality in the light of the constraints these behavior patterns impose.

A. The Killing Bite

In contrast to felids and mustelids, which have a killing bite oriented toward the neck of the prey animal, or canids and hyaenids, especially the cursorial social species, which appear to have no oriented killing bite, dwarf mongooses have an extremely stereotyped skull-crush bite oriented toward the eyes of the prey. Experimental attempts to change this orientation by moving the position of the eyes along the longitudinal axis of a mouse model have been largely unsuccessful (Rasa, 1973b). If eyes are lacking as an orientation point, as in the vast majority of invertebrates which form the main part of the dwarf mongoose diet, the bite is directed toward the anterior end of moving prey. The head bite has also been reported for *Herpestes sanguineus* (Baker, 1980), *Crossarchus obscurus*, and *Suricata suricatta* (Ewer, 1963), and may be typical of herpestids in general. This killing bite to the head is an extremely quick and efficient means of immobilizing prey, but the presence of such a stereotyped killing bite imposes restrictions on the size of the prey which can be captured and killed. Adult *H. undulata* were unable to kill an adult Norway rat in captivity, and the largest prey observed taken in the field was a multimammate rat (*Mastomys*, BL 12 cm). This contrasts greatly with observations on mustelids and felids which, by means of a neck-oriented bite, are capable of capturing prey many times their own body weight. No cooperative killing of large prey has been observed in dwarf mongooses, either in the laboratory or the field. This also contrasts with the social canids and hyaenids which, owing to their group hunting methods, are capable of capturing prey much larger than themselves. This phylogenetically fixed mode of prey capture has had far-reaching effects on dwarf mongoose social behavior and ecology and these effects can be considered as adaptations to compensate for a more efficient means of group nutrition. Two of the main constrictions imposed with their compensatory behavioral systems are considered here: space utilization in relation to group size and food provisioning.

1. Prey Size, Space Utilization, and Group Size

Since dwarf mongooses are not equipped with a bite capable of dispatching a large prey item and there is no cooperative hunting of prey, there is no prey sharing, except under certain circumstances which are discussed in Section A2. The prey normally captured is small, consisting almost entirely of arthropods, but occasionally small mammals, gecko lizards, and small birds are captured. This prey spectrum coincides well with that recorded for another group-living viverrid, *Suricata* (Roberts, 1981). Such particulate prey items are a scattered food source which is, to a great extent, unpredictable and requires extensive search in order for an individual to obtain a full meal. Owing to the behavioral restriction placed on the size of prey that can be overcome and its distribution, dwarf mongooses have adopted a seminomadic mode of life in which the group forages intensively over relatively long distances each day, each individual hunting and killing for itself. Only rarely do groups return to mounds they have visited just previously. A new sleeping mound is selected almost every night. This pattern of space utilization offsets prey depletion within sections of the territory and spreads the level of predation evenly over the entire area (see Rasa, 1986b, for foraging route maps).

During foraging, the group moves as a unit, usually through high vegetation, and cohesion is maintained by means of a vocalization, the contact call, a short nasal "peep" at 2 kHz (Meier *et al.*, 1983). The distance covered each day varies with group size (Fig. 1). Large groups (>5 individuals) traverse significantly greater actual and linear distances daily than do small groups (<5 individuals). Only when large groups have small young is their foraging distance

AVERAGE DAILY FORAGING DISTANCES

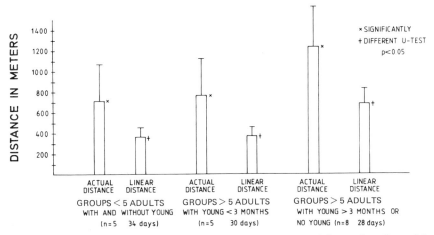

FIG. 1. Average daily foraging distances for small groups of fewer than five adults (over 1 year old) and large groups of 5 or more individuals, together with distances for large groups with small young. All data are from days with less than 15 min disturbance of foraging through external factors. Actual distance is the exact route followed by the animals. Linear distance is the straight line measured between the morning refuge and the midday refuge and from this to the evening refuge (all measurements made with a planimeter).

equivalent to that of small groups. The data shown are drawn from days on which disturbances resulting in a cessation of foraging (e.g., hiding from predators or herds of ungulates) did not exceed a total of 15 min. Foraging is initiated by the alpha female, which gives a "moving out" call (Meier et al., 1983) for the remainder of the group to follow her. She determines the route taken, the distance traveled, and the mounds used to rest in during the heat of the day and at night. In leading the group foraging, therefore, the alpha female must not only correlate the direction and distance traveled with the age of the anal-gland marking secretion at marking posts within the area, but also vary the foraging distance to compensate for the number of animals in the group. The differences in the distances large and small groups travel daily reflect the ecological pressure exerted on the group through its mode of nutrition, this being the relationship between energy output and energy input at the level of the individual.

a. Mechanisms Limiting Group Size. Territories appear to be stable over many years. The average distance traveled daily by a group in search of small, scattered prey has been shown to increase with group size. To prevent depletion of resources within the territory and the energy input/output ratio at the level of the individual reaching a negative balance, there must be a limitation on the maximum number of individuls that can be supported by the area. In dwarf mongoose populations, young remain with the natal group for up to a decade or more; no aggressive interactions resulting in group splits or individuals being chased away have been observed in either wild or laboratory-held groups. Other compensatory mechanisms have, however, developed to prevent group growth from continuing unchecked. Three behavioral mechanisms have been identified which aid in restricting group size.

i. Reproductive success of females.   Only the alpha female is able to raise young successfully. In 16 years, a total of 5 pregnancies in subordinate females have been recorded in the laboratory and 3 in study groups in the field. The young, in all cases but one, vanished within 24 hr of birth and were presumed eaten. Only once was a subordinate female successful in retaining her young. This occurred in a laboratory group of 18 animals, the subordinate female in question giving birth 3 days after the alpha female in the box that contained the alpha female's young, while she was babysitting these. A total of 7 young were recorded on the day following the birth and, judging by their disparate stages of development, 4 were those of the alpha female and 3 were from the subordinate female. The latter, however, did not appear to suckle the young as no suckling marks were visible around her nipples, while those of the alpha female were very obvious. By Day 18, when the young started to emerge from the nestbox, they showed extremely disparate body sizes. The smallest of the subordinate female's young became progressively weaker and died on Day 22. The remainder of the group showed a high level of agitation not observed with previous litters, and the young were continually carried about the enclosure by group members. The next smallest of the subordinate female's young was injured so badly by two subadults during such carrying that it finally died on Day 26. Only one of the subordinate female's offspring survived to maturity, while all 4 of the alpha female's young were raised successfully. This observation suggests that, even if the young of subordinate females are not killed at birth, they are less likely to survive than those of the alpha female.

ii. Estrus cycles.   Subordinate females cycle rarely and irregularly in comparison with the alpha female. In 3 laboratory-held groups over a period of 30 group years, subordinate females cycled only 8 times in comparison with 29 times for alpha females. The difference becomes more marked when the number of sexually mature subordinate females (12) is compared with the number of alpha females (3). Dividing the total number of estrus cycles in each class by the number of animals, the average frequency of estrus/subordinate female is thus 0.66 compared with 9.66 for alpha females. To date, all estruses in alpha females have resulted in pregnancies while, in subordinate females, only 62.5% of the cases resulted in pregnancy. The alpha male prevents copulation of subordinate males with subordinate females that are in estrus (Rasa, 1973c), but this prevention is not completely effective. He was not observed to mount these females himself in either captive or wild groups, and those becoming pregnant were known to be mounted by subordinate males.

iii. Splinter groups.   During the 6-year observation period on the 4 target groups in the field, splinter groups were recorded as detaching themselves from resident groups on 4 occasions. The splinter groups, with one exception, consisted of 1 adult female and 2 males. The exception was a group of 5, comprising 2 females and 3 males, which detached from a group of 28 individuals. The average size of the groups at the time of splinter-group detachment was 21 individuals (range 16–28). The mechanisms involved in splinter-group detachment are not known, but are not based on overt aggression between dominants and subordinates. They appear to be associated with increasing independence of the detaching female and her followers (Rasa, 1985). Splinter groups usually leave the territory of the resident natal group and become transients. Transient groups frequently become involved in fights with resident groups when they enter their territories and are chased away, usually over long distances (up to 2 km). Their fate is discussed in Section V.

2.   Food Provisioning

Since the majority of prey items captured are small, food provisioning is not typical of viverrids (see Ewer, 1973, for discussion). Dwarf mongooses have no behavior patterns analogous to prey-bringing to parturient or lactating females or young (as in felids, mustelids, and hyaenids) and do not regurgitate food for other group members (as in canids). The absence of such behavior patterns, together with the seminomadism imposed on the species through its restriction to small prey in scattered distribution, has had far-reaching effects on social organization, especially with respect to parental behavior, and on the ontogeny of the young.

a. Alloparenting.   Alloparenting has been recorded for both *Mungos mungo* (Rood, 1974) and the dwarf mongoose (Rasa, 1977a). In the latter species, depending on the size of the group, up to three group members (usually a female and two males) remain with the young while the remainder of the group, led by the mother, the alpha female, forage. Babysitters remain with the young until the group returns at midday, another set of babysitters taking over this activity during the afternoon when the first babysitters leave with the group to forage. No nest is built for the young since they are regularly moved from termite mound to termite mound, these moves taking place at an average interval of 1.6 days during the first 3 weeks of life. At this time, the young are unable to follow the group and the mother and subordinate females carry them in their mouths when the group moves to another mound. This pattern of infant transport is further evidence for the seminomadism imposed on the species through its mode of nutrition.

The young show an accelerated ontogeny of behavior patterns associated with orientation and mobility between 2.5 and 3.5 weeks of age and start accompanying the group much earlier than is known for other carnivore species, at about 3.5 to 4 weeks old. It is at this point in their development that food provisioning starts. A single young accompanies a single adult group member which, when it captures a food item, holds it in its mouth and growls softly. The young, vocalizing loudly (the food-begging squeal) then takes the prey from the adult's mouth and eats it. Similar feeding of the young by the parents has been described for *Suricata* (Ewer, 1963). During this period it is the alpha male and the high-ranking subordinate females which supply the majority of the food to the young. Food provisioning of the young during foraging continues until they are approximately 4 months old and capable of capturing prey for themselves, although attempts at prey capture start at about 6 weeks of age.

At the time the young start accompanying the group, they are still physicially relatively undeveloped. Their pelage is sparse and, although the young are capable of running short distances, they are incapable of traveling with the group for an average day's foraging. During this period, the group's movements are restricted (see Fig. 1). Figure 2 shows the distances traveled daily by a group in relation to the stages of maturation of the young. The data show that, when the young remain behind with the babysitters, there is only a slight restriction on the distance traveled by the group daily, although they must return to the point where the young have been left. However, during the period in which the young start accompanying the group but are still being carried, especially over open areas, the distance covered daily decreases significantly. As soon as the young are capable of following rapidly and no longer require carrying, the foraging distances increase significantly.

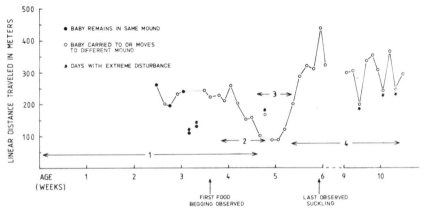

Fig. 2. Foraging distance data for a group of nine adults and two young. Measurements are the linear distance traveled/day. 1, Young left with babysitters during foraging; group returns to mound where young are left; young still immobile and carried between mounds. 2, Young start foraging short distances with the babysitters and group; still carried frequently. 3, Young foraging continually with the group and only carried in emergency or over open spaces. 4, Young foraging continually with the group and no longer carried.

The adaptive significance of this system of alloparenting is obvious. Since no behavioral mechanism is present to provide the mother with food if she stays with the babies, and since the food items are small and difficult to find, an alternative method of ensuring that the mother has sufficient reserves to support lactation has evolved. Subordinate group members remain with the young on a rota basis (Rasa, 1977a) while the mother leads the remainder of the group on typical daily foraging excursions, usually returning to suckle the young at mid-day and in the evening. It is also at these times that the young are usually moved to another termite mound.

In contrast to the majority of carnivores, a permanent den with a nest in which the young can remain while the parent (or group) forages would be maladaptive from two points of view. First, the presence of a permanent den would result in severe depletion of food reserves in the area surrounding it should the young remain stationary for their entire altricial period. The area must not only support the mother but the entire group as well. In addition, stationarity would mean that sections of the territory would not be visited for long periods of time and the marking posts there freshened. This could also lead to resource depletion should a transient group set up residence in such areas. Second, the presence of a permanent den used by a large number of small diurnal mammals would increase the chances of unguarded young attracting the attention of predators, especially ground predators (see Sections IV,B,2 and V).

b. Invalid Care. Food provisioning and restriction of daily foraging distance in dwarf mongooses has only been observed in one other context: when a group member is sick or injured (Rasa, 1976, 1983a). Invalid care has also been recorded for *Mungos mungo* (Pilsworth, 1977). Incapacitated animals are warmed, groomed, and afforded preferred access to food; they may even be fed if immobile. The group's foraging is restricted until the sick animal can accompany it again or dies. In contrast to the young, however, the sick individual is not left in the care of babysitters while the rest of the group seeks food. The entire group stays with the invalid until it either recovers or dies. This behavior is initiated and coordinated by the alpha female. Its adaptive significance is considered in the Discussion.

It is important to note that, in the five cases of invalid care observed (two in captive and three in free-living groups) all recipients of this have been subadult or adult animals (over 1 year of age). No care was evident in the cases of three sick or injured babies, all under 3 months old, although in two of these cases the groups in question had been previously recorded as having afforded care to older group members.

In summary, the absence of a killing bite allowing dwarf mongooses to capture large prey items which could provision the whole group, together with the absence of concerted pack hunting of prey, has resulted in the species having to adopt a seminomadic way of life in a territory large enough to support the entire group. Prevention of over-exploitation of this area and the necessity for the group to travel extremely long distances in order for all group members to obtain sufficient food have produced behavioral mechanisms which hinder the production of large numbers of young and restrict group expansion within certain limits. In addition, since prey items are so small, provisioning of potentially stationary individuals within the group would be impracticable, and an alternative means of ensuring that the lactating female receives sufficient nourishment has developed, this being alloparenting of the young from birth onwards by elder siblings. Similar care is afforded sick or injured individuals. In contrast to many other social carnivores, the only sharing of food that takes place is provisioning of the young during foraging or immobile invalids.

B. GROUP ATTACK

Dwarf mongooses attack all enemies as a closed group. Group attack occurs against intruding conspecific groups or individuals, predators on the ground, and an individual engaged in a fight within the group. Group attack in defensive or aggressive situations can be considered as both adaptive and maladaptive. It appears to be a phylogenetically fixed behavioral response, for no case of a single member of a group attacking a predator or strange mongoose group has been recorded. Its appropriateness and maladaptivity under various circumstances and the mechanisms evolved to counteract the latter are considered below.

1. Attack of Intruding Conspecific Groups

Dwarf mongoose territories border closely on one another with a slight overlap zone. Viable anal marking secretion on marking posts indicates that mounds are actively in use and also which group is using them. As stated in Section III, the territories of adjacent resident groups remain stable over several years. In addition to the resident groups in the area, however, there is also a population of transient groups which wander into residents' territories. The majority of such transient groups are small (2–5 individuals, $n = 8$). Only one record of an extremely large transient group (28 individuals) has been made in the area in 6 years.

a. *Interactions between Resident Groups.* When two mongoose groups meet, they fight. In all fights observed ($n = 16$), a spatial ordering of the combatants has occurred prior to attack. When an intruding group has been sighted, the animal that discovers them gives a high-pitched "Tsiiii" vocalization which results in all group members converging on it. This vocalization and its associated behavior has been observed in only one other situation, that of group attack on snakes. The group clumps together, giving the "excitement twitter" vocalization (Meier et al., 1983), while nibble-grooming and allomarking each other. The alpha male leads the attack, followed closely by the juvenile animals, with the rest of the group behind these and the alpha female bringing up the rear. This deployment of individuals in the attack on conspecifics has been experimentally tested in laboratory-held groups and does not appear to be a learned behavioral response (Rasa, 1977b). Under laboratory conditions juvenile animals have been shown to be more aggresive than older animals toward strangers to the group (Rasa, 1979). Individuals are rarely damaged during such group fights. Only one case of a juvenile animal subsequently dying of a wound inflicted during a fight has been recorded (Rasa, 1985). This is in contrast to *Mungos mungo* where such fights frequently lead to fatalities (Sadie, personal communication).

Aggressive interactions between resident groups take place when neighboring groups coincide temporally at mounds fringing their respective territories. Figure 3 shows the mounds where fights were observed between neighboring resident groups over monthly observation periods during the 6-year study. Fights are for *temporary* possession of a particular termite mound. In one observation, a single

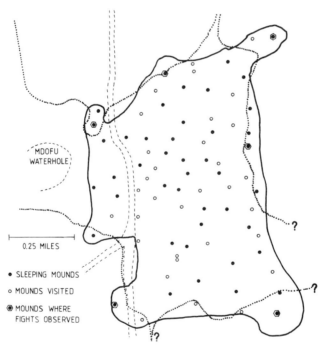

FIG. 3. Territory of one of the target groups in the research area showing mounds at which fights with neighboring groups were observed in the slight overlap between the boundaries of this territory and four adjacent ones.

mound was observed to change ownership eight times within a 5-hour period. At each conquest, the mound's marking post was vigorously marked by the capturing group. Hostilities between the groups ceased at nightfall and the group then in possession of the mound spent the night in it, the losing group in a mound about 30 m away in its own territory. The next morning, the winning group marked the marking post and moved back into its territory on a route approximately directly away from the mound occupied by the losers. As soon as the winners were no longer visible, the losing group moved to the mound, marked over the marks left by the winners, and returned over the route it had come. A similar pattern of events was recorded in interactions between neighboring groups on all other occasions. The outcome of these fights appears to be the demonstration of temporary, not permanent, rights to occupy the mound. The fact that the losing group waits until the winning group leaves and that the latter does not continue in the mound's defense on the following day suggests that such borderline mounds may be considered as neutral territory to be utilized by both parties. In addition, the frequent superposition of neighbors' marking secretion on the marking posts of such mounds suggests that these may combine to constitute a ''neighbor smell'' which would characterize such mounds.

It is difficult to determine the adaptive significance of the demonstration of temporary rights to a particular mound. The stronger, that is, numerically larger group, always wins such encounters. However, it is not this group's marks which are ultimately left on the mound's marking post, but those of the losing group, which covers the winner's marks with its own on the following day, so the mound cannot be considered as won by the actual victors of the encounter. A neighbor-smell hypothesis could, however, account for this anomaly. In these respects, interactions between resident neighbors differ markedly from those between resident and transient groups.

b. Interactions with Transient Groups. When resident groups encounter transient groups or single individuals within their territories, violent fights break out, especially if the transient group is small. These fights differ from interactions with neighbors in two respects. First, the fight is not associated with the tenancy of a particular termite mound, and no prolonged marking episodes at marking posts take place. Second, the transient group usually flees after the first encounter and is then chased out of the area. Resident groups check the marking posts of mounds used by the transient group during their retreat and mark over them.

As a result of the spatial organization of the attacking groups during fights, particularly in the case of small groups, individuals can be isolated from their natal group and chased far away. The farthest distance an individual was relocated away from its group directly after a fight was 1.7 km.

A total of seven cases of individuals becoming detached from their groups after a fight have been observed within the research area. Five of these were detached from transient groups. The identities and ultimate fates of these animals are shown in Table I.

Of the animals concerned, five were juveniles between 6 months and 1 year of age. These, although they are the most aggressive group members in intergroup altercations, are also the smallest and physically the weakest animals in the group. Their deployment directly behind the alpha male in group fights almost predestines them for detachment should they encounter a stronger adversary in the opposite group. This is especially the case if group size is small. This unusual fight formation and the subsequent loss to the group, predominantly of youngsters, together with a fairly high incidence of successful immigration of juveniles into other groups (42.8%) provides a means by which fresh genetic material can be introduced into an otherwise closed family unit.

Dwarf mongooses attempting to join a new group trail the group for an average of 36 days (range 29 to 42, $n = 3$) before acceptance, sleeping in termite mounds adjacent to the one used by the group. During this time they are especially vulnerable to predation. The two juvenile males predated in 1982 were both trailing groups when killed by raptors. Rood (1984) reports similar trailing prior to acceptance into the group for dwarf mongooses in the Serengeti. Acceptance into a group, however, is not equated with reproductive success in this species, since the alpha pair are the only group members to breed successfully. The immigrant must attain alpha status before it can breed. This occurred in the case of an adult male which immigrated into a group in 1981 and attained alpha status in 1985 after the original alpha male had been predated (see Section IV,B,3a).

TABLE I
Individuals Detached from Groups after a Fight[a]

Year	Detached from group	Fate
1980	J ♂	Joined new group
	J ♀	Not Known
1981	J ♂	Rejoined natal group after 3 days
	A ♂	Joined new group
1982	2 J ♂♂	Predated by raptors
1983	SA ♀	Joined new group
1984	None	
1985	None	

[a] J, Juvenile (up to 1 year old); SA, subadult (between 1 and 3 years old); A, adult (over 3 years old).

2. Group Attack on Predators on the Ground

In attacks on predators on the ground, the deployment of group members differs markedly from that observed in attacks against intruding mongoose groups. In the case of predators, it is the subordinate adult animals, especially the males, which are in the forefront, followed by the subadults, with the juveniles bringing up the rear. The alpha male only joins in occasionally, and the alpha female has not been observed to take part in such attacks unless group size is very small (about three animals). These two individuals usually remain several meters away from the attacking group where they bite objects and mark them vigorously with their cheek glands and perform threat scratching. This arrangement of the group in its approach to potentially dangerous stimuli has also been substantiated by experimental tests in the laboratory (Rasa, 1977b).

The main ground-living predators of dwarf mongooses in the Taru Desert are other, larger mongoose species, especially *Herpestes ichneumon* and *H. sanguineus*. Attacks have also been observed by black-backed jackals (*Canis mesomelas*) and the steppe monitor (*Varanus griseus*). All snakes are attacked, whether they are large enough to prey on a mongoose or not. Small snakes are killed and eaten, larger ones chased away. The most frequently encountered large snakes in the Taru are the puff adder (*Bitis arietans*), the spitting cobra (*Naja nigricollis*) and the black mamba (*Dendroaspis polylepis*). In addition to ground-living predators, however, dwarf mongooses also attack raptors on the ground or low in trees.

The majority of ground predators observed to have been attacked respond with evasion, defense, and finally flight. Of the 23 interactions observed, all except 4 (17.4%) resulted in the predator fleeing without having captured one of the group members. The response of the group toward snakes has been described in detail elsewhere (Rasa, 1973b). This basic attack strategy differs only slightly in response to the other predators, The "Tsiii" vocalization, however, is only given in the case of snakes. When attacked by large, agile predators (e.g., jackals, *H. ichneumon*), the group attempts to gain cover in a termite mound or under a bush or log; when the predator approaches, group members leap out, spit and bite at the enemy, and retreat immediately into cover again.

The most efficient mammalian ground predator is the African grey mongoose, *Herpestes ichneumon*. Against this predator, group attack appears to be a less efficient means of defense. In one observation, *H. ichneumon* captured one member of the group and ate it in the open while still being attacked by the remainder of the group. As soon as it had finished eating, it immediately sprang at another group member from the surrounding circle, captured it, and carried it away, followed by the rest of the group. Had the group scattered and hidden themselves after the killing of the first individual, it is unlikely that a second one could have been so easily captured. *H. ichneumon* is also the only predator, apart from large snakes, that has been observed to follow a dwarf mongoose group into a termite mound and attempt capture there.

In general, group attack on ground predators is an efficient means of defense. Most predators retreat after such attacks and are harried continually by the group until they leave the area. Harrying of a large snake has been observed in the kusimanse (*Crossarchus obscurus*) (Struhsaker, 1975) and may be typical for group-living viverrids. In some cases, vicious bites were seen to be inflicted on the predators by the mongooses. In one observation, a mongoose which had bitten into the leg of a marabou stork (*Leptoptilos crumeniferus*) which had swallowed a mongoose baby was carried almost 2 m into the air as the bird took off before it relinquished its hold (Rasa, 1985).

If a group member has been captured by a predator on the ground, the group increases the intensity of its attack and follows the predator carrying the captured group member over long distances. However, no case of freeing of an animal captured by ground predators has been observed. In the case of aerial predators which have not left the ground with their prey or have landed on accessible trees or logs, 37.5% of the captured animals ($n = 8$) have been seen to be released by means of this tactic. Similar behavior has been observed in the banded mongoose (Rood, 1983).

When dwarf mongooses are grasped firmly across the back or shoulders, their bodies become rigid, the pupils contract, and they remain motionless. A similar paralysis on attack has been observed in other species (Kaufmann and Rovee-Collier, 1978; Tortora and Borchelt, 1972; Sargeant and Eberhardt, 1975). As soon as the pressure is released, however, the mongoose regains full mobility. This physiological mechanism probably explains why all the animals observed to be captured by raptors and subsequently released were virtually unharmed. By remaining motionless when captured, they do not stimulate the raptor to increase the force of its grasp or to bite and kill the prey. A group attack in an attempt to free such a captured individual would therefore have high adaptive value, since the individual would be unlikely to be seriously harmed.

All raptors on the ground are attacked by the group as soon as they are seen. As an indication of the force of this attack, on two occasions pale chanting goshawks (*Melierax poliopterus*) were thrown onto their backs by mongooses which had leapt at them and thrust them backwards with their forefeet. On one occasion, group attack of a pale chanting goshawk which had captured a crested francolin (*Francolinus sephaena*) was observed and resulted in the bird's release. Group attack of predators on the ground, therefore, does not appear to be triggered by the stimulus of a caught conspecific, as has been described for jackdaws (Lorenz, 1965), but can initiated solely by the visual stimulus of an accessible predator.

It is interesting to note that the most efficient ground predator on dwarf mongooses is also a member of the same subfamily, the Herpestinae. The only records of members of one carnivore family killing other species of the same family come from the Felidae, where lions have been observed to kill the young of cheetah and leopards as well as young of their own species (Bygott *et al.*, 1979). Killing of young of their own species has also been observed in domestic cats (Liberg, 1981). However, there is as yet no record of one species hunting and killing adult members of a species from the same family as a food item.

Dwarf mongooses appear to be able to deal relatively efficiently with ground predators; losses are higher from aerial attack (see Section V). This appears to be mainly due to the fact that ground predators are attacked by the group as a whole, and continued attack by the group is also effective in gaining the release of already-captured animals, at least in the case of raptors. It is a highly adaptive group defensive mechanism except, perhaps, in the case of *H. ichneumon*.

3. Group Attack on Individuals within the Group

Within a dwarf mongoose group, very little overt aggression is shown between group members (Rasa, 1972, 1977a, 1979). Serious fights between individuals are rare and, should such an altercation break out, the entire group joins in. Attacked animals are not killed during the fight but usually die within a few days of stress-induced uremia, with blood nitrogen levels prior to death of up to 300% above control level (Rasa and van den Höövel, 1984; von Holst, 1969). Only five such attacks have been observed either in captive or free-living groups. In none of these cases was a definite cause for the altercation observed (e.g., rivalry over food, social partner, preferred resting site). If a fight between two individuals starts, the entire group converges on the combatants. Usually, only one is selected for mass attack and, in the five cases observed, this was always the lower ranking of the two. The attacked animal is surrounded by the group and bitten on any exposed part of the body, frequently with "shaking to death" movements. It emits high-volume protest screams and, once it has escaped from its attackers, hides in some easily defensible place (e.g., a nestbox or termite mound). Once the animal has escaped, the attack is not pressed, although the alpha pair may perform threat scratching in front of the animal's hiding place.

This tendency for the whole group to attack members engaged in aggressive altercation is maladaptive in that it can deprive the group of a valuable member. Its rareness is an indication that effective mechanisms must be present in social behavior to prevent it. The presence of a behavioral trait for group attack of group members has had far-reaching effects on the mechanisms for maintaining group stability and especially on those associated with the attainment of alpha position, which leads to personal reproductive success. Potentially aggressive situations are averted before they erupt into fights by the actions of other group members, especially the juveniles. These converge on the antagonists and perform "greeting," an appeasement gesture derived from the baby food-begging behavior, toward them. This has the effect of completely inhibiting aggression, and the two animals then separate (Rasa, 1977a). The vast majority of aggressive interactions, however, consist of the rivals pushing against each other with the shoulders and hips and giving loud protest screams. Actual bites or other damaging behavior patterns are not shown.

Observations of the behavioral mechanisms employed in the attainment of alpha position in both wild and captive groups illustrate other alternatives to overt aggression which prevent group disruption and the possible loss of a group member. These may be considered as adaptations to compensate for the maladaptivity of group attack in this context.

No case of an alpha animal being ousted aggressively from its position by a lower-ranking group member has been observed, either in captive or free-living groups. In captivity, known-age females up to 18 years old have retained their alpha position until death, and one individual bred successfully at 17 years of age. An alpha female in one of the free-living groups bred at an estimated 14 years of age. In contrast to other social carnivores such as wolves (Zimen, 1971) and lions (Bertram, 1976; Schaller, 1972), where rank changes take place through fighting, there does not appear to be a behavioral mechanism for the ousting of dominants on their reaching advanced age in dwarf mongoose societies. This may be associated with the fact that, of the six males and females that have been recorded as dying of old age, all have remained fertile for their entire lifespans. The only cases in which replacement of an alpha animal has been observed have been after the loss of this individual through its death or through experimental removal from the group. Since the entire group attacks group members engaged in a fight, overt aggression would not be an effective means of attaining alpha status or resolving rank altercations between rivals for this position. To avoid the costs of overt fighting, dwarf mongooses have evolved an alternative means of settling rank altercations.

a. Succession to Alpha Position in Wild Groups. In the population of dwarf mongooses studied in the Taru Desert over a 6-year period, three successions to alpha position have been recorded after the loss of an alpha animal. In two cases, adult daughters (4- and 5-year-old females) succeeded their mothers and formed successful breeding pairs with the fathers. In the third case, an immigrant male which had joined the group 4 years previously became the new alpha male and formed a pair with the alpha female after her mate had been killed.

In the first two cases, it was not possible to observe how, after the loss of their mothers, the two females attained the alpha position, since this occurred when the groups were not under direct observation. In the case of the immigrant male, however, the entire episode from the death of the original alpha male to the succession of the new one was observed. The following precis of the events taking place is extracted from field notes:

3/10/84 2:35 P.M.: Original alpha male killed and carried off by a Wahlberg's eagle (*Aquila wahlbergi*). The entire group hides in a termite mound after the attack.

3 P.M. Alpha female emerges from the mound followed by the rest of the group and sits on the mound vocalizing the "Where are you?" call (phonetically a "tsee-tsee-tsee-tsee-TSEE" at approximately 3.6 kHz, which is repeated rapidly in chains).

3:10 P.M. Alpha female leads the group in close formation to various surrounding mounds where she appears to be searching for the missing alpha male, peering into the ventilation shafts of the mounds. The "Where are you?" vocalization is repeated frequently at each mound, predominantly by the alpha female.

5:10 P.M. Alpha female leads the group back to the original mound and goes inside. (This is approximately 1¼ hours earlier than 6:37 P.M., the average time groups retreat into a termite mound for the night; see Rasa, 1983). No animal had emerged again from the mound by nightfall when observations ended.

3/11/84: The group remained at the original mound for the entire daylight period, only making short foraging excursions into the grass and bushes surrounding it. The subsequent night was spent in the same mound. The alpha female gave the "Where are you?" vocalization only sporadically but showed marked position indicating behavior.[1] With the exception of her 3.5-month-old young, none of the group members approached her during this time and performed amicable behavior with her (e.g., sitting in contact, grooming, or allomarking).

3/12/84. The same pattern of behavior was repeated and the group remained a third night in the same mound.

3/13/84, 6:35 A.M.: After group emergence from the mound, the immigrant male started to initiate amicable behavior with the alpha female, sitting next to her and performing neck-nibble grooming. The alpha female responded by standing up and moving position. This position moving in response to the male's attentions was repeated 14 times in 23 min.

6:58 A.M.: The group leaves the mound, the departure initiated by the alpha female immediately after the male had attempted to allomark her flank.

12:18 P.M.: No interaction on the mound the group used to spend siesta in was observed; the alpha female entered immediately, followed by the others. This mound lay 400 m in linear distance from the original mound.

4:45 P.M.: Alpha female leaves the mound, followed closely by the immigrant male and then the remainder of the group. The group foraged a linear distance of 40 m before entering a different mound for the night at 6:10 P.M.

3/14 and 3/15/84: Typical foraging behavior was resumed. The alpha female continued to move position whenever the immigrant male attempted to approach her closely and perform amicable behavior patterns.

3/16/84: Alpha female allows the immigrant male to groom her by neck-nibbling and sit in contact with her on the mound for the first time. She still responds to his attempts to allomark her flanks, however, by standing up and moving position and does not let him anal groom her. A 2-year-old and a 3-year-old subordinate male (both sons) also groomed and sat next to her. These were

---

[1]This consists of sitting conspicuously at the top of the mound with the head slightly raised. At the same time, the contact call is given at high volume. This visual and acoustical position-indicating behavior is most commonly seen when a group member, especially a young animal, has become detached from the group as a result of, for example, predator disturbance. The group does not search for such individuals and retrieve them, as is the case with young up to about 2.5 months of age, but remains stationary and seated conspicuously, giving high-volume contact calls until the missing group member rejoins them. The longest such waiting period recorded is 3 hr 40 min. After the loss of the alpha male, however, this behavior was continued for an entire day.

driven away by the immigrant male who performed threat scratching at the entrances of the termite mound ventilation shafts into which they had fled. This threat elicited protest screams from the animals inside the mound.

3/17/84: The immigrant male follows the alpha female very closely, continually attempting to sit near her and groom her. This pattern of behavior was continued over the next two days.

3/20/84: Alpha female comes into estrus and the male attempts to mount her. She blocks the attempt by giving the protest scream, snapping at him, and running away. Five subsequent attempts to mount were prevented in the same way. On the seventh attempt she passively allowed him to mount.[2]

3/22/84: End of alpha female's estrus. The new alpha male appears to be accepted by both her and the other group members since no further aggression is shown. He sits next to, grooms, and allomarks her without avoidance or protest.

These observations indicate that there is no open fighting between males in the group for alpha status. This position appears to be attained by a male attempting to form a bond with the dominant female through amicable behavior, a process which takes several days to complete.

b. Succession to Alpha Position in Captive Groups.   To determine the effect of the loss of the alpha animals on the behavior of other group members in detail, the alpha pair was removed from a stable family group of 11 individuals (7 males and 4 females) and the behavior of the other group members observed over the subsequent 5 weeks. It was not possible to remove each alpha animal individually to observe the effects of its loss on the group, as would be typical in the field, since previous attempts to isolate a single animal had resulted in the death of the individual concerned. Extreme stress symptoms were observed that resulted in death through uremia within 5 to 10 days. The removed alpha pair were housed in an enclosure where no visual or acoustical contact with the remaining group members was possible. The sex and age of the remaining group members was as follows, listed in order of rank for each sex: ♀2 (1.5 years, not sexually mature), ♀3 (3.5 years), ♀4 (5.5 years); ♂2 (2 years), ♂♂ 3 and 4 (3.5 years), ♂♂ 6 and 7 (4.5 years), ♂8 (5.5 years). One-hour observations were made three times daily as described in Section II.

A marked decrease in the general activity of the group occurred during the first 48 hours after the removal of the alpha pair. This period of immobility corresponds closely to that observed in the free-living group. During this period, the "Where are you?" call was emitted frequently by group members. On Day 3, however, ♀3 and ♀4, the two sexually mature females, started to groom each

[2]This estrus in the alpha female is unusual, since it is the only case of estrus recorded for the end of March (dry season) during the 6-year study period. In the Taru desert, females usually cycle between October and the first weeks of December. Corresponding records of estrus cycles for *Helogale parvula* are available from Botswana and Zambia (Smithers, 1971). It is not known whether dwarf mongooses have an induced estrus, since physiological data for the species are entirely lacking. The behavioral evidence given here, however, suggests that an induced estrus could be present.

other intensively. This grooming differed from the typical neck-nibble grooming in that the groomer attempted to stand with its forefeet on the back of the groomee and groom it along the top of the head and spine, not, as usual, at the sides of the neck and flanks. It was termed aggressive grooming. Both females produced copious saliva during grooming the rival, this resulting in the hair of both animals being thoroughly wet in the regions groomed. The roles of groomer and groomee changed frequently, the groomee moving out from under the forefeet of the groomer and climbing, in turn, on the groomer's back. Only one aggressive attack from ♀4 directed toward ♀3 was observed, and this was on Day 3. The altercation resulted in both females being immediately attacked by all the remaining group members as a body, on which they broke off the fight and hid in nestboxes. No further open attacks were recorded, although aggressivity was indicated by the rival females adopting the upright threat posture between grooming bouts.

The frequency of aggressive grooming between ♀3 and ♀4 exceeded that of any grooming interactions observed between dwarf mongooses under any other conditions. These frequencies are shown in Fig. 4 together with the frequency of upright threat during the same period. The aggressive altercation between the two females continued for 4 days, after which ♀3 assumed the alpha position.

Upright threat appeared to be indecisive as an indicator of dominance, since

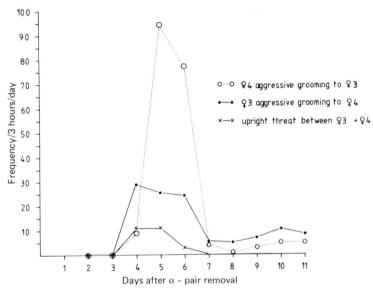

FIG. 4. The frequencies/3 hr of aggressive grooming and upright threat posture between the rival females over an 11-day period during which alpha status was assumed by ♀3 on Day 7.

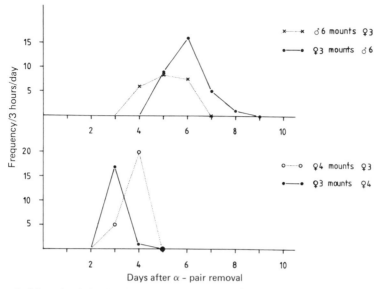

Fig. 5. Mounting behavior frequency/3 hr between ♀3 and ♂6, the subsequent alpha male, and ♀3 and ♀4, the rival females.

neither female showed tendencies to flee or be submissive after its performance. Aggressive grooming, however, was a good dominance-status indicator from the standpoint of which animal was most frequently groomer and which was groomee. On Day 7, ♀4 groomed less frequently than she was groomed, and this tendency was maintained for the rest of the experiment.

In addition to the grooming activity shown, both females mounted each other in the copulatory clasp. ♂6 was also frequently mounted by ♀3. The frequency of occurrence of mounting between these three animals is shown in Fig. 5. Concomitant with a decrease in her mounting of ♀4, ♀3 showed an increase in her mounting of ♂6, this ceasing by Day 9. ♂6 became the alpha male. His mounting of ♀3 started on Day 3, the first day of aggressive interaction between the rival females, and ended on Day 7, when aggressive interaction between the females also ceased. ♂6 was not seen to mount ♀4 nor she him.

A high rate of neck-nibble grooming also took place between the males of the group and the rival females. For the first 16 days of observation, the frequencies with which ♀3 and ♀4 groomed and were groomed by the males are shown in Fig. 6. Here, data have been lumped in 4-day intervals for clarity. During the first 4-day interval, only ♀3 groomed ♂6 frequently and was groomed little in return, except by ♂7. For ♀4, both ♂2 and ♂6 were preferred grooming partners. During the second 4 days, ♀3 increased her grooming of males, especially ♂♂ 4, 6, and 7 and was frequently groomed in return by all males

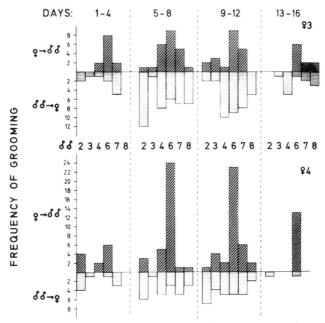

FIG. 6. The frequency/3 hr of neck-nibble grooming between various males in the group and the rival females and vice versa. The data are clumped in 4-day intervals. Stippled columns, the frequency with which the males groomed the females; crosshatched columns, the frequency with which the females groomed the males.

except ♂3. ♂2 showed the highest grooming frequency. For ♀4, by far the highest grooming activity was directed toward ♂6, but this was not reciprocated. This female was groomed significantly less frequently by all males during this period than was ♀3 ($p = 0.03$, Mann-Whitney U-Test). During the third 4 days, ♀3 maintained her high level of grooming ♂♂ 6 and 7 and was groomed frequently by ♂♂ 4, 6, 7, and 8. At the same time, ♀4 continued her high rate of grooming ♂6, again with low reciprocation, although all males groomed her. During the final 4-day period, however, although ♀4 continued grooming ♂6, she was hardly groomed by any of the other males in the group. These, however, with the exception of ♂♂ 2 and 8, continued to groom ♀3.

Over the entire 16-day period, ♀3 accounted for 40.1% of the total female grooming of males and received 61.7% of the total male grooming toward females. ♀4 groomed males more frequently than ♀3 (59.9%) but received less grooming in return (38.3%). 68% of her grooming was directed toward ♂6, but she was the recipient of only 16.1% of his grooming of females. It is of interest to note that, especially in the case of ♀3, the temporal sequence in the frequency with which individual males groomed this female followed relatively closely the priorities rank order in the group (Rasa, 1972, 1977).

This system by which animals in the group compete with one another for attainment of the alpha position appears to be unique for carnivores studied. Instead of open fighting to determine dominance status, what could be termed a "grooming tournament" lasting several days takes place, the outcome being decided by the change in status from groomee to groomer. This mechanism has probably evolved to prevent overt fights between group members, which would result in mass attack by the remainder of the group, thus preventing damage to the combatants while at the same time maintaining group cohesion. The mass-attack response of the group to the single overt fight observed indicates the importance of some alternative strategy to overt aggression. The absence of open fights may also be a means to avoid drawing the attention of predators, especially raptors, to the group (see Section V).

It is important to note that, during the entire period of rivalry between the females, the males remained passive. No aggressive interactions were observed between them, and grooming between males maintained a low level throughout (0.26 grooming episodes/male/3 hr). The succession of ♂6 to alpha position appears to be a case of female choice. This male was mounted and groomed by ♀3 as soon as hostilities began between the two females, and he responded by mounting and grooming her in return. As in the case of the free-living group, bonding appears to occur through amicable behavior. Mounting of the preferred male and the rival appear to have different social significance in dwarf mongooses. In the former case it appears to be a bonding mechanism, in the latter, a dominance display. ♀4's attempts to mount and groom ♂6, however, were either not reciprocated by him (in the case of mounting) or responded to at a relatively low level (grooming). The observed increases in grooming of ♀3 by other males in the group, correlating with their positions in the priorities rank order, may be interpreted as attempts by them to form a bond with the dominant female and thereby accede to alpha status. This amicable behavior, however, was not reciprocated either in increased grooming frequency or mounting of the male concerned by this female. Her choice of the new alpha male appeared to be already fixed by Days 3 to 4 of the altercation. A long-standing bond based on mutual preference as partners in resting in contact, grooming, and playing had existed between these two animals prior to the start of the female competition for alpha position (see Rasa, 1977a, 1979). The ranks of other group members remained unchanged with respect to one another after the new alpha pair was established.

Comparison of the time taken before the establishment of a new alpha animal in both wild and captive groups indicates that the process takes several days: seven for the wild group, six for the captive group. The high levels of grooming and mounting observed in the captive group probably reflect the fact that, in this case, both alpha positions were vacant and males also contested for alpha position through amicable and bonding behavior patterns directed toward the females.

In most species, allogrooming is considered a behavioral mechanism to form or cement bonds between individuals or to reduce aggresivity (Ewer, 1973). This is the first case recorded for mammals where it is used as a substitute for aggressive behavior. Grooming in viverrids, however, may include an aggressive component less obvious or absent in the other mammals (mostly primates) studied. Baker (1984) states that, in the slender mongoose (*Herpestes sanguineus*), an animal approaching another individual to solicit grooming assumes a submissive posture. For the majority of primate species, grooming is also associated with social status but, in this case, the groomer is usually subordinate in rank to the groomee (Kummer, 1968).

Dominance in other social carnivores is attained through overt aggressive behavior toward other group members. There is no record in the species studied (lions, wolves, African hunting dogs, jackals) of fighting rivals being attacked by the rest of the group as a whole. Since this appears to be typical for dwarf mongooses, it may explain why a modified amicable behavior pattern has been used as a substitute for overt aggression in this species and why partner selection appears to be conducted through female choice rather than rank altercations between the males as well.

V. Predator Pressure

Little is known about predator pressure exerted on vertebrates in the field. Sullivan (1984) is of the opinion that predator pressure is a negligible factor in the case of birds. The observation technique used in the dwarf mongoose field studies, however, has the advantage of not disturbing the predators present, especially the raptors, and the level of predation for this species was found to be extremely high. (For a list of avian predators and their success rates see Rasa, 1983b, in press.) It averaged 1.45 disturbances/foraging hour and 0.16 attacks/foraging hour based on 782 foraging hours of observation. It is only when the animals are foraging that they are vulnerable to attack, since predators have no chance of capturing them if they are already on a termite mound where they can hide immediately. Disturbances were considered as all behavior on the part of a predator which resulted in the mongooses warning, breaking off their foraging, and hiding.

Dwarf mongooses have an effective vigilance system, "guarding," performed predominantly by the subordinate males in the group. Females and the alpha pair are responsible for only approximately 10% of the total guarding performed (Rasa, 1986a). The effectiveness of this guarding behavior, however, is very much dependent on group size (Rasa, 1986b). The majority of animals killed are juveniles of 4 months old or less. The other category of group members suffering high predation rates is the guards themselves. This is due to the "leap frog" system of guard substitution utilized as the group moves along foraging. It necessitates the guard which has been left behind by the group having to run alone over distances of up to 80 m or more in order to rejoin it. It is during such solitary runs that these animals are captured by predators (Rasa, 1986a). Predator pressure, the effectiveness of guarding behavior, and predator efficiency have been dealt with in detail elsewhere (Rasa, in press).

Data gathered on the predator pressure exerted on groups of various sizes over a 6-year period have shown that groups with fewer than five individuals over 1 year of age are at a disadvantage compared with larger ones (Fig. 7). Although the disturbances resulting from predators are approximately the same for both large and small groups, small groups are attacked approximately 200% more frequently than large ones. This is due to the inefficiency of the guarding system in small groups, there being an insufficient number of individuals to maintain continual vigilance. Small groups also have a far higher level of predation than large ones, and approximately two-thirds of their young are killed within their first 4 months of life, compared with no young observed killed in groups with more than five older individuals. No young of small groups observed have survived their first year, and the small groups themselves have been eradicated within a maximum of 2 years (Rasa, 1986b).

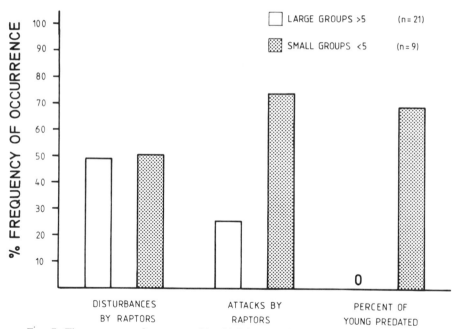

FIG. 7. The percentage frequency with which large and small groups were disturbed or attacked by raptors together with the percentage of the young killed by birds of prey within the first 4 months of life in large and small groups.

If large groups lose a high proportion of their members through disease or splinter-group formation so that their numbers drop below five, they are unable to survive (Rasa, 1986b). None of the nine splinter groups observed to have formed from groups in the study area existed for more than 2 years, since they continually lost members to predators. Splinter groups appear to be especially endangered since they have no permanent territories and are continually chased out of areas occupied by resident groups into areas with which they are not familiar. On two occasions, individuals from splinter groups were observed killed by raptors when fleeing after a resident group's attack. They appear to have no fitness since they cannot raise young of their own and also face extermination themselves. They can probably be considered analogous to the 'refugee populations' described by Carl (1971) for the Arctic ground squirrel (*Spermophilus undulatus*), where only animals on breeding territories have reproductive success, the refugee population facing extinction.

These data not only indicate the adaptiveness of group life for the dwarf mongoose but also offer an explanation for many of the behavior patterns whose proximate advantages at the level of the individual have been discussed in previous sections. The ultimate advantages of these behavior patterns now become understandable in light of the high predation levels on certain sections of the population.

VI. Discussion

In contrast to the majority of other social carnivore species studied, group life for the dwarf mongoose (Fig. 8) appears to have evolved as a protection against a high level of predation rather than as a means of more efficient prey capture or defense (see McDonald, 1983, for a review). Although Taylor (1976) is of the opinion that spacing out would be of advantage to a small cryptic animal in escaping randomly searching predators, this model does not hold true for dwarf mongooses, although they are both small and cryptically colored. His model, however, does not take into account that, in groups, it is possible for certain group members to actively reduce potential predation on other group members through group-protective behavior. This type of behavior is especially well developed in dwarf mongooses, a kin-based society, and can be considered as either an advantage or even a prerequisite for group life in this species. It is this mutual defense against predation which has probably shaped the evolution of altruistic behavior in this species.

A. Territoriality and Marking

Although the territory utilized by the group is independent of group size, as has been reported for several other carnivore species—badger (Kruuk and Par-

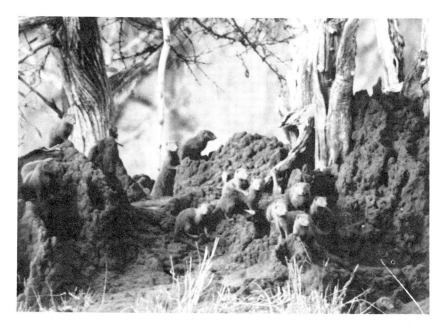

FIG. 8. The dwarf mongoose.

ish, 1982), domestic cats (Liberg, 1981), red foxes (Lindstrom, 1980), and black-backed jackals (Moehlman, 1983)—it is unlikely that habitat "patchiness" is a factor determing the size of the area, as has been found for badgers and red foxes. The Taru, a climax *Commiphora* woodland, is, in contrast to the agricultural land where the studies of badgers and red foxes were conducted, an extremely uniform biotope with little fluctuation in food availability (mainly insects), at least on a short-term basis. Two other more probable explanations may account for the noncorrelation of group size and territory size in dwarf mongooses.

The first appears to be a time factor commensurate with effective foraging and indication of active tendency. The group takes an average of 21.8 days to make a complete circuit of the area while foraging, this correlating with the duration of the anal marking secretion on marking posts distributed approximately every 25–30 m within it. In order to indicate active tenancy, these marks must thus be renewed within 20–25 days, the timespan in which the marks decayed to nonrecognition in laboratory experiments. Such regular renewal serves two purposes. First, it indicates to neighboring resident groups that a particular group is still present in the area. Although no expansionist tendencies have been observed between neighbors, this may aid in preventing permanent take-over of disputed neighbor mounds in the no-man's-land between territories (the regions of territory overlap). Here, knowledge of the relative strengths of neighboring groups may also play a part, these being recognizable from the group's combined anal secretions.

Second, although the presence of viable marks does not prevent transient groups from entering a resident group's territory, regular patrolling and checking of marking posts would betray their presence and result in their ejection from the area, since such transient groups utilize the resident group's resources. Although it has not been observed in the target groups studied, the lapsing of active scent control in a section of the territory could possibly result in a transient group gaining a temporary foothold there.

As mentioned in Section III, the presence of a group's "own smell" within its territory exerts a calming effect on group members, and the positioning of the marking posts upwind on mounds would result in the mounds themselves and, in effect, the entire territory being impregnated with the group's smell. No evidence of the odor of one group having an aversive effect on another group has been observed, in the sense of frightening away intruders. The discovery of marks from a strange group elicits high agitation, bottle-brushed fur, excitement twitter vocalizations, and immediate marking over by the group when it encounters such marks. The nonelicitation of fleeing responses appears to be true of many carnivores (see Ewer, 1973, for a review), and the reaction to such marks is to cover them with personal scent. This suggests that familiarity with the environment plays an important role in the selection and maintenance of living space.

It is this familiarity with the territory which is probably the greatest advantage that territoriality confers on dwarf mongoose groups. Data suggest that the group, or at least the alpha female which leads them, has a mental map of the territory. Although this may be of advantage in locating good food sources, its greatest advantage lies in the knowledge of the exact whereabouts of hiding places and the optimal routes to be taken to reach these. When threatened by an aerial predator, dwarf mongoose groups scatter and hide, usually singly, unless a termite mound is in the vicinity and can be used as a refuge by the entire group. Detailed knowledge of the entire surroundings is necessary for such an evasion technique to function efficiently. This detailed knowledge appears to be learned during ontogeny. It can be calculated that a young mongoose makes 13 complete circuits of its group's territory within the first year of its life and, presumably during this time, owing to the high frequency of predator disturbances (1.45/hr), learns where appropriate hiding places are by following experienced babysitters, at least for the first months. This aspect of territoriality has been largely neglected in studies of the subject.

A series of experiments conducted in the laboratory substantiate the importance of the knowledge of escape routes to the individual and emphasize the learned component of these. On four occasions, groups of two or three animals each were placed in familiar nestboxes in an unfamiliar room. When the boxes were opened, the animals emerged hesitantly, first for a few bodylengths, before fleeing into the refuge box again. These hesitant exploratory forays were continued in all directions from the box entrance, broken off for no apparent reason to dash to the box again, and slowly extended to encompass the entire area. Once the animals were familiar with the surroundings, obstacles such as logs and cardboard boxes were placed between 50 cm and 1 m in front of the nestbox entrance. After they had emerged from the boxes, the animals were frightened into precipitous flight and all collided with the introduced obtacles the first time they fled in the new situation. These experiments suggest strongly that routes to safe hiding places are learned during preliminary forays and that the interpolation of obstacles requires that these routes be learned anew. Obstacles do not appear to be recognized visually as such during flight, and fleeing routes seem to be based on previously learned directions and distances.

The deleterious effects of nonknowledge of the immediate surroundings can also be inferred from the observations on transient groups. As previously stated, these groups face extinction. One of the main factors contributing to this appears to be their inability to locate secure hiding places fast enough when attacked by raptors, owing to their lack of familiarity with the environment. The animals observed to be predated when stooped on by the bird of prey either hesitated or reversed direction during flight, resulting in their capture.

In addition to the learning component for routes within the territory, an olfactory component is also likely. Although no active marking of routes with the anal or cheek glands has been observed (e.g., marking of objects along the route or the ground itself by anal drag), passive marking is very likely to take place when the animals push through grass and underbrush, rubbing their flanks along the vegetation. The deposition of anal marking substance on the flanks of group members occurs actively, through allomarking, or passively through the animals' habit of clustering together to sleep or maintain body temperature when ambient temperatures are low, as in the early morning. Some evidence for the presence of such odor signals along routes has been gathered (Rasa, 1985). It is also possible that, like canids, mongooses may possess odor-producing glands on the soles of the feet, but no evidence for their presence is available. The presence of such passively marked routes within the territory together with the positioning of the marking posts upwind on mounds would result in the territory consisting of a network of odor pathways with centers of high odor concentration (the mounds), and this knowledge may be of great value for rapid orientation when in danger.

The territory of dwarf mongooses, therefore, is not only the smallest area capable of defense which encompasses sufficient resources for group maintenance and reproduction (Kruuk and McDonald, 1985), but also the area which can be effectively patrolled during foraging, efficiently searched for small scattered prey, and marked as being actively tenanted. Probably one of its most important features in this species is the intimate knowledge of the territory by all group members, especially from the point of view of the routes and refuges within it, and this knowledge plays a vital role in evading predation.

B. DWARF MONGOOSES AND BROWN'S THEORY
OF GROUP-SIZE OPTIMUM

Group life for the dwarf mongoose conforms very closely to Brown's (1982) model of optimization of group size and the factors underlying group territoriality. The latter he considers as one of the possible origins of helping behavior in vertebrates. His model is based on a single breeding pair living in a socially bonded unit with a variable number of nonbreeders which function as helpers in parental-care and group-protective roles. This model fits extremely closely to the condition actually found in dwarf mongoose groups, the alpha pair being the only animals able to reproduce successfully and the remainder of the group consisting predominantly of their offspring, the helping roles they engage in varying with the age and sex of the individuals concerned. Pulliam and Caraco (1984) emphasize that group size is the result of a net cost/benefit relationship at the level of the individual and that these costs and benefits may vary with status (Pulliam, 1976). In such cases, the optimal group size for a dominant animal may differ from that for a subordinate.

The factors Brown lists as determining optimal group size for an individual on a territory are concerned with optimizing this individual's fitness. He lists resource depletion, territory defense against conspecifics, vigilance, and reproductive success as the four factors playing major roles in the evolution of group territoriality. When the gains from the last three factors outweigh the loss from the first factor, then group territoriality would be of advantage.

Optimal group size would be determined jointly by the shared tasks and by the depletion function. Brown hypothesizes that group territoriality would evolve in a species when territorial defense costs are high. He shows, though, that the advantages gained by individuals, using this model of group territorial evolution, decrease with increasing group size and suggests that, owing to this, other factors may be involved. He puts forward resource depletion as a major variable in this context.

For dwarf mongooses, although territory defense is important, the finding that territories remain stable despite fluctuations in group size also suggests that territory defense is not a major determinant of group territoriality for this species. Brown only considers defense from the point of view of intruding conspecifics. Dwarf mongooses, however, also use group attack against predators, and dominant animals take little part in this. Although the theoretical advantage gained from increasing group size in groups of four or five animals may be less than that in smaller groups in the case of conspecific altercations, if the attack is directed toward a ground predator, then a larger number of helpers would be of advantage, at least to the dominant, since it would not have to take part in such attacks itself. For dwarf mongooses, the data suggest that vigilance and other group-protective roles are very likely to be the crucial factors leading to group territoriality in this species rather than resource depletion and territory defense.

Groups consisting of fewer than the reproductive pair and three helpers have no reproductive success and are themselves eliminated through predation. This indicates that a minimum of three helpers is necessary for group survival. If Brown's theoretical assumption that large unit size may not be disadvantageous under conditions where reduction of fitness due to the effect of a particular unit size on territory quality is low (as in the case of dwarf mongooses where territories are not expanded but appear to be traditional) then, theoretically, optimal group size would lie at about six individuals. For dwarf mongooses, however, the data show that fitness = 0 when group size = 5. Using Brown's formula and substituting 5 for 1 at fitness = 0, optimum group size for dwarf mongooses would be 11 animals before costs become equal to or exceed benefits. This optimal group size is close to the average group size actually recorded (12.3 individuals), and Brown's theory of optimal unit size may reflect real relationships between the factors he gives as influencing group territoriality in vertebrates.

As previously mentioned, Brown considers resource depletion an important factor influencing fitness in group territorial animals and states that it has received practically no attention in the literature. Although resource depletion is, of course, of ultimate importance to all territorial animals, the dwarf mongoose data indicate that the resource-related factor for this species may not be resource depletion itself but the effort, in terms of energy expenditure, required to exploit the resource, in this case food. Large groups must travel approximately half again as far daily as small groups during foraging. This suggests that it is not food availability itself which is limiting but the energy costs involved in searching for it, presuming that the food items are relatively evenly distributed. The foraging patterns observed suggest that food is fairly evenly distributed (Rasa, 1986b) and that large groups must simply search larger areas if all individuals are to obtain sufficient nourishment. "Local enhancement" (Crook, 1965) may play a role in the locating of food but, probably owing to the small size of the prey and its scattered distribution, not such a great role for dwarf mongooses as for frugivorous species (Ghiglieri, 1985) or other species where food distribution is patchy (Kruuk and Parish, 1982). For dwarf mongooses, it is postulated that the energy required to exploit the food source is the factor setting the upper limit of group size and not the limitation of the resource itself. It is likely that splinter groups are formed when the energy expenditure factor increases to the point that it outweighs the advantages of group territoriality, but no quantitative data are available on this topic.

As Pulliam (1976) suggests, optimal group size may differ for subordinate and dominant animals. For a dominant, the important factors are sufficient helpers to perform vigilance and group protective behavior efficiently and to help in raising and protecting the young so that they survive. Optimal group size for dominants probably is around 11 individuals, the point at which costs and benefits to the individual pay off. In addition, since dominants can take food from subordinates, resource depletion or availability may be less important for such animals than for subordinates. Dwarf mongoose groups, however, are often larger than this hypothetical optimum, and this increased size may reflect the optimum group size for subordinate animals. Since subordinates are the group members which are maximally engaged in group protection, vigilance, and babysitting, it would be to their advantage to have a larger group size so that these costs would be reduced per capita. As far as vigilance behavior is concerned, at least, the benefits of increased group size are minimal. The percentage of time spent performing vigilance behavior per individual in groups of different sizes does not vary significantly. What does change in larger groups, however, is the overlap time between guards, this resulting in increased security for the group as a whole and a reduction in the probability that a relieved guard will be predated (Rasa, 1986a).

More individuals participating in the attack on ground predators would also be of advantage to subordinates, since it would reduce the likelihood of a particular individual being killed in the interaction (Hamilton, 1971). More animals available for babysitting would also be of advantage, since more individuals could remain with the young, thus reducing the chances of their predation, especially by snakes and other herpestids, and also enabling shift changes to occur regularly. Finally, if food appropriation by dominants occurs frequently, as is the case, the costs of this to individual subordinates would be reduced in proportion to their numbers. All these factors would lead to a higher optimal group size for subordinate than for dominant animals.

Pulliam and Caraco (1984) make two assumptions regarding group size and predation: first, that attack rate is independent of group size, and second, that group life may exact a cost in terms of predation since groups are more conspicuous and predators are attracted to grouped prey. The data for dwarf mongooses, however, has shown that attack rate is not independent of group size but that small groups are attacked more frequently than large ones, probably because their vigilance system is less efficient. Both large and small groups, however, attract the same number of predation attempts so, for this species, attraction of predators is not a function of group size while attack rate is. This would tend toward the formation of larger groups to increase individual fitness. Since both males and females are actively engaged in group defense against predators, there would be no selection for sexual dimorphism where larger size is associated with the group defensive role, as is found in primates (Crook, 1972; Altmann, 1974).

In summary, therefore, group territoriality in dwarf mongooses appears to be distinctly advantageous, since the benefits derived by each individual outweigh the costs, at least in groups of approximately 12 individuals. Larger groups may reflect increased advantages to subordinate animals rather than dominant ones, since individual costs in such groups would be reduced. Large group size is also associated with a lower predation rate, which is of advantage to all group members. The constraining factor at extremely large group sizes is likely to be the individual energy expenditure involved in exploiting food resources rather than the depletion of these per se. It is when this cost outweighs the benefits incurred through the group protective factors that splinter groups are probably formed.

C. PROXIMATE AND ULTIMATE EFFECTS OF COMPENSATORY BEHAVIOR PATTERNS IN RELATION TO PREDATION

Within the framework of the ecological restraints of predator pressure, group size, and territory size, the dwarf mongoose has had to adapt its behavior to ensure maximum fitness at the level of the individual. We have already considered the adaptiveness and, in certain contexts, the maladaptiveness of two behavior patterns which appear to be phylogenetically fixed traits. Their proximate effects at the level of the individual have been shown. Their ultimate effects, however, can only be determined within the framework of the aforementioned constraints, especially that of predator pressure.

It is of significance that all the roles played by subordinate group members are associated with various aspects of group defense, either the defense of a certain age group (e.g., the babies), or the group as a whole. The fact that predator pressure on this species is very high has probably increased the adaptive value of such roles and has resulted in them being selected for in evolution, not only for the survival of the individual but that of the entire group, since small groups are exterminated. Survival of the group at near optimal size appears to be equated with reproductive success in dwarf mongooses, small groups being unable to raise their progeny owing to predation. Since group members are equally related from a genetic aspect (mother or father/full siblings, $r = \frac{1}{2}$), the survival of offspring of the alpha animals is of equal importance to all group members since these offspring represent an equivalent reproductive success to each individual. Only in this way can the presence of the various altruistic group-protective roles be explained from an evolutionary standpoint. In this context, the proximate effect of protection behavior is the survival of the individual. The ultimate effect, however, is the survival of the entire group as a reproductive unit. The data have shown that once group size drops below five individuals of 1 year old or more, the group loses all fitness and is itself eliminated through predation.

In this light, the adaptive significance of invalid care in this species becomes apparent. The proximate effect is the survival of the sick or injured group member. This behavior is altruistic only insofar as the group does not lose an adult member which could spell the difference between group survival and extinction at low group size. One would expect such behavior to be shown most frequently when group size is small. The data, however, do not suggest this. Of the five cases observed, the smallest group consisted of 19 individuals, the largest of 22 individuals; all groups exhibited invalid care. This behavior, however, may be preprogrammed in the genome as an adaptation whose greatest value is when group size is small. Its performance by large groups might be an atavism but could equally well be considered an insurance measure against sudden loss of several group members at once (e.g., through the formation of a splinter group or through disease).

The importance of only adult members to the group can be inferred from the fact that such care is *not* afforded to babies, at least those of 3 months old or less. Although this may be regarded as a case of investment and return (little having been invested in these young in comparison to adult animals), another interpretation would be that they do not contribute to group survival. Since they cannot contribute directly to the protection of the group, the group does not contribute to their protection. Whether such care would be afforded young in small groups where the survival of every individual is equivalent to the survival of the group has not been determined.

If the critical group size is five or more, then the question of group-member loss through intergroup fighting should be examined from the point of view of its ultimate adaptiveness. As previously described, the deployment of group members in such fights predestines the highly aggressive juvenile animals to such a fate. Their loss to the group may not be as severe as the loss of an adult animal, since they are not fully integrated into group-protective roles at this stage in their development. They form, however, a fairly effective method of gene exchange between groups, since almost half of them are successful in joining another group. During the time they live in such a group, however, they cannot be considered as increasing their inclusive fitness, since the members of the group are not related to them. Only on attainment of alpha position can they breed successfully and propagate their own genes. When within the group, they enjoy its protection and also play various group-protective roles, depending on their age and sex. This appears to be a case of reciprocal altruism (Trivers, 1971), these animals protecting nonrelated animals in return for their own protection.

The loss of juveniles is also most frequent in small groups. This reduces the natal group's survival potential, but since such groups have a low, or even zero, fitness, such juveniles may represent a means by which the group's genes are not irrevocably lost to the population as a whole, since they have an approximately 50% chance of joining another group and may achieve reproductive status there.

The difference in the deployment of group members in the attack of strange groups and predators on the ground can be considered as a balance between risk and benefit to the group as a whole. Although the mechanisms which result in such changes in deployment have yet to be determined experimentally (one possible key factor may be the behavior of the alpha male under the two conditions), the ultimate effect is that the animals most likely to be more efficient in coping with the danger inherent in the two conditions are the ones to confront this danger first. In the case of intergroup altercations, the alpha male and juveniles have a high aggressivity toward outsiders, over 200% higher than that of other group members. The risks involves in such fights, however, are low from the point of view of injuries received or group members killed. The only risk appears to be the loss of a group member by detachment (usually a juvenile), at least in resident groups. This loss, however, should not be equated with loss through predation, since these juveniles have a 50% chance of survival by joining another group and one group's loss is another one's gain. In cases where high risk of injury or death occur (e.g., attack of predators on the ground), it is the older, experienced males which initiate the interaction. Although they are valuable group members in the various group protective roles, their value to the group is very likely to be less than that of the alpha male. The nonparticipation of inexperienced juveniles in such interactions, or, at most, their participation in the background, is self-evidently adaptive in such circumstances where their inexperience would probably result in their being killed or injured. However, data are required to substantiate the hypothesis that there is a higher risk factor for inexperienced animals in interactions with predators. Since, however, juveniles have not been observed to attack predators first in either the field or the laboratory, their risk relative to that of experienced adults cannot be determined under normal group-living conditions.

The proximate effects of such defense strategies is that the risk of death to a member of the group is reduced. The ultimate effect is, as discussed previously, that the group itself is not brought to a point where the loss of one of its members could mean extinction for the entire group as a reproductive entity.

The importance of maintaining a group with five or more adult members may also explain the extremely low intrafamilial aggressivity shown by this species and the behavior patterns developed to substitute for overt fighting. The tendency for dwarf mongooses to attack as a group is of great advantage in interactions with group enemies but not when directed toward group members themselves. The attention of the animals is then directed toward the combatants and not toward potential predators. Although no cases of the predation of animals during a mass attack on one of the group members has been observed, such attacks being so rare, the potential risks may be inferred from observations of predation during intergroup fights. Three animals have been observed killed during such fights, all by brown harrier eagles (*Circaetus cinereus*).

Since it appears that intragroup fights may be risky situations since they allow predators to approach unseen, the adoption of behavior patterns allowing for altercations to take place without attracting predators and without disturbing the group's normal vigilance behavior would be of great advantage. The use of grooming, a relatively spatially static behavior pattern, in this context appears to be adaptive since it does not involve violent movements. During such altercations, the remainder of the group shows no tendency to participate, remains passive, and maintains its vigilance against predators.

The mechanisms inhibiting overt fighting within the group also appear to be in effect in the case of detachment of splinter groups. Here also, no obvious altercation between the females concerned has been observed. Such an altercation would not only be of danger to the parent group but of even greater danger to the newly formed splinter group itself. In the case of the latter, not only small group size but also the necessity to establish a new guarding rota as well as to learn a new living space would all be factors increasing predation liability.

Apart from the proximate effects of reducing predation at the time of the altercation, the ultimate effects of a strategy of reduced overt aggression within the group must also be considered. If the number of animals comprising the group is essential to the survival of the group itself, then a life strategy in which frequent overt aggression takes place could lead to a high rate of group-member loss through injury or expulsion from the group as well as through predation. Such a strategy would be of detriment to the group as a whole, especially since effective mechanisms are present to prevent rapid replacement of such losses, and would result in the group's extinction should the number of animals drop below the critical level.

D.   SELECTION MECHANISMS AND CONCLUSIONS

Dwarf mongoose group life and social structure, together with modifications in behavioral systems to optimize these, appear to be an adaptation for survival under conditions of high predator pressure. Groups consist predominantly of highly related individuals where the evolution of altruistic behavior patterns which enhance the survival of other group members can be attributed to kin selection (Maynard-Smith, 1964; Dawkins, 1976; Wilson, 1975). Personal genetic fitness in the sense of the rearing of own offspring is prevented by various behavioral means for the majority of the group members. However, since the reproductive unit consists mainly of direct family, each group member sharing half the genes of every other member, personal reproduction for every individual is not necessary from the point of view of individual fitness. It is not the actual production of young which is a measure of individual fitness, but their survival. By relinquishing personal reproduction and helping to rear their parent's offspring, siblings do not lose inclusive fitness but gain it on two levels. First, by their presence in the group and their performance of group-protective behavior patterns, they aid in the survival of the young directly. Second, simply by remaining in a reproductively efficient group (more than five animals) their own chances of survival are enhanced. Only when sufficient group members are present to share the costs of rearing young by assuming protective roles do dwarf mongoose young survive, since small groups have been shown to have zero fitness in this respect.

The production of young by all group members capable of doing so would be disadvantageous for the entire group. It would deplete territory resources and entail higher energy expenditure in the finding of food for all group members. The alleviation of pressure on the territory through the production of large numbers of splinter groups would also not add to the inclusive fitness of the natal group, since the splinter groups have a low survival rate as well. One possible means of increasing splinter-group survival rates would be the production of large splinter groups with more than five individuals. Although this may aid in a particular unit's survival, it must be remembered that the group would be genetically identical with the natal group. According to Darwin's (1859) hypothesis, the highest level of competition would be expected between genetically identical individuals. The presence of two genetically identical groups in the area would thus be of great disadvantage to the natal group if territories were contested.

The data have shown that selection in the dwarf mongoose operates on two levels: the level of the individual, when applied to single group members, and the level of the group as a reproductive unit once its membership drops below the critical level. According to Wilson (1975), a dwarf mongoose group can be considered a true Mendelian population, since it is a nearly closed society which exchanges only a small fraction of its members with other societies each generation. Since immigrants behave in the same way toward unrelated group members as do kin among themselves and vice versa, kin selection can be equated in this case with interdemic selection. The fact that entire groups become extinct once their numbers sink below the critical level of five suggests that interdemic selection may also be functioning at these population density levels. This could be the explanation for the fact that territories, once vacant, are not repopulated for several years (Levins, 1970).

Group life for the dwarf mongoose is thus an interplay of selection factors whose classification depends on the relatedness of the individuals in the group in question (i.e., number of immigrants present) and the size of the group at any one time. Whether or not group size is regulated by predation, disease, or behavioral mechanisms within it, its optimum appears to lie at approximately 11 individuals and its minimum at 5. Group life appears to have evolved as a means of protection against predators, not only of the young, as in many animals which form groups during the breeding season, but of the adult members as well. Behavioral mechanisms have evolved to counter both avian and ground predation, these being more or less effective depending on the predator concerned. Reduced conspicuousness in intragroup interactions also appears to be a means evolved to evade the notice of predators, and the whole system appears to be geared for group as well as individual survival.

Acknowledgments

I wish to thank the Deutsche Forschungsgemeinschaft for their continued financial support of the dwarf mongoose research project over the last 16 years and the Heisenberg Stipendium Commission for the opportunity to conduct the field studies. I should also like to thank Ray Mayers for kindly allowing me to carry out the fieldwork on his ranch in Kenya.

References

Abegglen, J. J. (1976). On socialization in hamadryas baboons. Ph.D. dissertation, University of Zürich.

Altmann, S. A. (1974). Baboons, space, time and energy. *Am. Zool.* **14,** 221–248.

Baker, C. M. (1980). Biology and behaviour of the slender mongoose, *Herpestes sanguineus* (Rüppel, 1934). M.Sc. thesis, University of Natal, Pietermaritzburg.

Baker, C. M. (1984). Social care behaviour in captive slender mongooses (*Herpestes sanguineus*). *Mammalia* **48,** 43–52.

Bertram, B. C. R. (1975). Social factors influencing reproduction in wild lions. *J. Zool.* **177,** 462–482.

Bertram, B. C. R. (1976). Kin selection in lions and in evolution. In "Growing Points in Ethology" (P. P. G. Bateson and R. A. Hinde, eds.), pp. 281–301. Cambridge University Press, Cambridge.

Brown, J. L. (1982). Optimal group size in territorial animals. *J. Theor. Biol.* **95,** 793–810.

Bygott, J. D., Bertram, B. C. R., and Hanby, J. P. (1979). Male lions in large coalitions gain reproductive advantages. *Nature (London)* **282,** 839–841.

Carl, E. A. (1971). Population control in Artic ground squirrels. *Ecology* **52,** 395–413.

Cheeseman, C. L., Jones, G. W., Gallagher, J., and Mallison, P. J. (1981). The population structure, density and prevalence of tuberculosis in badgers (*Meles meles*) from four areas in South West England. *J. Appl. Ecol.* **18,** 795–804.

Clutton-Brock, T. H., Guinness, F. E., and Albon, S. D. (1982). "Red Deer: Behavior and Ecology of Two Sexes." Chicago University Press, Chicago.

Crook, J. H. (1965). The adaptive significance of avian social organizations. *Symp. Zool. Soc. London* **14,** 181–218.

Crook, J. H. (1972). Sexual selection, dimorphism and social organization in the primates. *In* "Sexual Selection and the Descent of Man" (B. Campbell, ed.), pp. 231–281. Aldine, Chicago.

Crook, J. H., Ellis, J. E., and Goss-Custard, J. D. (1976). Mammalian social systems: Structure and function. *Anim. Behav.* **24,** 261–274.

Darwin, C. R. (1859). "The Origin of Species." John Murray, London.

Dawkins, R. (1976). "The Selfish Gene." Oxford University Press, Oxford.

Drickamer, L. C., and Vessey, S. H. (1973). Group changing in free ranging rhesus monkeys. *Primates* **14,** 359–368.

Ewer, R. F. (1963). The behaviour of the meerkat, *Suricata suricatta* (Schreber). *Z. Tierpsychol.* **20,** 570–607.

Ewer, R. F. (1973). "The Carnivores." Cornell University Press, New York.

Ghiglieri, M. P. (1985). The social ecology of chimpanzees. *Sci. Am.* **252,** 84–91.

Gosling, L. M. (1974). The social ethology of Coke's Hartebeeste, *Alcelaphus busclaphus cokei.* (Gunther). *In:* "The Behaviour of Ungulates and Its Relation to Management" (V. Geist and F. Walther, eds.), pp. 488–511. I.U.C.N. Switzerland.

Hamilton, W. D. (1971). Geometry for the selfish herd. *J. Theor. Biol.* **31,** 295–311.

Itani, J., Tokuda, K., Furuya, Y., Kano, K., and Shin, Y. (1963). The social structure of natural troops of Japanese monkeys in Takasakiyama. *Primates* **4,** 1–42.

Jarman, P. J. (1974). The social organization of antelope in relation to their ecology. *Behaviour* **48,** 215–267.

Kaufmann, L. W., and Rovee-Collier, C. K. (1978). Arousal-induced changes in the amplitude of death feigning and periodicity. *Physiol. Behav.* **20,** 453–458.

Klingel, H. (1969). Reproduction in the plains zebra *Equus burchelli boehmi*. Behavioural and ecological factors. *J. Reprod. Fertil.* Suppl. 6, 339–345.

Kruuk, H. (1972). "The Spotted Hyena." University of Chicago Press, Chicago.

Kruuk, H., and McDonald, D. (1985). Group territories of carnivores: Empires and enclaves. *In* "Behavioural Ecology" (R. M. Sidley and R. H. Smith, eds.), pp. 521–536. Blackwell Scientific Publications, Oxford.

Kruuk, H., and Parish, T. (1982). Factors affecting population density, group size and territory size in the European badger *Meles meles*. *J. Zool.* **196,** 31–39.

Kummer, H. (1968). "Social Organization of Hamadryas Baboons." Karger, Basel.

Kummer, H. (1971). "Primate Societies: Group Techniques of Ecological Adaptation." Aldine, Chicago.

Kummer, H., Gotz, W., and Angst, W. (1974). Triadic differentiation: An inhibitory process protecting pair bonds in baboons. *Behaviour* **49,** 62–87.

Levins, R. (1970). Extinction. *In* "Some Mathematical Questions in Biology," Lectures on mathematics in the life sciences Vol. 2, pp. 77–107. American Mathematical Society, Providence, RI.

Liberg, O. (1981). Predation and social behaviour in a population of domestic cat: An evolutionary perspective. Ph.D. dissertation, University of Lund, Sweden.

Lindstrom, E. (1980). The red fox in a small game community of the south taiga region in Sweden. *In* "The Red Fox" (E. Zimen, ed.), pp. 177–184. Junk, Den Haag.

Lorenz, K. (1965). "Der Kumpan in der Umwelt des Vogels." D. T.V., München.

McDonald, D. W. (1983). The ecology of carnivore social behaviour. *Nature (London)* **301,** 379–384.

Maynard-Smith, J. (1964). Group selection and kin selection. *Nature (London)* **201,** 1145–1147.

Mech, L. D. (1966). "The wolves of Isle Royale." Fauna of the Nat. Parks of the U.S.A. Fauna Series 7.

Meier, V., Rasa, O. A. E., and Scheich, H. (1983). Call-system similarity in a ground-living social bird and a mammal in the bush habitat. *Behav. Ecol. Sociobiol.* **12,** 5–9.

Moehlman, P. D. (1979). Jackal helpers and pup survival. *Nature (London)* **277,** 382–383.

Moehlman, P. D. (1983). Sociobiology of silverbacked and golden jackals (*Canis mesomelas, C. aureus*). *In* "Recent Advances in the Study of Mammalian Behavior" (J. F. Eisenberg and D. G. Kleiman, eds.), pp. 423–453. Special Publ. No. 7, The American Society of Mammalogists.

Pilsworth, R. (1977). Altruistic mongooses tend their sick friend. *New Sci.* **73,** 517.

Pulliam, H. R. (1976). The principle of optimal behavior and the theory of communities. *In* "Perspectives in Ethology," Vol. 2 (P. P. G. Bateson and P. H. Klopfer, eds.), pp. 311–332. Plenum, New York.

Pulliam, H. R., and Caraco, T. (1984). Living in groups: Is there an optimal group size? *In* "Behavioural Ecology, An Evolutionary Approach" (J. R. Krebs and N. B. Davies, eds.), pp. 122–147. Blackwell Scientific Publications, Oxford.

Rasa, O. A. E. (1972). Aspects of social organization in captive dwarf mongooses. *J. Mammal.* **53,** 181–185.

Rasa, O. A. E. (1973a). Marking behaviour and its social significance in the African dwarf mongoose (*Helogale undulata rufula*). *Z. Tierpsychol.* **32,** 293–318.

Rasa, O. A. E. (1973b). Prey capture, feeding techniques and their ontogeny in the African dwarf mongoose (*Helogale undulata rufula*). *Z. tierpsychol.* **32,** 449–488.

Rasa, O. A. E. (1973c). Intra-familial sexual repression in the dwarf mongoose *Helogale parvula*. *Die Naturwissenschaften* **60,** 303–304.

Rasa, O. A. E. (1976). Invalid care in the dwarf mongoose (*Helogale undulata rufula*). *Z. Tierpsychol.* **42,** 337–342.

Rasa, O. A. E. (1977a). The ethology and sociology of the dwarf mongoose (*Helogale undulata rufula*). Z. Tierpsychol. **43**, 337–406.

Rasa, O.A. E. (1977b). Differences in group member response to intruding conspecifics and potentially dangerous stimuli in dwarf mongooses (*Helogale undulata rufula*). Z. Säugetierkunde **42**, 108–112.

Rasa, O. A. E. (1979). The effects of crowding on the social relationships and behaviour of the dwarf mongoose (*Helogale undulata rufula*). Z. Tierpsychol. **49**, 317–329.

Rasa, O. A. E. (1983a). A case of invalid care in wild dwarf mongooses. Z. Tierpsychol. **62**, 235–240.

Rasa, O. A. E. (1983b). Dwarf mongoose and hornbill mutualism in the Taru Desert, Kenya. Behav. Ecol. Sociobiol. **12**, 181–190.

Rasa, O. A. E. (1985). "Mongoose Watch." John Murray, London.

Rasa, O. A. E. (1986a). Coordinated vigilance in dwarf mongoose family groups: the 'watchman's song' hypothesis and the costs of guarding. Z. Tierpsychol. **71**, 340–344.

Rasa, O. A. E. (1986b). Ecological factors and their relationship to group size, mortality and behaviour in the dwarf mongoose. Cimbebasia **8**, 15–21.

Rasa, O. A. E. (1987). Vigilance behaviour in the dwarf mongoose: Its costs and effectiveness in relation to inclusive fitness. Beh. Ecol. Sociobiol., in press.

Rasa, O. A. E., and van den Höövel, H. (1984). Social stress in the fieldvole: Differential causes of death in relation to behaviour and social structure. Z. Tierpsychol. **65**, 108–133.

Reich, A. (1981). The behaviour and ecology of the African wild dog in Kruger National Park. Ph.D. dissertation, Yale University.

Roberts, K. S. (1981). The foraging behaviour and strategies of the Suricate Suricata suricatta (Erxleben). M.Sc. thesis, University of Pretoria.

Rood, J. P. (1974). Banded mongoose males guard young. Nature (London) **248**, 176.

Rood, J. P. (1983). Banded mongoose rescues pack member from eagle. Anim. Behav. **31**, 1261–1262.

Rood, J. P. (1984). Pack life of the dwarf mongoose. In "The Encyclopaedia of Mammals, 1 (D. McDonald, ed.), pp. 152–153. Allen and Unwin, London.

Sade, D. (1972). A longitudinal study of social behaviour of rhesus monkeys. In "The Functional and Evolutionary Biology of Primates" (A. Tuttle, ed.), pp. 378–398. Aldine, Chicago.

Sargeant, C. B., and Eberhardt, L. E. (1975). Death-feigning by ducks in response to predation by red foxes (*Vulpes fulva*). Am. Midl. Nat. **94**, 108–119.

Schaller, G. (1963). "The mountain gorilla: Ecology and Behavior." University of Chicago Press, Chicago.

Schaller, G. (1972). "The Serengeti Lion: A study of Predator–Prey Relationships." University of Chicago Press, Chicago.

Sinclair, A. R. E. (1977). "The African Buffalo: A Study of Resource Limitation of Populations. University of Chicago Press, Chicago.

Smithers, R. H. N. (1971). "The mammals of Botswana." Mardon Printers, Salisbury, Rhodesia.

Struhsaker, T. (1975). Two Cusimanse mongooses attack a black cobra. J. Mammal. **56**, 721–722.

Sullivan, K. E. (1984). The advantages of social foraging in downy woodpeckers. Anim. Behav. **32**, 16–22.

Taylor, J. (1976). The advantage of spacing out. J. Theor. Biol. **59**, 485–490.

Tortora, D. F., and Borchelt, P. L. (1972). The effect of escape responses on immobility in bobwhite quail (*Colinus virginianus*). Psychon. Sci. **27**, 129–130.

Trivers, R. L. (1971). The evolution of reciprocal altruism. Rev. Biol. **46**,35–57.

van Lawick-Goodall, J. (1968). The behaviour of free-living chimpanzees in the Gombe Stream Reserve. Anim. Behav. Monogr. **1**, 165–311.

van Lawick-Goodall, J. (1973). The behaviour of chimpanzees in their natural habitat. *Am. J. Psychiatry* **130,** 1–12.

Vogel, C. (1976). Ökologie, Lebensweise und Sozialverhalten der Grauen Languren in verschiedenen Biotopen Indiens. *Z. tierpsychol.* Beiheft 17.

von Holst, D. (1969). Sozialer Stress bei Tupajas, *Tupaia belengeri. Z. Vgl. Physiol.* **63,** 1–58.

Wilson, E. O. (1975). "Sociobiology: The New Synthesis." Belknap Press of Harvard University Press, Cambridge, Massachusetts.

Winkler, P., Loch, H., and Vogel, C. (1984). Life history of Hanuman langurs (*Presbytis entellus*). Reproductive parameters, infant mortality and troop development. *Folia Primatol.* **43,** 1–23.

Zimen, E. (1971). Wölfe und Königspudel. *In* "Studies in Ethology" (W. Wickler, ed.). Piper Verlag, Munich.

Ontogenetic Development of Behavior: The Cricket Visual World

Raymond Campan, Guy Beugnon, and Michel Lambin

CENTRE DE RECHERCHE EN BIOLOGIE DU COMPORTEMENT
U.A. C.N.R.S. NO. 664
UNIVERSITÉ PAUL SABATIER
31062 TOULOUSE CEDEX, FRANCE

Research in ethology primarily concerns behavioral observations under natural or experimental conditions; that is, one begins inductively with an analysis of observed events and attempts to set up a causal system which accounts for the observations. Actually, the choice of the behavior patterns to be observed, and of the units of description, always involves implicitly or explicitly a more general preexisting conceptual framework, one which indicates that research also entails a deductive dimension. Even though some researchers do not admit it and claim they are objective when they record behavioral events, such objectivity remains relative; thus both the analysis and the ensuing scientific synthesis involve operations of the mind.

Therefore, more than in other more mechanistic biological disciplines, ethological data are images of a behavioral reality in which the inductive and deductive processes are combined in a subtle way to lead a particular observer to produce scientific claims. Unlike most ethological papers which present first the inductive aspects, such as the variables selected to be recorded along with the methods to be used for analyzing data, in this article the deductive principles are presented first by stating the theoretical framework of the research; the research is then presented.

I. Some Theoretical Principles

Let us start with Tolman's basic definition of observed behavior, "the motor activity of the animal as a whole." Such an operational definition can be improved by combining it with von Uexküll's classical point of view (1934) in which behavior appears as dialectic functional cycles of reciprocal interaction between an animal and its "own world" (*Umwelt*). The observed motor activity

165

both depends upon the environment and acts upon it. The action of the environment on behavior proceeds through a species-specific action system. Such an "own world" is then separated into two parts: a sensory world (*Merkwelt*) and an action world (*Wirkwelt*).

The basic concept of *Umwelt* is unavoidable, and it involves, in ethology, severe limitations which have to be stressed and cannot be bypassed. The moment it becomes a field of study, the animal's whole Umwelt becomes part of the observer's Umwelt. He or she describes the animal's Umwelt, does experiments on it, and conceptualizes it. Then the observer acts on it with his or her own action system and perceives it through his or her own specific sensory systems, often with the help of convenient technology. This means the observer is condemned to perceive the animal world, and its functional cycles, only as they overlap with the observer's world or what that world allows him or her to deduce about it. The observer will attribute to the form and description of these functional cycles no more than his or her own capacities allow. This is a fundamental limitation on the observer who can thus only build a partial description. Such an epistemological limitation must not prevent us, however, from continuing to use the concept of the animal's Umwelt.

Since 1963, when Tinbergen defined the future goals of ethology by four questions (What are the immediate causes of behavior? What are its functions? How did it develop during ontogeny? How did it change during phylogeny?), von Uexküll's initial viewpoint has been modified significantly. The world of actions, as well as the world of perceptions (limited by the sensory–motor capacities of the animal which are, at least partly, species specific), characterize an individual at a particular moment of its history. The Umwelt must take into account both the unique genotype of the animal (Jacquard, 1978) and its unique ontogeny. Moreover, the repeated behavioral performances by an animal are never identical, at the very least because behavior takes place at different times in its life. Also, the world of the animal has to be considered, in several respects, as modifiable: it can change objectively with time and with development of the sensory–motor capacities of the animal, as well as through changes in the actual meaning of that world according to the individual's experience and the effect of practice. This idea has been extensively developed by Schneirla (1965), who proposed that behavioral ontogeny rests on two historical processes: maturation and experience. A revision of von Uexküll's concepts in the light of those of Schneirla no longer leads us to consider functional cycles as species specific and timeless closed loops; by contrast, the concepts of individuality and chronology have to be introduced in order to stress historical rather than immediate interactions.

For a complete account the observer must describe the result of one or more dialectic processes, here and now, as well as the whole history of the relationship between the individual and its world, from the origin of that individuality, i.e., its genotype. Within such a theoretical framework (and phylogenetic limits), the behavioral concepts of developmental biology can apply. Concerning the embryology of structures and the emergence of functions, Beetschen (1984) writes that "the unrolling of a development program has to rely upon a permanent integration of genetic and epigenetic factors interacting with each other." Gottlieb (1973), in a book on behavioral embryology, distinguishes predetermined epigenesis, in which the developmental steps take place according to a pattern and a predetermined chronology, and probabilistic epigenesis, in which the feedback effects of behavior modulate the routes taken during ontogeny. In that case there would be a homologous relationship between the regulatory processes affecting differentiating structures during embryogenesis and the processes which affect behavioral ontogeny through both functional cycles and the dialectic between an individual and its world. The concepts of developmental biology are also used by Schneirla (1965) to describe behavioral development in terms of processes of maturation and experience which are not only correlated but coalescent at each stage.

Von Uexküll's concept of Umwelt as we have modified it fits, of course, within the framework of probabilistic epigenesis (Campan, 1980). Through it we get closer to a set of ideas concerning behavioral development which have been independently proposed in both ethology and child psychology. Such a trend could be characterized as *constructivist*. This word was used to describe the A/W theory of Schneirla by Richard (1974): an individual's experience is established through approach processes (A) aroused by any low-intensity stimulus source and withdrawal processes (W) by any high-intensity stimulus source. The term *constructivisim* has also been used by Piaget (1977) to define genetic epistemology; the development of intelligence in the child is a construction following successive steps through assimilation processes, which occur when a new element is incorporated into a structure, and accomodation processes, which occur when this new element modifies that structure. Constructivism could also be applied to another giant of child psychology, Wallon, who is very close to Schneirla and who considered behavior holistically as a continuous "édification et construction de la personne" running from the earliest stage in child development through the action of internal and external factors in which maturation and experience are combined. He writes (Wallon, 1941): "D'étapes en étapes, la psychogenèse de l'enfant montre à travers la complexité des facteurs et des fonctions, à travers la diversité et l'opposition des crises qui la ponctuent, une sorte d'unité solidaire, tant à l'intérieur de chacune qu'entre elles toutes. Il est contre nature de traiter l'enfant fragmentairement. A chaque âge, il constitue un ensemble indissociable et original."

Through such constructivism, which represents one particular conception of behavioral development, the dialectic processes of animal–world interaction and the coaction of maturation and experience become systems and dynamic totalities. Such a point of view was presented by Gautier *et al.* (1978) as a cybernetic model. The individual–environment system is included as one of several self-regulated "homeorhetic" systems. The use of Waddington's term *homeorhetic* stresses that development is progressive and not static, as connoted by "homeostatic." The dialectic opposition of organism and environment appears as a temporal patterning of homeorhetic adjustments, the result of the coevolution and coadaptation of organisms and their environments. These authors refer to assimilation and accomodation processes as described by Piaget to account for such adjustments.

We have taken a similar stand (Campan, 1980), defining behavior as the dynamic expression of dialectic relationships between an individual and its world. The theoretical interpretation that we are defending leads us to consider two subsystems partially overlapping and combined: the individual and its world. Each subsystem consists of many interacting elements combined to constitute a whole system, giving rise to a unique emergent which, here and now, is behavior. This individual–world system is dynamic as a result of its autonomy (Vendryès, 1981); its ontogeny is then an individual adventure proceeding according to the model of probabilistic epigenesis and following, because of its autonomy, the rules of self-organization (Varela, 1983).

Our work lies within such a theoretical framework which is, at once, constructivist, systemic, and self-organizing with respect, necessarily, to a limited behavioral target: the ontogenic construction of the visual world of the cricket. In the first part of this article we deal with the developmental changes of some psychophysiological conditions controlling the selection of visual information; these factors are only parts of the various interacting elements within the individual subsystem. In the second part, we study, from the same ontogenetic viewpoint, some complex, interactive, and highly variable ecological conditions within the environmental subsystem. Of course such an approach cannot be exhaustive. However, we may consider that the eventual involvement of new factors of a psychophysiological or environmental nature, which remains possible at any time, would affect only slightly the general processes of behavioral ontogeny.

In the third part, the history of a number of behavioral emergents within such a developing visual world is reported. Finally, we attempt to derive the consequences of our model by drawing several possible general rules governing the behavioral changes in the course of individual development.

Five different species of crickets were studied, depending on the questions asked and the techniques required: *Nemobius sylvestris* (Ns), *Pteronemobius lineolatus* (Pl), *Pteronemobius heydeni* (Ph), *Gryllus campestris* (Gc), and *Gryllus bimaculatus* (Gb).

II.   Psychophysiological Factors Involved
in the Selection and Use of Visual Information

Psychophysiological factors are considered at two interactive levels: competence of the visual and motor systems, on the one hand, and performance, i.e., the perceptive and motor capacities revealed by visual orientation, on the other. We cannot pretend to cover the field exhaustively, but can only propose a model, with its general rules of development, that can be applied to the whole subsystem.

A.   Development of Competence

In the successive larval instars in Ns (Goulet *et al.*, 1981), the number of ommatidia within the compound eyes increases progressively from about 300 to around 1200, which, of course, improves the precision of the spatial analysis of the visual world. Rather irregularly distributed at first, the ommatidia eventually are organized in very regular rows. Such growth is correlated with an increase in the interocular zone, a slight reduction of the total visual field, and, above all, an important broadening of the binocular field (Fig. 1A); these changes should improve relief and depth perception. Each ommatidium with its fused rhabdom modifies its own structure during ontogeny, at first by thickening the corneal lens and lengthening the crystalline cone, thus improving the convergence of refracted light on the rhabdom end. The increase in the number and length of the ommatidia during ontogeny consequently reduces the ommatidial angle from 11 to 5° on average (Fig. 1A), thus allowing a more precise spatial analysis of forms in the visual world. We also know, by recording the receptor potential from individual retinula cells, that the extent of the receptive field of the rhabdom in adults (acceptance angle) does not exceed the value of the interommatidial angle (Lambin and Jeanrot, 1982).

Campan and Honegger (1986) reviewed some data concerning Gb. In this species, the ommatidia from the posterior and ventral sides of the eye have larger diameters than the central ones, but with flat corneal lenses. Furthermore, the cells from the dorsal edge of the eye are more sensitive to blue, and they have visual fields ranging from 10 to >35°; they also are very sensitive to polarized light (Labhart *et al.*, 1984). By contrast, the neighboring cells from the rest of the dorsal area respond to green and UV with a narrow acceptance angle (5.9 ± 2.2). The number of ommatidia in adult Gc is about 3100. Finally, Fig. 1B compares the general structure of the visual field in Gc and Ns.

Only limited data are available concerning the neural structures integrating the visual information (Campan and Honegger, 1986). As in other insects, crickets have three neuropiles (the lamina, the medulla, and the lobula) connected

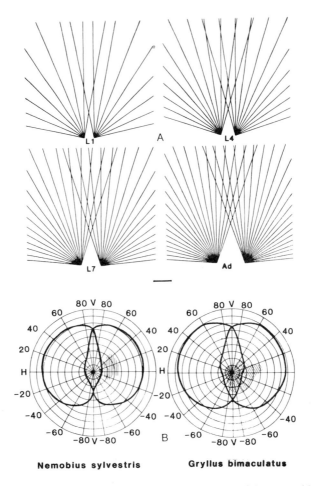

Nemobius sylvestris   Gryllus bimaculatus

FIG. 1. (A) Ontogenetic changes in the optic axis geometry of the ommatidia from both eyes in *Nemobius sylvestris*. L1, L4, L7, larval instars 1, 4, 7; Ad, adults. Bar, 1 mm. (B) Extent of the cricket visual field in polar coordinates (V, vertical plane; H, horizontal plane). The hatched area corresponds to the fixation zone of the eye determined by behavioral experiments in *N. sylvestris* and by electrophysiology in *Gryllus bimaculatus*.

through chiasmas. The optic tract of Gc contains about 1500 afferent fibers. If we compare that number with the 3100 ommatidia, each including eight retinule cells, the information reaching the brain is already very convergent, even if the columnar organization within the neuropiles suggests that the spatial projection of visual information is preserved. Interneurons lying between the two optic lobes should be able to perform some binocular comparison (Honegger and Schürmann, 1975). There are also projections into the protocerebron (calix of the mushroom bodies, central complex), connections with the ocellar nerves, and projections into the deutocerebron, as well as possibilities of comparison with other sensory modalities; as a matter of fact, many multimodal interneurons respond jointly to acoustical, mechanical, and chemical stimulation, whether they are intrasegmental or intersegmental, such as, for instance, the descending interneurons connecting the brain to the motoneurons responsible for orientation behavior (Richard *et al.*, 1985). The neuronal structures and mechanisms underlying locomotion, particularly those controlling leg movement, were studied in Gb by Laurent (1985). However, none of the nerve structures involved in the neuroethology of visual orientation has been, as yet, studied during ontogeny. Nevertheless, at the very least, motor competence for orientation behavior must improve during development because of the growth of legs.

B.   DEVELOPMENT OF PERFORMANCE

Perceptual capabilities improve during ontogeny along with the development of competency of the sense organs. Campan and Honegger (1986) reviewed the relevant data.

1.   Visual Acuity

Visual acuity was measured in Ns by the spontaneous choice method. The *minimum visible* was defined as the minimum angle at which an object has to be seen to be perceived; that is, the minimum angle at which a black target induces a scototactic response (Campan and Médioni, 1963). This threshold is 1° for the first larval instar and much lower for the adult (Fig. 2); it is in any case much smaller than the ommatidium opening angle. The threshold rises with target distance (Fig. 2) as well as when contrast conditions between the target and the background are impaired. The effect of contrast is stronger for young animals. The *minimum separable* is the minimum angle between two objects allowing them to be perceived as visually separated. It has been evaluated in adult Ns by measuring the spontaneous preference for checkboards of different sizes. We found an approximate value of 4°30', which fits both the ommatidial angle and the receptive field of the rhabdoms. One can imagine that the first larval instar in which the interommatidial angle is almost twice that of the adult will have a much poorer *minimum separable,* which is, of course, an important limitation on form perception.

2.   Form Perception

An animal has to perform visual scanning to see an object whose angular size is greater than the visual acuity threshold. As a matter of fact we know that in mammals, as well as in insects (Diptera), relative movement between the target and the retina is necessary to prevent receptor adaptation and to enable form

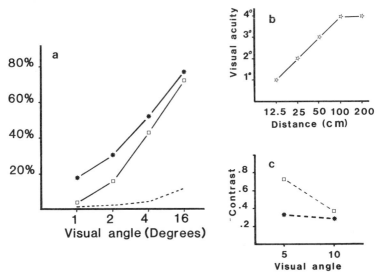

FIG. 2. Visual acuity in *Nemobius sylvestris*. (a) Percentage of scototactic orientation depending on the angular width of the black vertical target. The short dashes indicate the theoretical random level of orientation toward each screen. *, Adult; □, larval instar 1. (b) Changes in visual acuity with the distance of the target (adults). (c) Threshold differences for a significant scototactic response according to the contrast between the target and the background. Comparison between two values of target angular size for two different developmental stages (□, 5–6 larval instar, *, adult).

perception. Figure 3A shows the results when a tethered Ns, allowed to indicate its orientation by turning a polystyrofoam ball held with its legs, walks toward a black target and scans visually by moving its head. When its head is waxed to the thorax, the orientation disappears. However, orientation is again possible if the target is illuminated with a flickering light whose frequency is kept below 4 to 5 Hz. The same low critical frequency is also found in other physiological responses which could be functionally associated with visual scanning. Thus, the intracellular "on" response of the retinula cells is a large spike which disappears at 5 Hz when the eye is stimulated with a variable frequency flickering light (Lambin *et al.*, 1985). In the same vein, a tethered animal performs head oscillations with a 2–3 Hz frequency; a freely moving cricket keeps its head motionless relative to the thorax, but its orientation walk toward the target is broken by very short stops whose frequency is 2–3 Hz. Finally, in a study of interneurons carrying visual information in Gb down to the thorax where the motor commands lie, Richard *et al.* (1985) found that when the eye is stimulated with a flickering light of increasing frequency, the individual cutoff frequencies range from 4 or 5 Hz to 40 Hz. The amplitude of the head oscillation of a tethered animal and oscillation of the body axis of a freely moving cricket are both around 5° and

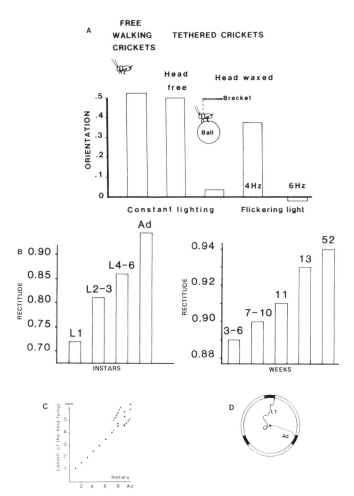

FIG. 3. (A) Variation of the orientation index according to different conditions of relative movement between an animal and a target (*Nemobius sylvestris*). (B) Change of the rectitude ($0 < R < = 1$; R, radius of the platform/length of the trail) of target orientation routes according to age in two different situations: field orientation (left) and classical scototaxis (right). Ad, Adult. (C) Corresponding growth of femur length. (D) Examples of scototactic orientation routes for a first instar larva and an adult.

cover 1–2 ommatidial rows (Lambin *et al.*, 1981). Visual form perception, therefore, requires visual scanning which is performed by either head or body oscillations whose amplitude corresponds to at least one ommatidial row and whose frequency approaches 2–3 Hz. Obviously, given such conditions, the perceptual performance of a first instar larva will be different because the interommatidial angle is approximately 11° and the legs and body are much smaller

than in adults; thus, visual scanning requires larger amplitude oscillations. This
might account for the fact that, in experiments of orientation toward a target, the
routes of young animals are much less direct and straight (Fig. 3D) (Campan *et
al.*, 1975; Campan and Gautier, 1975; Beugnon *et al.*, 1983).

Form perception also implies the use of a fixation area on the retina. As a
matter of fact, in Ns, precise analysis of the position of the body axis (including
the head) relative to the target shows that during the orientation walk the insect
eye fixates one of the two edges of the target with a particular area of the retina
(Lambin, 1985) located around 20° lateral to the sagittal plane (Fig. 4). This area
corresponds to a part of the field which lies at the edge of the binocular field.
Such a functional heterogeneity of the retina has also been demonstrated by
measuring the orientation performance of a tethered cricket when the target is
successively presented to every part of the visual field. This functional exploration reveals a retinal area particularly effective in releasing a positively oriented

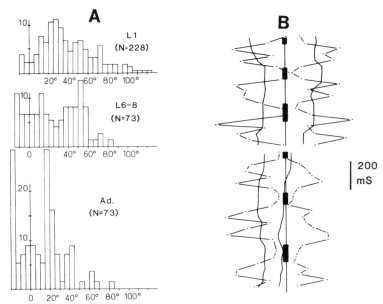

FIG. 4. Visual fixation in *Nemobius sylvestris* (A) Variation during ontogeny of the
horizontal angular projections of a black target edge on the visual field during an orientation walk. 0°, Position of the sagittal axis; the negative values correspond to the con-
tralateral part of the binocular field. Vertical axis indicates percentage of total. (B) The
vertical straight line represents the body axis during orientation toward a black target. The
animal's path runs from the lower part of the diagram to the upper. The continuous lines
on both sides of the sagittal plane indicate the successive angular positions of the projections on the retina of the two target edges during the orientation walk, and the points show
the successive angular positions of the tips of both antennae. The thickening of the vertical
axis schematizes the plane of the pauses interrupting the walk for some hundred msec.

response (Jeanrot *et al.*, 1981); this zone ranges from 10 to 90° lateral to the sagittal plane, with a particularly sensitive area approximately 30° slightly above the horizontal plane [that is to say, less than 10° outside of the binocular field (Fig. 1B)]. In Gb, study of the spatial distribution of individual receptive fields of the visual interneurons descending within the neck connectives also shows an area of functional heterogeneity, while the part of the total field which is best represented is also located laterally at the limit of the binocular field close to the horizontal plane (Fig. 1B) (Richard *et al.*, 1985).

In young crickets, the necessity of visual scanning dictates less direct orientation routes, and the fixation area is not functionally as effective as in the adults. In fact, if one compares the angular positions of the cricket body relative to the target during an orientation walk, these are widely scattered in first instar larvae and remarkably centered around 20° from the sagittal plane in adults (Fig. 4) (Lambin, 1985).

A final mechanism involved in visual form perception must be mentioned; lateral inhibition, demonstrated within the Ns retina (Lambin and Jeanrot, 1982). Its function is to improve form perception by increasing contrast effects. It is not known if the effectiveness of this process is different in larvae compared to adults.

The visual exploration of forms in Gc as well as in Ns occurs at the same time as antennal exploration of the target edges. Such antennal scanning associated with visual scanning was first described by Honegger (1981) then by Lambin (1985) (Fig. 4).

Form perception, limited by visual acuity, is, therefore, an active, complex process involving visual scanning, the use of a fixation area, and correlation with nonvisual sensory information. Perceptual activity in such conditions is also the result of developmental changes from the gross and poorly defined world of the young larvae into the world of forms and of much more precise visual signals of the adult.

3. Relative Distance Perception

It has often been suggested that, in insects, depth perception beyond several centimeters from the animal is impossible and that the world is flat and devoid of relief. In Ns we studied the perception of the relative distance between two objects (Goulet *et al.*, 1981; Campan *et al.*, 1981). If Ns has to choose between two black targets with the same visual angle but located at different distances from it, it orients consistently towards the nearest one. The cricket is thus able to assess the relative distance of two objects and the spontaneous choice method allows us to measure the performance of the visual system in that field.

For an object whose angular size lies above the visual acuity threshold (11° × 56°), we performed two series of tests. In the first experimental situation, called "short distances," two vertical screens were placed at 5 and 10.9 cm, respectively, from the choice point; in the second situation, called "long distances," the vertical screens were placed at 52 and 130 cm. In each situation, we varied the angular distances between the internal edges of these targets. The preference was evaluated with an index varying from −1 (exclusive choice of the farthest target) to +1 (exclusive choice of the nearest). If the angular distance between the internal edges of both targets was larger than the extent of the binocular field slightly enlarged by the head movement, the discrimination between targets became impossible. The performances decreased as the targets were placed farther away, and the capacities of the larvae in that case were far below the adult capacity (Fig. 5).

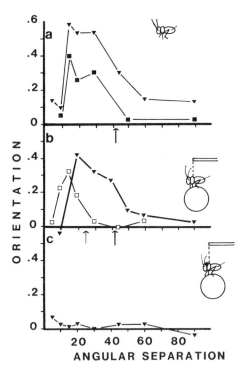

FIG. 5. Relative distance perception by *Nemobius sylvestris*. (a) Free-moving adults; ▼, long distance; ■, short distance. (b) Tethered crickets; ▼, adults; □, larval instar 3–4. (c) Tethered adults, fixed head, flickering light. A pair of vertical bars are presented with identical visual angles but different distances from the animal. The angular distance of the inner edges of the two targets (x axis) is consistently varied from 10–100° visual angle; their radial distances in relation to the animal remain constant. On the ordinate the index measures the ratio of orientation runs of the cricket toward the nearest target minus the orientation toward the distant target divided by the total number of orientation runs. For the short-distance situation the closer stripe is 5 cm away from the cricket; it is 52 cm away for the long distance.

To permit such discrimination, specific visual scanning is essential, and if we wax the head to the thorax, the spontaneous selection of the nearest target disappears even when form perception remains possible (with a low frequency flickering light) (Fig. 5). Here again we were able to demonstrate some of the functional limits to perceptual performance, where the effects are clearly stronger for young animals than for adults.

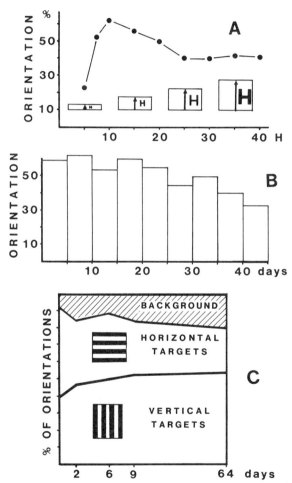

FIG. 6. (A) Percentage orientation of adult *Nemobius sylvestris* toward a black target of constant width but increasing height (from Jander, 1965). Height is given in degrees. (B) Habituation of the scototactic response by an individual *N. sylvestris* (10 trials each day for 40 days). (C) Variation in the relative proportion of animals preferring, respectively, vertical stripes, horizontal stripes, or white background during 64 training trials in which only an approach to the vertical stripes was continuously rewarded.

4. Discrimination of Visual Forms

Visual perception capacities related to form discrimination can be shown by results of spontaneous choice or learning experiments. Jander (1965, 1968) measured the spontaneous preferences of Ns presented with vertical black rectangles of the same width but of various heights. The crickets walked very systematically toward the shortest targets up to 10° high, after which the preference decreased and remained constant between 20 and 40° (Fig. 6). The same behavior was found in other cricket species, particularly Gc and Gb. According to Jander, this means that form perception is performed by limited surface detector systems which are excitatory at their center and inhibitory at their periphery.

Other geometric forms which were spontaneously chosen could be functionally related to the animal's natural ecological conditions. Thus, Ns which hide below the dead leaves in woods choose horizontally oriented forms (horizontal black stripes), whereas another species, such as *Oecanthus pellucens* which climbs up bushes, prefers vertical stripes (Jander, 1968, 1971).

Although we did not study the development of these preferences exhaustively, we tried to modify them through learning experiments. Thus, for an individual cricket, daily repetition of experiences of scototaxis induces habituation, the orientation toward the black target decreasing regularly during the 40-day tests (Fig. 6) (Campan, 1978). In discrimination learning experiments in a terrarium where two figures are presented simultaneously, the approach to only one being positively reinforced by food and drink, crickets greatly modify their preferences. Thus, we are able not only to reverse the scototactic preference, which is a very strong one, but to induce a preference either for vertical or horizontal stripes (Fig. 6), or for many other more complex stimuli tested in pairs, as well (Campan *et al.*, 1975). The same kind of experiments were successfully repeated with *Acheta domesticus* by Kieruzel and Chmurzynski (1982).

III. ECOLOGICAL CONDITIONS AND ORGANIZATION
OF THE VISUAL WORLD

These conditions were mainly studied in Ns. This cricket lives primarily in the oak and pine forests of the temperate regions of the Old World but, more and more, has been colonizing hedges and embankments where the litter of dead leaves is as thick as that of the forest.

Morvan and Campan (1976) and Morvan *et al.* (1977, 1978) studied cricket distribution. Sampling several areas using the quadrat method, they found the insects' distribution to be heterogeneous and aggregative. As shown in Fig. 7, the distribution depends on the position of the sample area in relation to the forest edge. This position reflects, from the edge into the forest, decreasing thermal and light levels and increasing humidity. Furthermore, the peculiar spatial location of each tree also affects some characteristics of the distribution. Occupation of space is rather different from one site to the other, even if the sites are close. Moreover, the distribution is not exactly the same for larvae and adults, with wide fluctuations according to the seasons.

At the edge between wood and field or forest trail, the distribution of the animals varies daily in a systematic way (Campan and Gautier, 1975; Lacoste *et al.*, 1976; Morvan and Campan, 1976; Beugnon, 1980). Figure 8a shows one example of the fluctuation of the occupation of space between wood and field during the day based on quadrat samples. The direct observation of the cricket locomotion at the wooded edge of a forest trail reveals that this daily variation results from movements that are rather systematically oriented toward trees in the morning and away from them in the evening (Fig. 8b).

In an attempt to understand the biological function of these movements in the natural habitat, and thereby to understand ecological factors affecting cricket development, we studied the daily sequence of activities by direct observation both in the natural habitat and in seminatural laboratory conditions (Lacoste *et al.*, 1976). The basic activities, feeding and reproduction, are conducted late in the afternoon and at nightfall during the evening migration into the open. By contrast, morning movements toward trees and the forest edge are correlated with the search for more humid conditions, thus avoiding desiccation during the hottest hours of the day.

These observations suggest the existence of some attachment to the sites where the crickets live, sites they are able to leave and then find again. This was systematically proven in the field by successive captures and recaptures of marked individuals (Morvan and Campan, 1976) that demonstrated the site attachment of most individuals. In the experimental area, 98% of the recaptured population did not move more than 10 m away from the release point, and none of the marked crickets was recovered over 40 m away when the maximal distance sampled was 65 m. Following a marked population reveals that 50–60% of individuals are found after 1 or 2 days, 30–55% after one week, 20–40% after two weeks, and approximately 20% three weeks later. In the spring, some of the individuals that were marked in the late fall are still present.

Attachment to the site was also evaluated in an experiment done on both sides of a forest trail. By marking the two opposite populations differently, one can show that the trail is never spontaneously crossed. However, when insects are passively displaced to the opposite side of the forest path, about 6% of the marked animals cross it and regain their original site (Morvan and Campan, 1976).

Very young Ns, after hatching at the beginning of the summer, are immediately confronted by a natural world where they must migrate perpendicularly to the

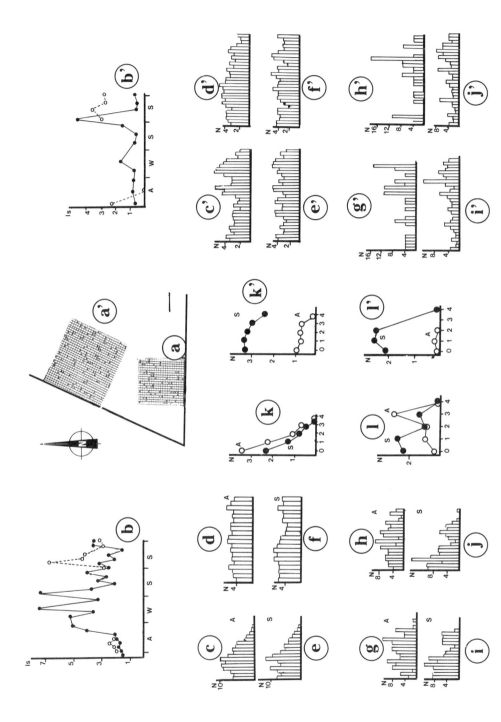

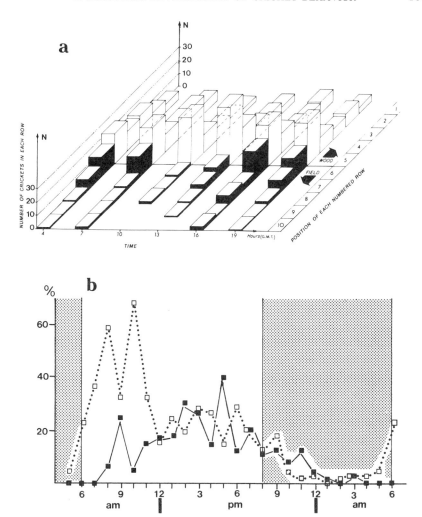

FIG. 8. Daily variation in the distribution of *Nemobius sylvestris* in their natural habitat. (a) Distribution in the rows parallel to the edge between wood and field. (b) Direct observation of crickets' movements at the edge of a forest path. □, Orientation toward forest; ■, orientation toward path. The y axis indicates percentage of population.

FIG. 7. Seasonal distribution of two samples, a and a', of *Nemobius sylvestris* studied by the quadrat method. The following explanations apply to both. (b) Seasonal variation in the aggregation index (Is) during the autumn (A), winter (W), spring (S), and summer (S) in adults (●) and larvae (○). Distribution in the rows parallel to the edge of the trails is given for larvae (c,e), males (g,i), and females (h,j). Distribution is also given for larvae in the rows perpendicular to the edge (d,f). (k,l) Cricket distribution according to the distance (m) from a nearby tree. A, Autumn; S, spring. Bar, 10 m.

edge of forest trails or fields. They need to guide themselves to their appropriate habitat.

In other species studied, the ecological conditions prevailing where they develop were not as systematically studied. Pl and Ph species often dwell in damp grassy areas alongside lakes or ponds; however, a small number of insects occur at the edge of nearby forests even though the conditions prevailing are very different. The shores of lakes or ponds, however, constitute an edge between two habitats, an edge comparable to the forest edge for Ns, and, when subjected to predation, the *Pteronemobius* crickets readily jump onto the lake surface and then return to the bank when out of danger.

Pl and Ph are two sympatric species and often present the same characteristics (Beugnon 1985, 1986a). The bank on which they live is also a place to which each cricket is attached, a place each is capable of finding again; such navigational skills must develop during its ontogeny.

Gc adults and larvae dig holes in different types of meadows: some sloping, with high or short grass, and with or without rocks, bushes, trees, and undergrowth. Individually marked animals move 15–20 m away from their burrows and return in a few minutes. Site attachment, especially in males, can last for more than several weeks. In this case the young need to develop a system of cues in order to return to their burrows.

So, regardless of species, at a microecological level the individual niche of a cricket during its ontogeny may differ among individuals even if they live in close proximity. The animal may live, by preference, at some distance from an edge, more or less close to a tree, in isolation or in a dense group, in an open meadow under perennial or deciduous cover, in high grass, or under more or less thick litter.

Moreover, the conditions encountered fluctuate, daily or seasonally, sometimes drastically, according to human activities (forest exploitation, forest fires, digging or drying out of natural or artificial lakes). Each individual cricket is exposed to a unique and complex combination of conditions varying in both their spatial and temporal distributions. Furthermore, in each case the animal exhibits a more or less strong attachment to its site, returning to it with variable accuracy and faithfulness. These sites of aggregation are areas between woodland and field, forest trail, or meadow for Ns, the shore of a lake for Pl and Ph, and a burrow for Gc.

Evidently, it is in their particular habitat, or in the immediate vicinity, that the crickets reproduce and lay their eggs, thus determining the place where the next generation will hatch. The young become attached to some of the characteristics of this habitat which serve as useful cues to guide their outbound and return trips.

By studying only the information conveyed by the visual channel, our analysis may ignore other possible cues, such as those related to olfaction or gravity. Nevertheless, vision does reveal some general rules of organization that must apply to all the sensory systems.

IV. ONTOGENY OF BEHAVIORAL EMERGENTS

Perceptual abilities expand as development proceeds within the constraints of the ecological demands set by attachment to the living site in each of the species studied. Within this conceptual framework, we have chosen to study the development of visually guided movements in the natural habitat as an example of behavioral development which may shed light on general processes.

A. BEHAVIORAL TARGET

Ns will serve as a model; the relevant data were collected by Beugnon (1983).

Crickets living at the eastern edge of a forest (Fig. 9a) make daily migrations oriented woodward in the morning and fieldward in the afternoon and evening (Beugnon, 1980). The basic experiment was devoted to the investigation of the visual cues that the insects may use during these movements.

All of the orientation studies reported in this section were based on a technique described by Campan and Gautier (1975). The insects, collected generally a few minutes before use, were individually released at the center of a circular wooden platform placed 40 cm above ground level. The walking surface could be maintained horizontally or inclined in any direction, and the setup could be surrounded by an opaque screen where artificial targets could be placed. The length, directness, and speed of the path taken by crickets were recorded. Finally, the direction of escape, as the angular position of the individual when it reached the periphery of the platform, was noted.

The mean value of orientation for each group is represented by the mean vector, the length of which (between 0 and 1) is a measure of concentration of the sample (Batschelet, 1981). The level of statistical significance of this vector is computed by the nonparametric Rao's test or by the parametric V test when a theoretical escape direction can be predicted a priori. Comparison between two samples is realized using the nonparametric two-sample Watson's test (Le Bourg and Beugnon, 1985).

Crickets from the area in Fig. 9 were released at the center of the setup located at point 1, 3 m inside the field beside a NW/SE-oriented edge. The observed escape directions, while variable, were significantly concentrated perpendicular to the closest edge (area b). If, on the other hand, all the possible terrestrial and celestial cues including polarized skylight pattern were hidden, the distribution of crickets did not show a significant mean escape direction (area c).

Another series of releases conducted at point 2 revealed, independent of the time of day, a strong negative correlation between the light distribution reflected by the surroundings and the sample distribution. This was regardless of current sun position (Fig. 9, area d). In overcast weather conditions, latency and trial duration were three times longer and less direct, though individual variation was great.

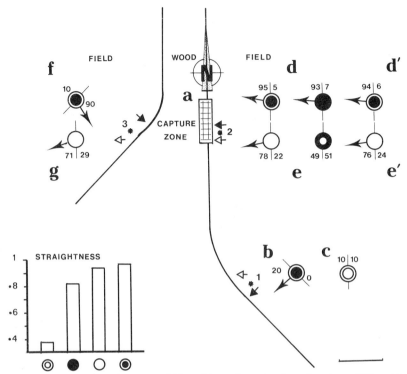

FIG. 9. Spatial orientation tests of *Nemobius sylvestris* released at three different locations (release points numbered). Experimental conditions were as follows: ◉, terrestrial and celestial cues; ●, terrestrial cues only (releases under overcast sky); ○, celestial cues only (opaque screen hiding landmarks under blue sky); ◐, no definite visual cues (opaque screen under overcast sky); ◎, no visual cues (opaque screen and cover). The number of individual angular positions at the periphery of the platform is indicated on both sides of the diameter line parallel to the edge axis. The mean angular orientation of the samples is illustrated by the black external arrow (if statistically significant, at least at $p < 0.05$). White triangular arrows indicate the theoretical escape direction (TED) given by celestial cues. In this experimental situation, TED corresponds to the westward returns in the direction of the capture zone (a). Black triangular arrows indicate the direction of the closest dark forest, perpendicular to the edge axis as seen from the release point. All tests were conducted in the morning except for d′ and e′ which were from afternoon sessions. See text for further discussion. Bar, 10 m.

When the experiment was done with every surrounding landmark hidden (Fig. 9, area e), the sample distribution at the periphery of the platform was more scattered. Nevertheless, a significant preferred direction appeared under a blue sky, in the morning as well as in the evening. Under an overcast sky, on the contrary, the same random distribution appeared as in the situation shown in area c.

Thus, two kinds of visual cues appear to be important in these experiments.

They were clearly distinguished in the following test (Fig. 9, area f). When the experimental platform was located at point 3 under natural conditions with all visual cues present, most of the crickets fled directly woodward, showing a positive correlation with the distribution of weakest reflected light from the panorama. If, on the other hand, terrestrial landmarks were hidden (area g), escapes were more scattered but there was still a very significant general flight woodward. Therefore, if a choice of terrestrial or celestial visual information is allowed, most of the animals will rely on landmark cues.

In the next section we consider how, through development, crickets gradually organize their visually guided behavior and integrate the information given by terrestrial and celestial cues according to the ecological conditions to which they are exposed. We start by analyzing their first reactions.

B. From Scototaxis to the Use of Terrestrial Cues

In an early paper (Campan and Médioni, 1963) we showed the existence of a strong scototactic tendency in Ns. It appears in larvae soon after hatching. In an experimental arena, crickets flee very systematically toward black targets (Table I). This spontaneous tendency lasts into adulthood with progressive improvement of orientation accuracy. A study of the ontogeny of the daily rhythm of scototactic orientation, with crickets of different ages collected in the wild, does not reveal any daily rhythm in younger larvae (Fig. 10b) apart from a slight decrease in the tendency at nightfall.

By the second and third larval instars, a morning peak (acrophase) appears; then, throughout the day, the tendency decreases to a nocturnal minimum which is especially accentuated in the fourth and fifth larval instars (Campan et al., 1965). This rhythm corresponds quite well to those rhythms observed during daily migrations (Fig. 10c) to and from trees. Finally, the rhythm also corresponds to the daily variations in orientation toward the trees in the platform experiments.

In another natural site, a N/S forest trail (Fig. 11a), Campan and Gautier

TABLE I
SCOTOTACTIC TENDENCY IN CRICKETS

	Light intensity	
Orientation away from light	2000 lux	1 lux
Theoretical[a]	13	13
Observed[a,b]	68	52

[a] Data are percentages.
[b] $p < 0.01$

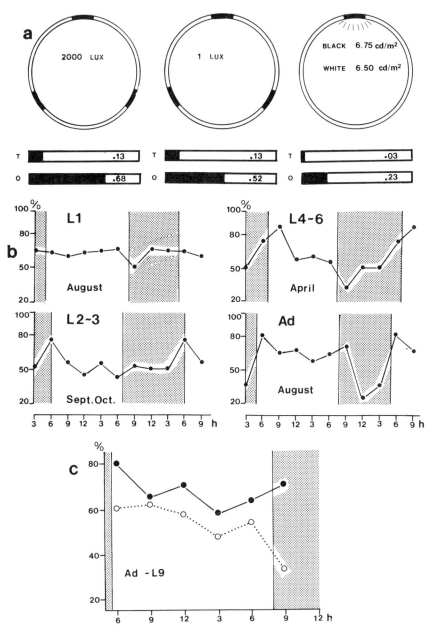

FIG. 10. Scototactic orientation of *Nemobius sylvestris*. (a) The observed frequencies (O) of crickets attracted by black targets are significantly higher ($p < 0.01$) than the theoretical frequencies (T), even with a black stripe reflecting more light than the otherwise white background (right). (b) Daily variation of scototactic orientation rhythm in the course of development. Percentages (y axis) are of orientation toward black stripes in laboratory conditions. Stippling indicates darkness. (c) Rhythm of orientation toward trees in the field (○) plotted alongside the scototactic rhythm (●).

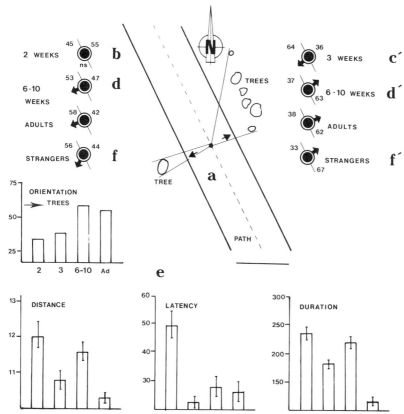

FIG. 11. Development of visual orientation on a forest trail (a). Left and right polar graphs indicate results with crickets collected on the left and right sides of the trail, respectively, and released in the center of the forest path (Bar, 2 m). Because of the observed bimodal distributions, the computed values of the mean vector are not biologically relevant. Thus, the black external arrows indicate the direction of each mode after grouping of values in 20° classes. (e) Orientation is toward trees, expressed as percentages. Mean distance (m) is that covered from the center to the periphery of the platform for each age group. Latency is the time (sec) before the crickets start walking. Mean duration of the tracks is expressed in seconds ± SE.

(1975) studied the ontogeny of visual orientation. In this situation, 2-week-old larvae, which are very scototactic, present a very diffuse, weak, and not statistically significant orientation toward trees (Fig. 11b). This tendency increases and becomes significant as soon as the larvae are 3 weeks old (Fig. 11c'). Six- to ten-week-old larvae escape in the same way as adults (Fig. 11d and d'). Measures of the characteristics of the paths also (Fig. 11e) reveals a sharp increase in the accuracy of orientation during ontogeny, mainly at the beginning. This reflects an orientation toward trees which becomes more and more systematic. It suggests that this orientation to terrestrial cues gradually emerges from the initial scototaxis. Moreover, familiarization with the pattern of environmental features occurs. Morvan and Campan (1976) have shown that adult crickets living at the edge of a straight forest trail which were released 80 m farther up the same forest trail, out of range of their living area, displayed an orientation toward the closest trees under a sunny sky that is less accurate than that of the native crickets (Fig. 11, 11').

This was also demonstrated in another experiment done by Beugnon at point 2 of Fig. 9a. Young (2- to 3-week-old) larvae, native to the site and so already familiar with it, exhibit escape directions which are highly positively correlated with the darker zones of the surroundings (Fig. 12a). In the same situation, naive 5-month-old larvae hatched and reared in the laboratory (Fig. 12b), or adults collected as larvae in the field but reared in the laboratory for 6 months (Fig. 12c), have a more scattered distribution of escape paths than native larvae. This was also verified with various other measures of orientation (Fig. 12).

In adult Ns, in general, orientation toward patterns giving little reflection in the surroundings appears at a significant level in various populations living in a great diversity of habitats such as forest trails, clearings with trees of different heights, clumps of trees, or isolated trees. But this is not always the case.

C. From Photonegativity to Astroorientation

Beugnon (1984) demonstrated the basic photonegative tendency of young Ns larvae to flee westward, i.e., opposite to the sun azimuth in the morning (Fig. 13a). This occurs independent of visible landmarks. An apparent change of sun position, with the help of a mirror when direct view of the sun is prevented,

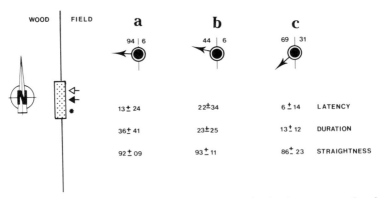

FIG. 12. Development of visual orientation at the N/S edge between wood and field. (a) 2- to 3-week-old larvae native to the site; (b) 5-month-old larvae bred in the laboratory; (c) Adults reared in the laboratory during their last larval stages for a 6-month period.

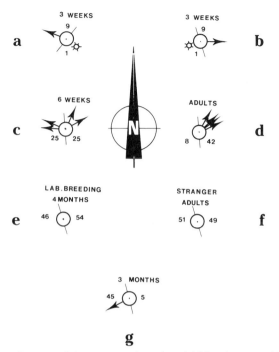

FIG. 13. From photonegativity to astroorientation. (a) Morning test with true azimuthal sun position. (b) Sun reflected by a mirror. (c) Mean individual menotaxis after five successive releases of four cricket larvae. (d) As in (c) but with adults. (e), (f) Adults strange to the area, laboratory bred and wild. (g) 3-month-old larvae native to the site.

confirms the systematic photonegativity of the crickets (Fig. 13b). Formerly, this photonegativity was suggested only under laboratory conditions by Campan and Médioni (1963). A study of orientation of 6-week-old larvae in their natural habitat (Fig. 13c) reveals that individuals show a menotaxis, each adopting an angle to the direction of the light source (Beugnon *et al.*, 1983). Later in ontogeny, one direction becomes common to all the individuals in the same population (Fig. 13d). Naive crickets or those from other populations do not show any preferred escape direction (Fig. 13e and f). This suggests that photonegativity can shift to a menotaxis that can be learned later on as a mnemotaxis and can induce an astroorientation system using either the sun's position or polarized skylight with time compensation (Fig. 13d and g).

These experimental data illustrate rather well Viaud's proposals (1955) concerning the gradual evolution from phototaxis to astroorientation; initially light phototaxically guides the animals and then the animals use light as a guide.

In complex natural systems, of course, terrestrial and celestial cues may be positively or negatively associated to insure that the insects move appropriately through development. Each insect is affected by individual experience, but the cues used are also very dependent on the structure and localization of reinforcing factors in the habitat of its species.

D.   DEVELOPMENT AND HABITAT

Behavioral differentiation varies greatly with ecological conditions.

1.   Forest Edge

In the forest edge situation of Fig. 7, we have seen that the accuracy of orientation toward dark areas of the panorama increases during ontogeny. We have also demonstrated that crickets learn a particular astronomical direction, which guides them naturally toward the closest edge; this is due to the learning of a positive association between terrestrial and celestial cues. If one follows the development of this association it can be shown that native larvae from 2 to 3 weeks of age, already familiar with the site and capable of directing themselves toward the dark zones, do not yet know how to use the astronomical component (Fig. 14a). Neither do older larvae nor adults which are naive or strangers to the site (Fig. 14b and c). In the local population, the use of a common astronomical component (Fig. 14d) almost comparable with the adults appears at 2 months of age.

2.   Forest Trails

In the case of a N/S-oriented forest trail, experiments performed by Campan and Gautier (1975) show that Ns crickets, in the course of ontogeny, learn to associate a definite astronomical direction with the side of the trail on which they live. As already mentioned, orientation toward trees is scattered for 2-week-old larvae but more accurate at 3 weeks; significant orientation toward the familiar

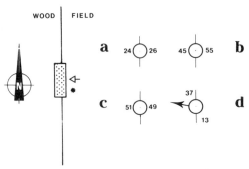

FIG. 14. Development of celestial orientation at the N/S edge between wood and field. (a) 2–3 weeks; (b) naive adults; (c) strange adults; (d) 2 months.

edge similar to that in adults appears only between 6 and 10 weeks (Fig. 15a). Whenever the platform is placed closer to the trees, the influence of the astronomical component decreases (Fig. 15b).

In the case of trails with different orientations such as, for example, E/W (Fig. 15c) or NE/SW (Fig. 15d), the adult crickets flee, on the experimental platform, only by using landmarks guiding them toward the darkest zone of the panorama.

3. Lake Shores

Beugnon (1985, 1986a) studied the spatial orientation of the riverine crickets Ph and Pl when they return to the shore after escaping onto the water. In the natural site shown in Fig. 16a, the pH adult crickets, when they can use visual cues, swim toward the bank closest to the point where they jumped off.

Even when the surrounding landmarks are experimentally hidden and the sky is clear, return to the familiar shore is possible with the same accuracy (Fig. 16a–c). Under overcast conditions, the homeward direction disappears. As soon as they are able to swim, riverine crickets use celestial cues under blue sky, whereas non-shore-dwelling crickets, living in a wet wood, do not display astroorientation when tested in the same way (Fig. 16d).

On the other hand, whatever the site of capture, a single trail of forced-escape swimming behavior on the lake surface allows a cricket to learn celestial cues associated with the closest bankward return (Fig. 16e–g). Learning seems to be more difficult if the bank lacks conspicuous landmarks like bushes and trees. In the latter case, some individuals with previous experience of celestial orientation still behave according to it.

This is a situation where return toward the inhabited site depends on the direction of the outward trip, sometimes influenced by past experience.

4. Return to the Burrow

The same type of problem occurs in Gc species. Any active outward trip (spontaneous or forced) can be followed by an accurate return. On the other hand, when the animal is passively transported over 60 cm away from the burrow, it is unable to return directly. However, within 30 cm the probability of return is high after passive transport (Fig. 17). So, as with spiders (Görner, 1972), Cataglyphis ants (Wehner, 1981), and beetles (Frantsevitch et al., 1977), learning the return direction occurs during the outward trip. In these situations, spatial information is stored as a "volatile memory orientation" (Beugnon, 1986b).

5. Choice among Terrestrial Cues

In some situations the panorama is rather complex, and the use of some cues is only revealed by experimental choice tests. As shown in Fig. 18, top, crickets are collected along a N/S forest edge and then released 300 m away. Their

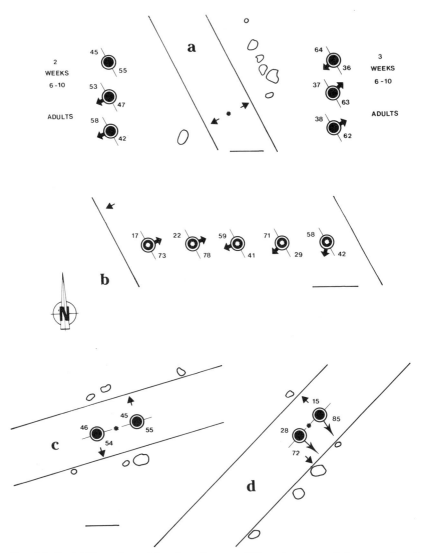

FIG. 15. Variability of spatial orientation on differently oriented forest trails. (a) Crickets collected on a nearly N/S forest trail. Bar, 3 m. (b) Variations of the sample distribution according to the point of release and the distribution of the incident light. Bar, 1 m. (c), (d) Independent of the side of capture, crickets escape toward the darker zones on either side of a nearly E/W forest trail or on the same side of a NE/SW forest path. Bar, 3 m.

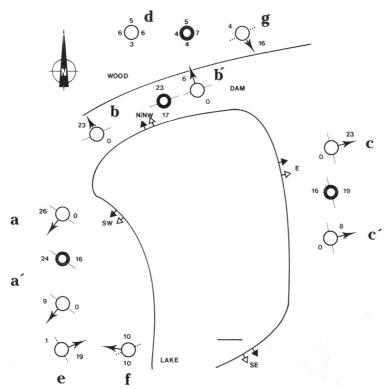

FIG. 16. Use of celestial cues in escape swimming in *Pteronemobius* species. (a), (b), (c) Celestial cues allow accurate bankward return in shore-dwelling adult crickets except under overcast weather conditions (darker circles). (a'), (b'), (c'), Astroorientation in young larvae. (d) Non-shore-dwelling adult crickets do not use celestial cues in their wet wood habitat. (e), (f), (g) After a single trial of forced evasive swimming on the lake surface, adult crickets learn the last bankward astronomical direction, regardless of capture site (riverine or not). Bar, 10 m.

theoretical escape direction (TED) is toward the west (Fig. 18b). When released on the platform near a NW/SE forest edge, they generally move toward the dark zone of the panorama, approximately matching their TED (Fig. 18c); the direction of the mean vector is similar to the one observed at their home site.

By contrast, when crickets are tested close to the NE/SW or NW/SE edges, they escape toward the closest dark forest edge (Fig. 18d and e). However, a certain number of individuals keep on fleeing in their TED, that is, toward the most distant westward forest edge.

This must mean that Ns crickets do not rely systematically on the closest landmarks as described earlier, but sometimes use astronomical cues to guide them toward distant forests. In a similar way, in fine weather, it was shown that Pl rely preferentially on celestial cues.

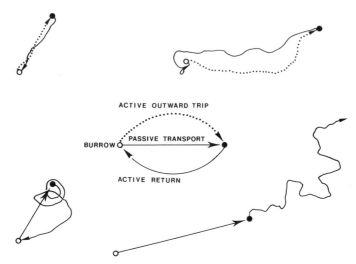

FIG. 17. Homing in *Gryllus campestris*. Straight-line distance was 50 cm. See text for further discussion.

In a situation where there are little square woods (Fig. 18, bottom), Ns were tested at different depths inside their native forest (Mieulet, 1980). In each experiment, dark areas were distributed inside the forest where the incident light was coming from different directions according to the distance of the release point from the forest edge.

The distribution of these stimuli in the visual panorama led to escape behavior toward the inner forest. This orientation is away from the resultant of all incident light, as in studies of phototaxis (Fig. 18g–i).

6. Sloping Forest

Another set of ecological factors characterizes the N/S edge of a sloping forest. A series of experiments with Ns were performed by Mieulet (1980) (Fig. 19).

Under blue sky, when the platform is kept horizontal, adult crickets escape toward the lowest reflecting part of the panorama (Fig. 19b). The guiding system is visual, as shown by the very large scattering of the escape reactions when all visual cues are masked (Fig. 19c). If the landmarks are hidden (Fig. 19d), crickets flee, contrary to previous findings, significantly more often away from the dark edge of the forest. This flight direction appears both in the morning and the afternoon (e).

The opposition between the location of dark areas and direction given by "distant" cues reveals that the former guides the insects toward trees whereas the latter, if they are the only visible ones, guides them in an opposite direction.

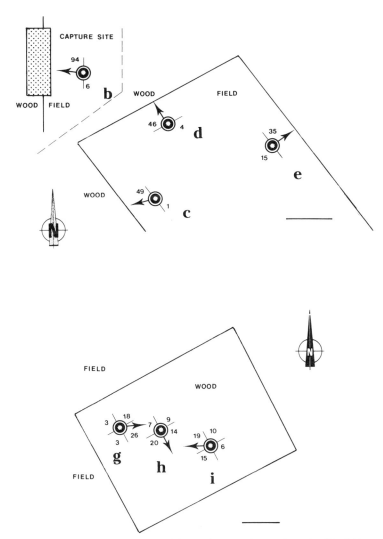

FIG. 18. Competition among terrestrial cues in *Nemobius sylvestris*. (Top) Escapes are directed toward the closest trees (c, d, e), but some individuals (e) flee in their westward TED (b). (Bottom) The mean angular orientation depends on the location within the wood of the release point. Bars, 10 m.

This is certainly associated with some unknown ecological features peculiar to the site.

The learning of this directional component appears rather late in the course of ontogeny. Even 3- to 4-month-old native larvae do not yet display a common escape direction (Fig. 19f). Also, another point remains obscure: what is the

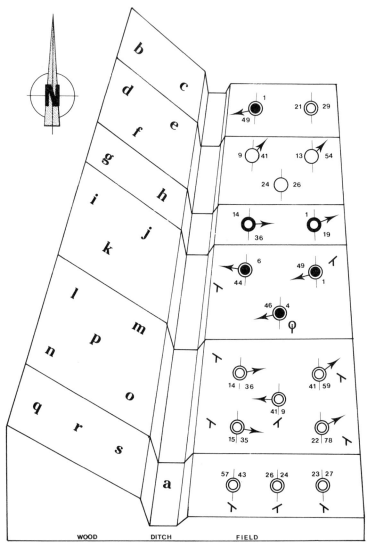

FIG. 19. Spatial orientation at a sloped forest edge. (b)–(h) Releases during morning. (e) Afternoon release with adults or (f) 3-month-old larvae. (i)–(s) Use of gravitational cues.

nature of the "distant" cues? Under overcast conditions, when all landmarks are hidden, a significant orientation still remains possible, and this is approximately in the same direction as under a blue sky (Fig. 19g, h); the use of a visual guiding system is demonstrated by the random distribution of escape directions recorded when all visual cues are hidden.

Finally, at the same site, we have looked for the role of gravitational information in orientation. The platform was inclined 40° in four different directions corresponding to the natural slope: opposite or perpendicular to the axis of the slope, north, and south. With all visual cues available, whatever the direction of the slope, crickets flee westward toward the forest edge (Fig. 19i–k). But when the panorama is entirely hidden, native adult crickets escape systematically in the direction of the inclined plane) (Fig. 19l). If inclination corresponds to the natural slope, without visual cues the insects are able to leave the slope of the forest and reach the neighboring field. Native 1-month old larvae display a gravitational orientation which is just statistically significant. This tendency increases with age (Fig. 19m–p). On the other hand, 7- to 9-month larvae from other areas do not use gravity information (Fig. 19q–s).

7. Deep-Woods Situations

In a clearing (Fig. 20a), 2-month-old larvae, already familiar with the site, exhibit a significant orientation toward the darker parts of the visual panorama

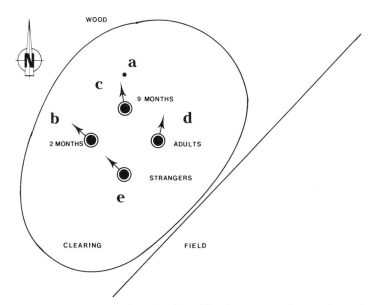

FIG. 20. Spatial orientation in a clearing. All releases were from point a. Strangers were all adults.

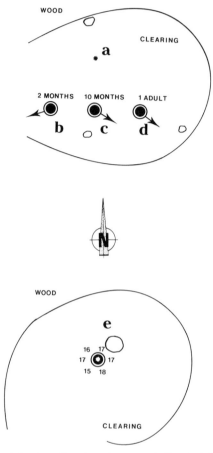

FIG. 21. Spatial orientation deep in a wood. See text for discussion.

(Fig. 20). With age, even though the relative reflected light distribution changes little, the mean vector shifts gradually northward (Fig. 20c, d). At the same time, adult crickets unfamiliar with the site have a preferential orientation very similar to that of young native larvae (Fig. 20e). These data suggest that the direction taken has been gradually learned, by native larvae according to microecological characteristics of the site, characteristics that adults from other areas have not learned.

In another underbrush habitat within a clearing (Fig. 21a), 2-month-old larvae show a highly significant orientation westward, but the correlation with the reflected light distribution is not significant (Fig. 21b). Ten-month-old larvae from the same population display a significant SE orientation (Fig. 21c) so that their flight directions are positively correlated with the brightest areas of the panorama. This was confirmed during a series of trials with the same adult cricket (Fig. 21d). Finally, in a deep wood situation where light from the reflected surroundings is rather scattered, crickets do not show any common preferred escape directions (Fig. 21e).

V. RULES OF BEHAVIOR ONTOGENY

Although many pieces of the puzzle are still missing, the data we have presented in this article, with the support of some speculations, allow us to propose both the outline of a possible scheme for ontogeny and some general rules for behavioral development. The first two aspects of the scheme are as yet unknown in crickets but can be imagined from work on other species.

Though we have not studied this aspect, we accept the widely held view that phylogeny fixes the general frame for each individual's development. The data we have presented are also concordant with the idea that the unique genotype, particular to each individual (Jacquard, 1978), delimits a field of competence wide enough to allow the expression of a wide behavioral diversity. Our results support the conception of the actual ontogeny which is the result here and now of the mutual constraints of ontogeny and phylogeny (Richard, 1979). The limits of the framework within which behavior develops are, therefore, finally drawn during development itself.

We also know that when young Ns larvae (for instance) hatch, they are already 1 year old (dating from the laying of eggs) (Campan, 1965), a year during which self-produced epigenetic effects would have been possible. The earliest stages of development occur throughout a kind of individual "prehistory" that we cannot observe during the development of the embryo, the time of hatching, and the hours after hatching.

Nevertheless, the youngest larvae, even as early as we have studied them, already have an action system including a repertoire of possible responses to the intensity and direction of simple stimuli. Thus, Ns is at the same time photonegative and scototactic, which means that it exhibits withdrawal reactions in response to strong direct light and approach reactions to the lowest reflections. Such a description fits the A–W theory of Schneirla (1965) for any animal at the beginning of its behavioral development. Nevertheless, since the first steps remain unknown in crickets, one cannot exclude the hypothesis of a scototaxis which could be a consequence of photonegativity. Such an idea is supported by data from a study on the vision of several caterpillar species (Bui Huy Binh and Campan, 1982). We have demonstrated that the most primitive photoreceptors are correlated with phototactic responses, not with scototactic ones. Scototaxis requires a more powerful visual system, an intermediate position being fulfilled by the contrast response that Michieli (1959) called perigrammotaxis. In the same way, scototaxis could be only a step toward true form perception. Such considerations, at once ontogenetic and phylogenetic, suggest the following hierarchy of visual capacities from the primitive to the most advanced and complex: phototaxis, perigrammotaxis, scototaxis, and form vision; these grades could represent the successive steps of early development depending on both maturational and experiential processes. The fact that the hatching cricket must leave its egg in the darkness of the soil and that it must then climb up to the surface could be a reason for the very early development of its responses to light and gravity.

But in our scheme of development, since data on the earliest period are missing, we limit ourselves to considering posthatching development of three basic components involved right after hatching in approach and withdrawal reactions: phototaxis, scototaxis, and geotaxis. We could also deal with other components, possibly even more primitive ones, such as those concerned with the chemical or vibratory world or with responses to magnetic fields.

Phototaxis, mainly negative, contributes to synchronizing insect movements during the day, leading them toward the forest in the morning so that they hide in the daytime. The thermal and hygrometric consequences of natural sunlight could play a major part in this. In the evening, on the contrary, if the surroundings of the forest remain relatively bright, light intensity is progressively reduced until it reaches the threshold value for the change from photonegativity to photopositivity, thus inducing movement in the opposite direction.

Scototaxis, on the other hand, could determine the orientation responses to reflectance of the natural panorama surrounding the insect. During the daily regular migrations in the first weeks of its larval life, a cricket might learn an association between some reflectancy pattern and the main stimuli important to its survival, such as those concerned with foraging activities, avoidance of dry areas, etc. The data we have reported here support this idea, since young larvae, although already scototactic, do not yet orient toward the low reflecting areas of the panorama; this is not the case one week later. Simultaneously, such an orientation becomes progressively synchronized with the daily migrations, the scototaxic tendency increasing in the morning, when the insects walk toward the forest, and decreasing during the afternoon and at sundown, when they walk in the opposite direction. Later, the young larvae are able to discriminate between the particular familiar pattern of reflected light and an unknown one. Such cues guide their routes in a way comparable to that proposed by Guthrie (1983) for fish. At the same time, obviously, the maturation of the visual system of each larva occurs with increasing individual experience; its competence then enlarges by improving contrast sensitivity, form perception, and relative localization at least. Scototaxis could, therefore, be the basis of the construction of a functional network of perception of terrestrial cues which is part of a complex and unique system of relations between an individual and its world.

By the same token, phototaxis need not be the only factor responsible for the daily synchronization of movements at the forest edge. The recurrence of the sun's position in relation to the surroundings and the negative reactions initially induced, combined with orientation toward the darker areas of the panorama, could induce a systematic angular orientation in relation to the light source. The individuality of this has already been demonstrated, each animal choosing a particular flight direction relative to the sun's position. Nevertheless, owing to the ecological conditions of a particular habitat which are almost the same for each individual of the local population, photomenotaxis soon develops into a mnemotaxis, the learned direction being common to all. Later on, changes with time and the sun's position are compensated for. As suggested by Viaud (1955), such phototaxis could then be at the origin of astroorientation. In our particular case, the main direction is common to all individuals of a population living in a given area. It is the result of interwoven changes affecting the ontogeny of both basic components, phototaxis and scototaxis, while an individual combines them and associates them with its experience. Thus the learned astronomic direction is toward some areas of the reflectancy pattern characteristic of the visual panorama at a given site. This is particularly obvious in relation to the whole network of visual cues which guide return to a forest border or the bank of a forest trail. More subtle arguments also support such a hypothesis. Thus, as can be predicted, it is easier for crickets to learn an astronomical direction needed to return to a known site when they live at a N/S forest edge facing the sun at dawn than it is if the edge faces west. For the same reasons, the relative importance of astroorientation in the case of a N/S trail is stronger when the insects must return to the west rather than to the east. In the same way it should be more difficult for the crickets to learn a return direction when they live at an E/W border whether they face north or south. This is shown by experiments performed on E/W forest borders; either they return to the edge or their return is independent of the edge where they normally live, thus revealing that no learned astronomic direction is involved (Beugnon, 1984).

Concerning geotaxis, the third of the three basic components we chose to follow during ontogeny, what little data we have so far suggest the following speculative scheme. Geotaxis could be the basis of a geomenotaxis using gravity cues when crickets live in a slanting area. Otherwise, the basic tendency could decrease and even vanish, at least temporarily. The experiments we have reported here reveal that the slope cue is used by crickets only when no visual cue is visible. In natural conditions this can occur at night (or in dense fog), which could explain why the insects tend to walk down the slope in the area studied where the forest border was located downhill when they leave the forest mainly in the evening and at night. Gravity is, as demonstrated, a learned cue which, if it is taken into account independently of the visual ones, should be associated with the same events for each individual cricket; then it becomes common to most animals of the local population.

Finally, although we have limited our work to the use of some visual and gravitational cues, our hypotheses could be extended to other sensory modalities such as chemical cues, which could be associated with the direction of the main winds [as with the pigeon (Papi, 1976)], or cues derived from features of the earth's magnetic field.

The various transitions we have hypothesized for the ontogenetic construction of the animal's own world—from scototaxis to visual cues, from phototaxis to astroorientation, from geotaxis to slope orientation, as well as the combination of all this information—could involve the same behavioral mechanisms. Experimental psychology proposes a wide range of possible models. The rhythmic occurrence of trips back and forth in the home area or around the burrow places the insect in an operant conditioning situation (Morvan and Campan, 1976). The approach to or withdrawal from some areas of the reflectancy pattern of the panorama, in a particular astronomical direction, occasionally climbing up or down a slope, are associated with many daily events of the individual's life which may constitute reinforcements: feeding, exploration, and warmth outside the forest or in the clearings; humidity, shelter from predators and climatic conditions, or presence of conspecifics inside the forest. In such a context, each cricket is also in a situation to experience exposure learning or latent learning and, insofar as it is faced with the whole panorama repeatedly during its movements, it is able to memorize particular features. Finally, all animals, and especially young larvae, are in a topographic learning situation, learning topography and routes like the rat in its maze. These are situations where spatial information is stored as a constant memory orientation (Beugnon, 1986b).

The results from Pl, Ph, and Gc also show other types of learning, taking into account the occasional and variable orientation paths of crickets returning to their burrow or to the last bank where they jump off. The proposed model from experimental psychology, then, is that of one-trial learning because the cricket learns on each trip the direction of its return by integrating the information it gets from the outward journey [see Beugnon, (1986b) for a more detailed discussion of spatial information processing and memorization].

Laboratory experiments with Ns (Campan and Lacoste, 1971) have been used to imitate the natural situation. They show that repetitive presentation of some visual forms associated with food rewards or, alternatively, with no reward can foster either discriminative learning or habituation (Campan, 1978). This last point means that the insect constructs its relationship with its own world by learning the functional value of the cues it is able to detect. When we assess this process within the framework of biphasic approach/withdrawal theory, it corresponds to the transition proposed by Schneirla (1965) from responses to stimulus intensity to responses to stimulus quality, a functional consequence of the interaction between maturation and individual experience.

The scheme we have proposed sets forth the history of the complex individual–world system, comparing successive stages which constitute a series of snapshots of the relationship of the individual to its universe within this system. Each stage represents a step in the construction of the functional competence of the system to accomplish a performance, to express a relationship, i.e., to beget a behavioral emergent. The mechanisms proposed to account for the interactions among the elements, as well as for the changes from stage to stage and the diversity of recorded performances, reveal the variety and richness of possible individual–world relationships.

The diversity of possibilities is evident even when the analysis is at the level of a population of individuals living in the same area. Thus, the prevailing astronomic direction for a given site may be associated with the reflectance distribution within the panorama and result in approach to a dark area. In contrast, at another site it may indicate a completely different direction, at times the opposite one. In the same way, orientation with regard to the slope of the area may be associated with the same reinforcements as those guiding the insects in relation to the darker areas of the panorama. This may be in concordance with the astronomic directions or, conversely, be associated with completely different reinforcements located elsewhere within the environment.

On the basis, initially, of simple interplay among primary components, most individuals of a given cricket population in a given location construct, during the course of ontogeny, relational animal–world systems which are genuinely their own. The result is that, in each of the systems involved, there is the capability to generate functionally comparable behavior products which result from the interplay of the same network of spatial information.

Of course the scheme proposed thus far has some predictive value; that is, if we know enough about the ecological characteristics of a given site and about the local population, it is possible to assess with reasonable probability the nature of the network of cues involved in the orientation performance of most of the animals. This reveals some aspects of the image of their environment which the individuals from that population may have and the status, at that time, of their relationship to the world.

Nevertheless, this probabilistic prediction applied in detail to a particular individual could be completely false. This can be seen in Fig. 22; all of the results we have reported demonstrate a huge diversity of orientation durections among different individuals and large variation in the chosen direction for the same animal from one route to another. Thus, when the general properties of the system allow us to predict the main orientation direction as N/E, there are always some individuals orienting S or W. In the same way, whereas the main orientation direction should guide the crickets toward the darker areas of the panorama, some crickets, nevertheless, systematically flee from them and go toward the brightest parts. As another example, if we predict a very straight route for a known, preferred direction, some animals exhibit a very winding one while other

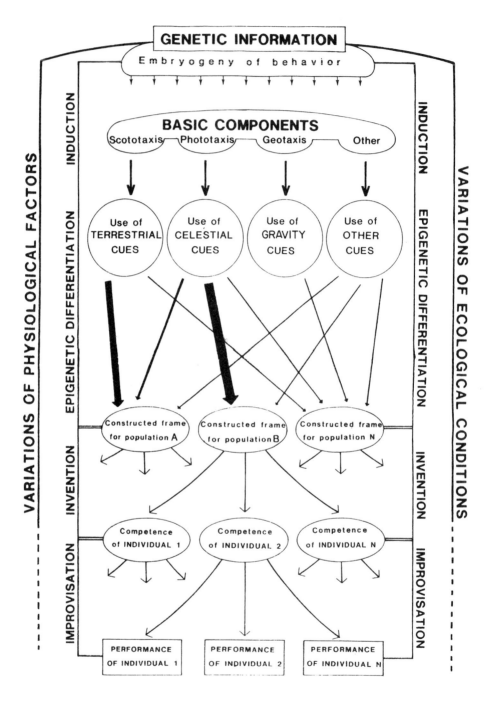

FIG. 22. Historical and present stages of the individual–world system illustrating the whole scheme of behavioral ontogeny.

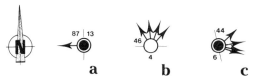

FIG. 23. Variations in orientation in three situations. (a) Mean angular orientation of crickets living at a N/S forest edge. (b) Individual orientations of four animals tested with 10 successive trials each (northward TED). (c) Individual orientations inside a square poplar wood; the nearest borders of the forest are located to the northwest and southwest.

crickets flee straightaway in the opposite direction. Finally, an individual consistently orienting, in successive trials, in a precise direction can all at once choose a completely new one.

As Weisskopf (1984) stated in a paper on the borders and limits of science, "We must avoid one misunderstanding, however. The occurrence of unpredictable events does not mean that the laws of nature are violated. On the contrary the actual causes and the mechanism of amplification are no 'miracles' from the scientific point of view; they are comprehensible but unpredictable."

Because the knowledge of the general capabilities of a sample of individuals within a population does not allow us to predict individual behavior with all its variability, we have to describe this with other rules and other concepts. This is what Marler (1983) did to account for the variations observed in the structure of bird songs. The first of his concepts, *invention,* illustrates the fact that a particular individual possessing capabilities peculiar to a population to which it belongs may go beyond them and invent new ones in the course of its ontogeny and the unique interaction it has with its own world. This concept could, for example, apply to the few crickets which are still able to maintain a distant orientation using information which is at yet unclear under conditions where most of the individuals within a population no longer orient significantly because both terrestrial and celestial cues are hidden. We have to conceive that, through their unique, individual experience of the particular network of ecological conditions with which they are faced, they have invented a new strategy.

In the same way during an orientation trip, the decision the cricket expresses by the choice of observed direction takes into account the complexity of the interactions within the network of elements of the individual–world system in which it is involved. Its relationship to the world at this instant is expressed by a *hic et nunc* action which is unique and unpredictable, a result of *improvization,* the second concept proposed by Marler (1983).

Therefore, as stated in the beginning of this section, individual behavioral performance appears as a result of the relation of the subject to its world, and the *hic et nunc* emergence of the dynamic individual–world system expresses the complexity of the interactions among all of its elements. Figure 23 presents various historical and current stages of this system, illustrating the whole scheme of behavioral ontogeny until the *hic et nunc* instant.

VI. CONCLUSION: THE GENERAL RULES

The ontogeny of the orientation behavior we have described appears comparable to other developmental phenomena. Even if it requires its own concepts and specific mechanisms, it is similar to other developmental processes. Thus, to describe behavioral development in embryological terms is a useful attempt at generalization.

Modern embryology tells us that development begins with first a transcription and then a translation of the genotype leading to a differential compartmentalization of the embryo into a fate map. This preserves a very broad potential and, for some time, the organism remains very sensitive to epigenetic influences (Lemoigne, 1979; Beetschen, 1984). Later, through a process of differentiation which limits and defines their capability, the prospective groups of cells are transformed into a morphogenetic field of determined groups of cells. Induction phenomena are involved in this process, and they can be defined as the transformation of a cell group, cell layer, or organ through the influence of another cell group, cell layer, or organ (Wolff, 1963).

Epigenesis can be described as a succession of inductions resulting in a progressive determination of the whole embryo in all of its compartments. For Wolff (1963), differentiation and determination is an adaptation of the embryo to the current external conditions. Therefore, it appears as a metastable state of an individual–world system, responsive to the interactions among its components. The determined state should, therefore, result from a probabilistic, and not very precise, programming. Modifying inductive and regulatory processes are superimposed upon determination in the way described by Changeux (1983) for the selective stabilization (functional validation) of synapses during neurogenesis. Finally, this developmental dialectic can be accelerated or delayed according to conditions of stimulation; in this field neurogenesis also provides several examples. After stabilization and determination, the structures formed are no longer reversible, and they are functionally protected by many conservative regulatory processes. Nevertheless there remains, in their functioning, some limited adaptive plasticity which is able to adjust both structures and functions to the particular needs of an individual.

In the field of ethology, we know that very early in ontogeny the range of potentialities is usually diverse. During many sensitive periods, different for various types of behavior, an animal is particularly open to specific epigenetic influences which contribute to the determination and stabilization of individual behavior patterns.

The model that we have presented here does not take into account the embryonic period. Yet one may consider the fundamental components of orientation present at hatching (phototaxis, scototaxis, geotaxis, etc.) as analogous to inductors which could come into play early enough in the chain of successive differentiations. From these inductors will develop particular behavioral abilities of the individual–world system which will first be metastable and destined either to be stabilized or to disappear according to the nature of interactions between both the elements of the system and the consequences of these interactions. The ontogenetic transformations are therefore constructed analogously with the model of the chain of induction–differentiation which constitutes many successive stages of the same individual–world system; the complexity and wealth of epigenetic influences determine the range of stabilized capabilities. Thus, depending on the environment, some crickets will either use no particular cue, or, on the contrary, direct their movements by visual, astronomic, or gravitational cues in combinations of increasing complexity. Finally, in the behavioral field as well, the level of stimulation to which the individual–world system is subjected, whether it is of external or internal origin, speeds up or slows down the differentiation process.

Homologies between the ontogeny of the individual–world system we have described and embryology are therefore quite numerous; they may lead us to consider the differentiation of structures and behavioral capabilities as two aspects of the same developmental process. Probabilistic epigenesis furthermore stresses the role of reciprocal function–structure interactions in the development of both structures and functions; behavioral embryology (Gottlieb, 1973) presents numerous examples illustrating these interactions. Thus, constructivism, which was basic to our conception of ontogeny, may also apply to embryogenesis.

However, the final behavioral capabilities, unlike structures for the most part, are actually only metastable and also differ in the nature of regulatory processes ruling interactions among the elements of the individual–world system. Piaget (1977) has stressed the role of conservative physiological regulation in maintaining the system in a balanced state; the individual–world system includes many mechanisms of this type. Nevertheless, behavioral emergence has a regulatory function for the individual system from which it sprang. Behavior is, therefore, what was termed "innovating regulation" by Piaget because, through the memory of events, it introduces new elements to the system and transforms its balanced state. After behavioral performance, the metastable state of the system differs from what it was previously, its capability is modified, and it is usually increased.

Thus, when some subjects are inventive and acquire new capacities, they will introduce them into their own individual–world system. Improvization, once it is stabilized either directly or through repetition in some other way, might become invention and so improve the system's capability.

Furthermore, as shown in Scheme 1, any new capacity introduced into an individual–world system contributes, as a result, to the population–world dynamic, which is itself involved in the species–world system, and results in the phylogenetic dynamic through the interplay of these nested systems as proposed by Gautier *et al.* (1978).

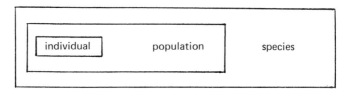

This logic greatly enlarges the field of constructivism and leads us to place it in the more general systems framework.

In this regard a paper by Varela (1983) on the mechanism of self-organizing systems is relevant. A system is a type of gestalt defined by its own unity relative to the background. Such a concept allows us to describe systems at several levels, provided that all the constituent elements have enough interactions in common to appear as a unit. We have described here the basis of behavioral emergents by the individual–world system dealing with the dyad individual and world, both of which may be considered as systemic gestalt systems.

The developing individual, as studied in embryology, as well as the individual–world combination, are both characterized by a strong internal determination; the external influences to which they are open are only disturbing or modifying, but not determining, ones. Such peculiarities define autonomous systems (Varela, 1983). Although it exhibits some points of external coupling, an autonomous system is defined by its internal coherence and is mainly characterized by a "coupling by closure." On the contrary, when external determination is essential, the appropriate term would be "coupling by input." Under these conditions, an autonomous system should be considered as operationally closed even if it is completely so. The progressive modifications of such a system, its dynamic, resulting mainly from its internal mechanisms, is described as self-organization.

This argument applies to any autonomous systems and therefore it applies to those we have considered so far, i.e., the developing individual, its transformation, and the individual–world dyad. Ontogeny as well as dynamic behavior follow the rules of constructivism and appear as a self-organizing process generating novelty and unpredictability. This should lead ethologists to view fields such as behavioral phylogeny, ecoethology, and neuroethology in a new light.

Finally, if the constructivism that we have already generalized to the whole field of developmental biology also characterizes the working of autonomous systems, then it should apply equally to population dynamics and species evolution.

Acknowledgments

Since 1961, when the cricket work began in Toulouse, so many people have been involved that it is impossible to list and thank them all. Nevertheless, C. Beca, T. Chalumeau, A. Pechou, and V. Preteur were principally involved in the preparation of the present article. Many thanks are also due to the editor and the associate editors of the volume for their critical reading of an earlier draft of the English manuscript.

References

Batschelet, E. (1981). "Circular Statistics in Biology." Academic Press, New York.

Beetschen, J. C. (1984). "La génétique du développement." PUF, Coll. Que sais-je?

Beugnon, G. (1980). Daily migrations of the wood cricket *Nemobius sylvestris* (Bosc). *Environ. Entomol.* **9**, 801–805.

Beugnon, G. (1981). Orientation of southern mole cricket, *Scapteriscus acletus,* landing at a sound source. *Fl. Entomol.* **64**, 463–468.

Beugnon, G. (1983). Terrestrial and celestial cues in visual orientation of the wood-cricket. *Nemobius sylvestris* (Bosc). *Biol. Behav.* **8**, 159–169.

Beugnon, G. (1984). De la photonégativité à l'astroorientation chez le Grillon des bois *Nemobius sylvestris* (Bosc). *Monit. Zool. Ital.* **18**, 185–197.

Beugnon, G. (1985). Orientation of evasive swimming in *Pteronemobius heydeni* (Orthoptera: Gryllidae, Nemobiinae). *Acta Oecol. Oecol. Gen.* **6**, 235–242.

Beugnon, G. (1986a). Learned orientation in landward swimming in the cricket *Pteronemobius lineolatus. Behav. Processes* **12**, 215–226.

Beugnon, G. (1986b). Spatial orientation memories. *In* "Orientation in Space" (G. Beugnon, ed.), pp. 9–19. IEC, Privat, Toulouse.

Beugnon, G., Mieulet, F., and Campan, R. (1983). Ontogenèse de certains aspects de l'orientation du grillon des bois, *Nemobius sylvestris* (Bosc), dans son milieu naturel. *Behav. Processes* **8**, 73–86.

Bui Huy Binh, and Campan, R. (1982). Etude comparative de quelques aspects de la vision des formes chez deux espèces de chenilles de Lépidoptères: *Arctia caja* et *Galleria melonella. Bull. Soc. Hist. Nat. Toulouse* **118**, 199–222.

Campan, R. (1965). Etude du cycle biologique du Grillon *Nemobius sylvestris* dans la région toulousaine. *Bull. Soc. Hist. Nat. Toulouse* **100** 371–378.

Campan, R. (1978). l'utilisation des repères visuels terrestres dans l'orientation des insectes. *Ann. Biol.* **17**, 61–90.

Campan, R. (1980). "L'animal et son univers. Etude dynamique du comportement." Privat, Coll. Bios.

Campan, R., and Gautier, J. Y. (1975). Orientation of the cricket *Nemobius sylvestris* (Bosc) towards forest-trees. Daily variations and ontogenetic development. *Anim. Behav.* **23**, 640–649.

Campan, R., and Honegger, H. W. (1986). Neurobiology of vision. **In** "Behavioral Strategies of Crickets and Underlying Physiological Mechanisms" (F. Huber, W. Loher, and T. E. Moore, eds.). In press.

Campan, R., and Lacoste, G. (1971). Les préférences visuelles spontanées chez le Grillon *Nemobius sylvestris* et leurs modifications sous l'effet de l'experience. *96ème Congrès National des Sociétés Savantes, Toulouse* **3**, 465–483.

Campan, R., and Médioni, J. (1963). Sur le comportement "scototactique" du Grillon *Nemobius sylvestris* (Bosc). *C. R. Soc. Biol.* **157**, 1690–1695.

Campan, R., Gallo, A., and Queinnec, Y. (1965). Détermination électrorétinographique de la fréquence critique de fusionnement visuel: Étude comparative portant sur les yeux composés de dix-sept espèces d'insectes. *C. R. Soc. Biol.* **159**, 2521–2526.

Campan, R., Goulet, M., and Lambin, M. (1976). Le rôle du mouvement relatif dans la perception visuelle des formes chez le grillon *Nemobius sylvestris*. *Biol. Behav.* **1**, 57–68.

Campan, R., Goulet, M., and Lambin, M. (1981). L'appréciation visuelle de l'éloignement relatif entre deux objets chez le grillon *Nemobius sylvestris* (Bosc) et l'aptérygote *Lepismachilis targionii* (Grassi). *Bull. Soc. Hist. Nat. Toulouse* **117**, 41–50.

Campan, R., Lacoste, G., and Morvan, R. (1975). Le rythme journalier de l'orientation scototactique chez le grillon des bois *Nemobius sylvestris* (Bosc): Approche de la signification biologique. *Monit. Zool. Ital.* **9**, 119–136.

Changeux, J. P. (1983). "L'homme neuronal." Fayard.

Frantsevitch, L. I., Govardovski, V., Gribakin, F., Nikolajev, G., Pichka, V., Polanovsky, A., Shevchenko, V., and Zolotov, V. (1977). Astroorientation in *Lethrus* (Coleoptera, Scarabaeidae). *J. Comp. Physiol.* **121**, 253–271.

Gautier, J. Y., Lefeuvre, J. C., Richard, G., and Trehen, P. (1978). "Ecoéthologie." Masson.

Görner, P. (1972). Resulting positioning between optical and kinesthesic orientation in the spider *Agelena labyrinthica* (CP). *In* "Information Processing in the Visual System of Arthropods" (R. Wehner, ed.). Springer, New York.

Gottlieb, G. (1973). "Behavioral Embryology," Vol. 1. Academic Press, New York.

Goulet, M., Campan, R., and Lambin, M. (1981). The visual perception of relative distances in the wood-cricket, *Nemobius sylvestris*. *Physiol. Entomol.* **6**, 357–367.

Guthrie, D. M. (1983). Visual central processes in fish behavior. *In* "Advances in Vertebrates Neuroethology" (J. P. Ewert, R. R. Capranica, and D. J. Ingle, eds.), pp. 381–412. Plenum, New York.

Honegger, H. W. (1981). A preliminary note on a new optomotor response in crickets: Antennal tracking of moving targets. *J. Comp. Physiol.* **142**, 419–421.

Honneger, H. W., and Schürmann, R. W. (1975). Cobalt sulphide staining of optic fibres in the brain of the cricket *Gryllus campestris*. *Cell Tissue Res.* **159**, 213–225.

Jacquard, A. (1978). "L'éloge de la différence." Seuil.

Jander, R. (1965). Die Phylogenie von Orientierungsmechanismen der Arthropoden. *Verh. Dtsch. Zool. Ges. Jena*, 266–306.

Jander, A. (1968). Uber die Ethometrie von Schlüsselreizen. Die Theorie der telotaktischen Wahlhandlung und das Potenzprinzip der terminalen Cumulation bei Arthropoden. *Z. vergl. Physiol.* **59**, 319–356.

Jander, A. (1971). Visual pattern recognition and directional orientation in insects. *Ann. N.Y. Acad. Sci.* **188**, 5–11.

Jeanrot, N., Campan, R., and Lambin, M. (1981). Functional exploration of the visual field of the wood-cricket, *Nemobius sylvestris*. *Physiol. Entomol.* **6**, 27–34.

Kieruzel, M., and Chmurzynski, A. (1982). Visual preferences for certain flat patterns in the house cricket and their conditionally acquired changes. *Biol. Behav.* **7**, 119–135.

Labhart, T., Hodel, B., and Valenzuela, I. (1984). The physiology of the cricket's compound eye with particular reference to the anatomically specialized dorsal rim area. *J. Comp. Physiol.* **155**, 289–296.

Lacoste, G., Campan, R., and Morvan, R. (1976). l'enchaînement journalier des comportements chez le grillon *Nemobius sylvestris*. *Acrida* **5**, 27–44.

Lambin, M. (1985). Ontogenèse de la fixation visuelle au cours de la marche orientée chez le grillon des bois *Nemobius sylvestris*. *Behav. Processes* **11**, 31–38.

Lambin, M., and Jeanrot. N. (1982). Données électrophysiologiques sur la rétine et le système visuel périphérique chez *Nemobius sylvestris*. *J. Physiol.* **78**, 310–316.

Lambin, M., Campan, R., and Richard, D. (1985). Aspects fonctionnels de la vision en lumière intermittente chez un insecte, le grillon. *Ann. Biol.* **24**, 105–128.

Lambin, M., Jeanrot, N., and Campan, R. (1981). Rôle des mouvements de la tête et du corps dans la perception visuelle chez un insecte: *Nemobius sylvestris*. *Bull. Soc. Hist. Nat. Toulouse* **117**, 51–62.

Laurent, G. (1985). "Organisation du programme locomoteur prothoracique chez le grillon. Biomécanique, neuroanatomie, physiologie." Thèse 3ème Cycle, Toulouse III.

Le Bourg, E., and Beugnon, G. (1985). Apple II programs in circular statistics. *Behav. Res. Methods, Instruments and Computers* **17**, 141.

Lemoigne, A. (1979). "Biologie du développement." Masson.

Marler, P. (1983). Some ethological implications for neuroethology: The ontogeny of birdsong. *In* "Advances in Vertebrate Neuroethology" (J. P. Ewert, R. Capranica, and D. Ingle, eds.), pp. 21–52. Plenum, New York.

Michieli, S. (1959). Analiza Scototakticnih (perigramotakticnih) Reakcis Pri Artropolih. Acad. Sci. et Atrium Slovenica, Cl IV: Historia, Naturalis et Medicina, pp. 237–286.

Mieulet, F. (1980). "Etude de la variabilité des modes d'orientation chez le grillon des bois, *Nemobius sylvestris*, selon des biotopes différents." Thèse 3ème Cycle, Toulouse-III.

Morvan, R., and Campan, R. (1976). Les déplacements du grillon des bois: Conditions d'acquisition et de maintien d'une orientation dominante. *Terre Vie* **30**, 276–294.

Morvan, R., Campan, R., and Thon, B. (1977). Etude de la répartition du grillon des bois *Nemobius sylvestris* (Bosc) dans un habitat naturel. I. Les larves. *Terre Vie* **31**, 637–659.

Morvan, R., Campan, R., and Thon, B. (1978). Etude de la répartition du grillon des bois *Nemobius sylvestris* (Bosc) dans un habitat naturel. II. Les adultes. *Terre Vie* **32**, 611–636.

Papi, F. (1976). The olfactory navigation system of homing pigeon. *Verh. Dtsch. Zool. Ges.* **69**, 184–205.

Piaget, J. (1977). L'épistémologie des régulations. In "L'idée de régulation dans les sciences," pp. 1–9. Maloine, Paris.

Richard, D., Prêteur, V., Campan, R., Beugnon, G., and Williams, L. (1985). Visual interneurones of the neck connectives in *Gryllus bimaculatus*. *J. Insect Physiol.* **31**, 407–417.

Richard, G. (1974). Réflexions sur les sciences du comportement à propos des travaux de Schneirla et de ses continuateurs. *J. Psychol. Norm. Pathol.* **71**, 135–148.

Richard, G. (1979). Ontogenesis and phylogenesis: Mutual constraints. *Adv. Study Behav.* **9**, 229–269.

Schneirla, T. C. (1965). Aspects of stimulation and organization in approach withdrawal processes underlying vertebrate behavioral development. *Adv. Study. Behav.* **1**, 1–74.

Tinbergen, N. (1963). On aims and methods of ethology. *Zeits J. Tierpsychol.* **20**, 410–433.

Uexküll, J. von. (1934). "Streifzüge durch die Umwelten von Tieren und Menschen." Springer-Verlag, Berlin.

Varela, F. (1983). L'auto-organisation: De l'apparence au mécanisme. *In* "Colloque de Cerizy. L'auto-organisation de la physique au politique" (D. Dumouchel and J. P. Dupuy, eds.), Seuil, Paris.

Vendryes, P. (1981). "L'autonomie du vivant." Maloine, Paris.

Viaud, G. (1955). Taxies et tropismes dans le comportement instinctif. *In* "L'instinct dans le comportement des animaux et de l'homme," pp. 5–43. Masson, Paris.

von Bertalanffy, W. (1973). "Théorie Générale des Systèmes." Dunod.

Wallon, H. (1941). "L'évolution psychologique de l'enfant." Paris, Colin.

Wehner, R. (1981). Spatial vision in arthropods. *In* "Handbook of Sensory Physiology" Vol. VII/6a, Vision in Invertebrates" (H. Autrum, ed.), pp. 287–616.

Weisskopf, A. (1984). Frontiers and limits of science. *Alexander von Humboldt Stiftung Mitteilungen* **43**, 1–11.

Wolff, E. (1963). "Les chemins de la vie." Hermann, Paris.

Index